Experimental Brain Research Supplementum 7

Neural Coding of Motor Performance

Edited by J. Massion J. Paillard
W. Schultz M. Wiesendanger

With 88 Figures and 7 Tables

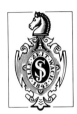

Springer-Verlag
Berlin Heidelberg New York 1983

Dr. J. Massion
Professor Dr. J. Paillard
Centre National de la Recherche Scientifique
Institut de Neurophysiologie et de Psychophysiologie
B.P. 71, F-13277 Marseille, Cedex 9

Dr. W. Schultz
Professor Dr. M. Wiesendanger
Institut de Physiologie, Université de Fribourg
Pérolles, CH-1700 Fribourg

ISBN 3-540-12140-4 Springer-Verlag Berlin Heidelberg New York
ISBN 0-387-12140-4 Springer-Verlag New York Heidelberg Berlin

Library of Congress Cataloging in Publication Data. Main entry under title:
Neural coding of motor performance. (Experimental brain research supplementum ; 7) Includes bibliographical references and indexes. 1. Motor cortex.
2. Efferent pathways. I. Massion, J. II. Series: Experimental brain research.
Supplement ; 7. [DNLM: 1. Nervous system–Physiology–Congresses. 2. Motor activity–Physiology–Congresses. W1 EX485B v.7 / WL 102 N491 1982]
QP383.N48   1983   599'.0188   83-364

Offsetprinting: Beltz Offsetdruck, Hemsbach/Bergstr.
Binding: J. Schäffer OHG, Grünstadt

2125/3140-543210

Preface

This volume covers the proceedings of a symposium held in Marseille in March 1982 as a satellite meeting of the IBRO First World Congress in Lausanne. About 70 participants from more than ten countries attended the symposium, whose central theme was "Neural Coding of Motor Performance."

Whereas coding within the sensory systems has been discussed widely, coding in the field of motor control has been analyzed much less. Over the past 10 years an impressive amount of information has been assembled combining recordings in central and peripheral neural structures during the performance of simple and complex motor tasks. Data such as those relating the behavioral phenomena of the awake animal to single-cell recordings from various cerebral areas have been carefully worked out by a number of investigators. It was thought at the symposium that the time had come for this information to be collected and reexamined, and presented in one volume. The present book was conceived to cover the scope and significance of coding throughout the nervous system.

What is meant by "coding" in the central nervous system? This question can be answered in general by bringing together data and viewpoints from many disciplines – behavior, neurophysiology, neuropharmacology – and clinical observations. Generally speaking, one may call coding a method of communication, i.e., the language that brain cells use for exchange of information. The complex issue of coding in the context of motor behavior is considered in the Introductory Lecture.

The contributions to the symposium have been grouped under four section headings. The first section is introductory, including those presentations which give a survey of the functional organization of neural networks involved in motor functions.

The second section deals with the steps in the motor act that precede movement execution. Each step brings into play specialized brain circuits, some of them being activated long before the onset of movement. Relation of unitary activity with motivation, preparation, attention, signal detection, etc. and their possible significance in terms of coding are reported.

The third section presents the pre-established connections ("wiring") that subserve motor patterns, and the fourth centers on the coding seen with movement execution, both in the command pathways for the control of movement and in the feedback loops which are active during the performance.

The 35 contributions included in this volume were presented either orally in sessions or as posters and were subsequently submitted to referees. The organizers wish to thank all those who contributed to this work. They are particularly grateful for the assistance of Dr. P. Levin in editing.

The symposium received financial support from the Centre National de la Recherche Scientifique and the Université de Luminy, whose help is gratefully acknowledged.

J. Massion   J. Paillard   W. Schultz   M. Wiesendanger

Contents

List of First Named Authors*

---

* The address of each first mentioned author is indicated below the according contribution heading

1 Page, on which contribution commences

Introductory Lecture: The Functional Labelling of Neural Codes

J. Paillard

C.N.R.S., INP 4, B.P. 71, 13277 Marseille Cedex 9, France

INTRODUCTION

When considered as a communication machine, the nervous system is assumed to deal with "information". The potential "information" gathered by sense organs impinges in the form of various energies and substances ; and the impinging events are converted into a form that the nervous system can handle. Following transduction of the stimulus by the receptors, further transformations occur at many levels within the nervous system before the centrifugal command signals affect the motor machinery and finally manifest themselves in overt behaviour.

Once identified by electrophysiological methods, the train of nerve impulses was recognized as a universal carrier of nervous information over transmission channels. ADRIAN (1928) first used the term "message" to qualify this kind of nervous activity which is clearly related to the communicative function of the neural apparatus. The question immediately arose as to the content of such messages and the code in which they are transcribed and transmitted for interpretation by competent "readers".

Neural coding has been investigated mainly at the sensory stage where controlled physical changes can be directly correlated with corresponding changes in the receptor's neural response. In contrast, the coding of motor commands has attracted less attention (PAILLARD, 1978). The purpose of this introduction is, therefore, to identify some of the problems arising specifically when dicussing "coding" in the context of motor control.

1 - FORMAL VERSUS EMPIRICAL APPROACHES TO CODING PROCESSES

1.1. The term "coding", that has two different meanings in common parlance, has also been widely used in various specialized fields from genetics to computer technology. The common use of the term envisages a code either as a set of signals conveying meaningful information between distant points (i.e. the morse code) or as a system of principles that constrains the behaviour of the individual to rules commonly shared by the members of a community (i.e. the penal code). Both meanings are broadly appropriated to describe the presumed properties of neural "messages".

The difficulties emerge, however, when trying to specify and compare the properties of "neural codes" with those of computer language where the term "code" or "coding" has acquired several different and rather loosely related meanings. It may either describe the repertoire of elementary instructions that the computer is called upon to execute (the "command code") or be used as a synonym of a "program" - a preorganized set of instructions designed for performing a specific operation (the "algorithm"). Furthermore, they can designate the set of rules ("coding scheme") by which numerical quantities, instructions, alphabetic symbols etc. are· electrically represented within the workings of the computer (i.e. binary codes). Whatever our assumptions about the nature of the discrete symbols which may compose the elements of a putative "neural" code, the obvious multiplicity and the arbitrariness of such descriptions (see below) lead us to believe that there is probably no single universal neural "coding scheme" comparable for instance, to the "genetic code" or to other kinds of technological code than can be easily "cracked" and dissected into their elementary components.

1.2. Addressing this difficulty, an earlier work session of the Neurosciences Research Program (NRP) on "Neural coding" (PERKEL and BULLOCK, 1968) recognized two fundamental approaches to the investigation of "neural codes". The first emphasizes an empirical approach that tries to correlate either measurable physical properties of the stimuli with relevant features of the sensory messages, or quantifiable characteristics of the behavioural performance with relevant features of the command signals, in order to attach a functional label to presumptive neural codes. The second or formal approach considers the neural code as a working scheme of representation in the nervous system and tries to set out the formal requirements of such a code.

The Brooklyn NRP meeting chose the second line of approach and attempted to described codes as "forms of representation of information in the nervous system" considered as a general communication system. Such a system is described, in terms of Shannon's information theory, by four basic components and functions : (i) the referent which consists of the relevant features abstracted from the flow of input signals and supposedly represented by means of the "coding scheme". (ii) the transformation which characterizes the encoding process or the editing of output signals whereby the referents are represented. (iii) the transmission or conduction process whereby the encoded information is preserved and channelized to its anatomically specified addresses. (iv) the interpretation of the encoded information by a reaching structure which operates either a recoding by a higher set of neurones or a decoding by an effector organ.

Avoiding any a priori commitments to any particular class of substrate of the neural coding process, this broad and formal definition of a "neural coding scheme" allows both the application of the concept at various levels of neural organization - whether intracellular, cellular or neural ensemble, and its extension to a multiplicity of putative "coding schemes".

No less than thirthy four discriminable neural events were identified at the NRP meeting as having the required formal properties of a coding scheme (see Table 1). Undoubtedly, the recent identification of new classes of neurochemical signals (see SIGGINS and BLOOM (1981) and the contributions of NIEOULLON and of SCHULTZ to this Symposium) has further increased the number of what could be considered as "candidate" codes.

In fact, the obvious question, clearly raised at the Brooklyn meeting, is whether a "coding scheme", identified and recognized as such by neurophysiological tools, is actually used at all as an information-carrier by the living organism. In contrast, we may suspect that signals that "make sense" to the nervous system and convey useful information may be indistinguishable from random noise by investigators within the limited range of sensitivity of their observational tools.

1.3. Thus, a code perceived by the neurophysiologist as one presenting the formal requirements of a "coding scheme" can, at best, only be considered as a "candidate code". It can become an "established code" only if it is shown to have, in addition, some significance with regard to the animal's behaviour. But "significance" is not easy to evaluate and can only be empirically assessed. An event generally gains its significance from the context in which it is interpreted. For instance, information transfers which organize behavioural activities at the macroscale of the organism may have themselves

A TABLE OF CANDIDATE NEURAL CODES
OR
FORMS OF REPRESENTATION OF INFORMATION
IN THE NERVOUS SYSTEM

I. NEURONAL EVENTS OTHER THAN IMPULSES
   A. Intracellular Events
      1. *Receptor potential: amplitude*
      2. *Synaptic potential: amplitude*
      3. *Synaptic conductance change: amplitude*
      4. *Synaptic conductance change: spatial distribution*
      5. *Membrane potential: spatial and temporal distribution*
      6. *Graded potential in axonal terminals*

   B. Intercellular Events
      1. *Transmitter released*
      2. *Potassium ion released*
      3. *Neurosecretion released*
      4. *Electrotonic coupling between specific cells*
      5. *Electrotonic interaction via extracellular space*

II. IMPULSES IN UNIT NEURONS
   A. Representation by Identity of Active Fiber
      1. *Labeled lines*
   B. Codes Based on Temporal Properties of Impulses
      1. *Time of occurrence*
         a. *Instant of firing*
         b. *Phase locking to stimulus*
      2. *Interval statistics codes*
         a. *Frequency: weighted average*
         b. *Frequency: instantaneous*
         c. *Frequency: increment above background*
         d. *Frequency: rate of change*
         e. *Frequency of firing/missing at fixed intervals*
         f. *Coefficient of variation*
         g. *Higher moments; interval histogram shape*
      3. *Temporal pattern of impulses*
      4. *Number of impulses or duration of burst*
      5. *Velocity change in axon*
   C. Codes Based on Other Properties
      1. *Amplitude change in axon*
      2. *Spatial sequencing*

III. ENSEMBLE ACTIVITY
   A. Representation by Spatial Array
      1. *Topographic distribution of active fibers*
   B. Codes Based on Temporal Relations Among Active Channels
      1. *Latency distribution*
      2. *Phase distribution*
      3. *Probability of firing after stimulus: PST histogram shape*
   C. Representation by Form of Composite of Multiunit Activity
      1. *Evoked potential shape*
      2. *Slow waves in ongoing EEG*

Tables of neural codes. From PERKEL and BULLOCK (1968).

other requirements (i.e. metabolic) at the microscale of synaptic and cellular levels. These requirements are fulfilled by local or more distant
mechanisms of regulation. Signals involved in such regulation might therefore
be time-locked to behavioural events although not directly related to those
events as of information - carrying value at that level. It is generally
considered that the "communicative" compartments of the nervous system combine a hierarchical emboxing of interacting levels of organization with a
distributed mode of processing of information in parallel channels. This
raises considerable problems for the interpretation of the meaning of nervous
signals at the various stages of the transformation of encoded sensory
messages in a complex network. A description of interpretation (meaning) of a
neural code must include a specification of the target sites, the rules of
the decoding process and considerations of noise and reliability. The most
widely investigated class of neural codes is that in which information is
carried by nerve impulses in a single channel where the characterization of
"coding schemes" in their four formal aspects is sometimes possible. The use
of impulses in parallel channels is much more difficult to investigate and to
characterize formally. Moreover, codes based on topographic distribution of
active fibers are still poorly understood.

1.4. The coding of motor commands offers new opportunities in that the
final target sites as well as the functional meaning of the output signals
are well specified. The mechanisms of decoding of efferent messages and of
their transformation in muscular force by the servo-motor unit are broadly
known (cf. PAILLARD, 1976). Motor performances can usually be well controlled
and their behavioural meaning empirically evaluated. In contrast the referent
input signal are generally more difficult to identify as resulting either
from converging messages issued for many different sources or from signals
having only a triggering function that resolves in the releasing of prewired
output programs.

The approach of neural coding in the context of motor control will therefore
be concerned with "empirical", "operational" rather than with "formal" codes.
Thus, operationally, two main features of the organization of nervous activity have to be taken into account. First, the precise wiring plan of the
involved neural structure ; and, second, the temporal sequence of the train
of impulses transmitted as "messages" within the distributive network of
nervous tissue.

2 - SPATIAL VERSUS TEMPORAL CODES

It has been known for almost 150 years that the most "meaningful" elements of neural information are those that are built into the structure of the nervous system. In 1833, Johannes MULLER formulated his "law of specific energies" whereby the modality within which sensation is experienced is independent of the nature of the stimulus itself and is determined only by the central connections of the nervous fibres by which the "message" is conducted : a train of nervous impulses carried by an auditory fibre will give rise to a sensation of sound whereas a similar train of impulses carried by an optic fibre will be interpreted as a visual event. Different "meanings" are then attributed to formally identical "messages", depending on the location of the reading structure in the nervous system. Moreover, a change in the frequency of the nerve impulses in either message would be interpreted as an increase in the intensity of the perceived sound or of the perceived light. Thus, we are led to attribute a coding function to the spatial distribution of messages and to distinguish it from the temporal coding of nervous messages.

2.1. It is now accepted that the most elementary yet most pervasive form of neural coding is that accomplished by the so-called "labelled lines". They realise a specificity of addressing that constitutes a "coding function". Each neurone has its receptive field or its qualified configuration of inputs and distinctive addresses for the further distribution of its efferences that narrowly define the type of information it may accept, process and emit. This can be extended at the level of neuronal ensembles and of cortical areas. The important advances made by nineteenth century neurology were based on the attempt to understand the functional relevance of circumscribed cerebral areas. In fact, the functional significance (semantic content) of information that is spatially distributed in this way can be known only through the interpretation that is given to it by its reader - that is, by the organiza-tion of structures that are capable of receiving and interpreting it.

These structures are represented on a scale of several dimensions : that of the neuronal cell with its polysynaptic assortment, that of the polyneural columnar field with its internal laminar architecture, and that of the polycolumnar fields that characterize the various cytoarchitectonic areas identified in the cortex. At all these levels, as FESSARD (1969) already emphasized, the operation of reading incoming information is isomorphic to a process of "pattern recognition", to a matching operation that resolves in the editing of an output message or in the triggering of a latent program. It is the very existence of such an output programme which testifies that a given spatially coded form has been "recognized" and interpreted as functionally meaningful. ARBIB (1981) speaks of "layered control surfaces" to designate the cascade of "mapping operations" involved in perceptual activity - for example, to extract from first order sensory messages signals at a sufficiently abstract level to specify the representation of the object perceived and allow its subsequent recognition by higher order "control surfaces". The same can be said, in the motor sphere, to enable the transition from an abstract representation of the goal to be attained (goal image) to a plan of action and then to the even more precise specification of the several parameters of the program of action, including those controlling the sequential ordering of polyneural activity (cf. PAILLARD, 1982).

2.2. Candidate-codes based on temporal properties of impulses have certainly been the most extensively investigated class of neural codes owing to computer facilities. The representation of stimulus intensity or of amount of muscular force by means of rate of impulses comprises the basic classical code of neural messages. Many other parameters have been shown to be operative and potentially available for use as candidate-codes (see Table 1). The time of firing ("Go!" signal) is probably basic for the coding of motor command as well as the temporal patterning of triggering signals. Coding of serial order still remains a major unresolved issue in the study of nervous activity (see however GROSSBERG, 1978 ; MOROWITZ, 1979 ; ARBIB, 1981). To infer the identity of afferent codes by observing a neuronal output requires generally of the experimenter the computation of probabilities or the use of cross-correlation techniques. As stressed by MOORE et al. (1966), however, this does not imply "that the assumptions and methods used by experimenters in their own decoding efforts bear any resemblance to processes employed by the nervous system itself". Temporal patterning and representation by configurations of multiunit activity constitute "ensemble codes" that are still poorly understood in spite of their presumed importance for the organization of nervous activity at its higher levels.

2.3. Are we then able to interpret the local activity of single neurones as coded information having a demonstrable relevance for the behavioural outcome to which it is temporally related ? The recording of single-cell activity in unanaesthetized animals during prescribed behavioural tasks has opened the way for relating some "candidate codes" to the characteristics of motor performance. Promising data have been provided by recent neurophysiological studies and this meeting will certainly make a further contribution in this area. Two major difficulties, however, emerge in the course of their functional interpretation : the first concerns the difficulty of precisely identifying the place of a given neurone in its structure·of connectivity and of assessing its presumed "coding function" ; and the second involves the attribution of some functional labelling to its temporal coding that could be related with the nature of the task, the movement characteristics or other identifiable features of the performance.

3 - THE LABELLING OF NEURAL CODES

3.1. The structural specification of unicellular activity is defined by the pattern of connectivity that links the neurone studied with other neurones belonging to a local module. The module itself gains its functional specificity from its connections with adjacent and more distant modules with which it composes functional, interacting areas that are themselves inter-connected, in higher order ensembles. The only direct proof that a spatial configuration of interconnected neurones has an identifiable coding property is to activate the circuit and observe the resulting behavioural effect. Fortunately, many stereotyped behavioural activities can be triggered that way by stimulating some focal structures that control the whole "coming into play", in prescribed order, of the muscles composing the movement. But it is difficult to extend the concept of "command neurones", derived from the study of simplified networks in invertebrates, to more complex nervous organiza-tions. "Decision points", representing structures that release an entire programme of action, are probably the rule at lower stages of nervous organization where electrical stimulation triggers biologically meaningful programmes, usually belonging to the innate repertoire of the species. At higher processing stages, however, it has never been possible to elicit electrically skills that are newly learned, as if the coding of such new programmes requires either the reading of a pattern of input that is too complex to be generated by electrical stimulation or some other still unknown generative rules (cf. PAILLARD, 1982a). We are moreover still far from being able to locate the "speaking" neurones of electrophysiological studies within the neuronal circuitry of the modular units to which they belong, in order to decipher its structural coding function. Broad regional mappings of functio-nal specialization have, however, been achieved during the last decade and the columnar approach has been promising. It is to be hoped that this exacting line of research will yield fresh insights into the logic of structural coding in the nervous system (MOUNTCASTLE, 1978) and into the identification of the existing repertoire of "latent programmes" that provi-des the circulatory "information" with its very "meaning". For the time being, our main resources still lie in the temporal analysis of neural activity.

3.2. The time-locking of neural activity with behavioural events is certainly the prerequisite of neurobehavioural research. This chronometric approach has been fruitful in specifying the place and time at which neural activity may procede, accompany or follow identifiable phases of behaviour. Such timing makes it possible to investigate more precise properties of the recorded activity than hitherto. Thus, the possible relationships between neural activity and the parameters of force, position, speed or direction of a given movement have been investigated. This is a valid attempt to attribute a functional label to presumptive coding properties of neuronal activity. But, as such, it is fraught with new difficulties. Although it is comparatively easy to specify the content of neurosensorial signals in terms of information about force, position, length and speed, the fact that these signals soon converge on common neurones in the processing chain and then combine in various vectorial operations makes it extremely hazardous to identify the coding function of the resultant central activity.

The same is true for the efferent chaining of command operations : there are numerous examples from recent studies of motor control showing that the parameters controlled by nervous command are not, in general, those that would have been expected from physical descriptions of the kinematic properties of the movement. For example, HENN and COHEN (1976) identified neurones in the rostral paramedial zone of the pontine reticular formation that have distinct frequency changes prior to and during quick saccadic eye movement but, conversely, little or no tonic activity associated with eye position. They showed that eye movement - related neurones of this region seem to describe the change of position (Δ pos) resulting from an horizontal saccade by a vector having an amplitude A and an angle α. These two parameters are related to positional changes by the equation Δ pos = A. cosα. In each of the 80 cells recorded in this area, the activity could be related to one of the above three parameters. Units coding the change of position (Δ pos) and the amplitude (A) conveyed the information by number of spikes whereas units coding the cosine of the angle between the direction of movement and a reference direction did so by frequency. This clear demonstration of a vectorial description of movement suggest the possibility of similar modes of coding elsewhere in the central nervous system.

3.3. Another line of investigation stems from control system theory. The principles of control systems, when applied to neural systems, leads to the prediction that some invariant characteristics may be used as a stable reference relative to which the state control of the system can be organized. In fact, time invariance has been designated, mainly by experimental psychologists, as a regulator of action. The amplitude of a movement can easily be changed by changing speed while preserving the same duration. Contemporary studies have focussed on the identification of the invariant characteristics of movement on the assumption that such invariance in timing relations may reflect the logic of operations by means of which central processes participate in the organization of movement.

Such an approach has, for example, been successfully applied to the study of locomotion. It has been shown that the duration of the swing phase of the step cycle is invariant with the speed of locomotion and that the onset of activity in all of the physiological extensors of a given leg is approximately synchronous (ENGBERG and LUNDBERG, 1969 ; GRILLNER, 1975 ; SHIK and ORLOVSKY, 1976). Interlimb coordination in locomotion or in the activation of functional synergists in postural activity is known to present consistent patterns of activity that are preserved as a basic invariance when the conditions of execution are changed (NASHNER, 1977). A similar approach has been used to study the movement of the arm when pointing to a visual target. SOECHTING and LACQUANITI (1981) have shown that the trajectory of the wrist in space is independent of the speed with which the movement is executed. Moreover, an invariant relationship exists between the rates of shoulder flexion and elbow extension, especially in the terminal phases of the movement. These findings raise the question as to whether movement is organized in terms of the intrinsic coordinates of the body and they point the way towards specific hypotheses regarding the manner in which movement is planned and controlled (GROSSBERG, 1978).

By the same token, MORASSO (1981) carried out a similar investigation but with added restrictions as to the number of degrees of freedom to be controlled. By means of an articulated device, movements of the arm were reduced to flexion - extension of the elbow and of the shoulder. The subjects received no particular instructions other than to reach the target position. The results showed that, for different types of reaching movement, the joint angular velocities exhibit quite different patterns whereas the tangential hand velocity for different movements has a single peaked curve that varies little in shape between movements. The duration of movement was relatively constant for each subject whatever the shape of the joint angular patterns. Consequently, the author suggested that the central commands, which underlie the observed movements, are more likely to specify (i.e. to code) the spatial trajectory of the hand than the relative position of the joints' angle. This is in accordance with earlier studies by VIVIANI and TERZUOLO (1980) who provided a detailed kinematic description of hand movement during handwriting, showing that the basic kinematic variable (peak tangential velocity and curvature of the trajectory) preserve the invariance of their temporal pattern when speed of writing and size of letters are changed.

3.4. These findings emphasize the fact that it can be misleading to try to correlate single cell activity with parameters of movement that are evaluated in the extrinsic coordinate system of physical measurement. The invariances revealed by the experiments cited above are all expressed in some intrinsic coordinate system. This implies the existence of a coordinate transformation between the two frames of reference if the location of the target is mapped psychophysically in some extrinsic coordinate system. The need for such transformations has recently been stressed, for both the organization of spatially oriented movement (PELLIONISZ and LLINAS, 1980) and the transformation of spatial motor commands into coordinate joint angular patterns (BENATI et al., 1980). The mapping of local sensorimotor spaces and their integration within supramodal maps of extrapersonal and body space could well provide a "spatial code" potentially able to serve as a common language for organizing spatial motor commands within intrinsic coordinate systems of which the descriptive rules are only beginning to emerge (PAILLARD, 1982b).

3.5. Undoubtedly, the present impetus in the robotic field (BENATI et al., 1980) and the need for new principles of control for "task-oriented" systems will stimulate the search for new coding or organization principles in living systems. Such principles have evolved in response to the environmental pressures to which a species must adapt in order to survive and are translated into the layered neural networks that constitute the complex information-processing machine which we have to decipher. We certainly have to be prepared to encounter - depending on the evolutionary level of the nervous structures involved - different processing capacities, different degrees of sophistication or of abstraction in the internal representation of the physical reality and then different descriptions of that reality using different languages. We have finally to take into account, in our search for the coding properties of neural messages, the idea - now pervasive in neurobiology - of a hierarchy of levels of control superimposed upon a distributed control of the coordinated activation of interwoven subsystems.

4 - LEVELS OF CONTROL AND LEVELS OF CODIFICATION

Research on the motor system is now providing detailed knowledge of the local circuitry and functioning of the different parts of the motor machinery of which the general organizational principles were clearly recognised a century ago by JACKSON (reedited 1932).

4.1. The three-stage model of control developped by ALLEN and TSUKAHARA (1974) has been influential in contemporary neurophysiological thinking (see Fig. 1). At the lowest stage, we find the so-called executive level that is controlled by the motor cortex with the contribution of the paleocerebellar loop to update the evolving movement in accordance with the prescribed motor command and the context of postural requirements. This level is dominated by the structural codification of the genetically prewired circuitry of the primary repertoire of basic motor programmes. The servo-assistance of such programmes depends also on prewired feedback loops. The information circulating in the more peripheral reflex loops is probably directly translated into the original code of the sensory transduction, the loop gain being controlled by central command. However, as soon as we try to follow the message in second-order elements of the transmission chain, it seems that the original codification has lost its initial clarity and the content of the message is difficult to identify.

4.2. A taxonomy of classes of "empirical" codes is clearly required to guide our effort to elucidate the functional labeling of neural activity. Time and force and their combination for speed specification are the most usual labels encountered in motor control research (BROOKS and STONEY, 1971, and this symposium). Direction, end position of moving body segments or place in the external environment are clearly less well identifiable in terms of neural coding. Two examples may serve to illustrate how such an operational approach can be based.

4.2.1. William POWER (1973), who has developed an interesting control model for the nervous system organized in a "tangled" hierarchy of reference signals, envisaged the first five levels of sensori-motor control as each being associated with a dominant rule of codification. (i) The intensity control is the basic mode for representing state variables of the system using the frequency code in the first and last order neurones. (ii) Second-first and second-last order neurones weigh and integrate information from several sources and realize a kind of vector control. A vectorial measurement is then coded in their output signals. (iii) The configuration control that intervenes at the next level relies basically on a structural code : recognition of patterned input belongs to this kind of control as well as the patterned distribution of efferent messages to prescribed neuronal pools ; the direction of a movement is typically under the aegis of this kind of control (see the contribution of GEORGEOPOULOS in this symposium). (iv) The control of change, by the use of the first or second derivative of state variables (rate of change), is the most commonly coded dimension encountered

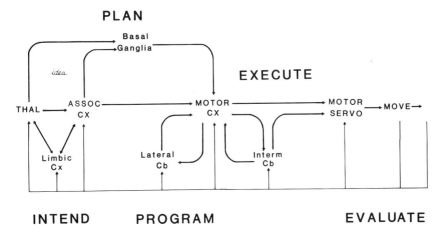

Fig. 1. Revised schema of ALLEN and TSUKAHARA (1974) by J. PAILLARD (1982b)

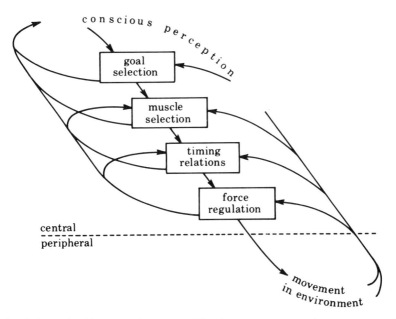

Fig. 2. Schematic diagram of a generalized motor program (MAC KAY, 1980)

in the organization of central commands, as it is encoded by a special class
of sensory transducers (dynamic versus static encoding). (v) Finally, the
control of sequences belongs to the last category of basic neural coding
properties. Higher order coding processes are of course to be considered.

4.2.2. In the same line but in another context MAC KAY (1978) recently
proposes to view the nervous system as organized in several hierachically
interwoven loops each characterized by the control of a given class of
parameters defining a program of action with the corresponding classes of
neural codes . They comprise : force regulation, timing relations, muscle
selection, goal specification and conscious control (Fig. 2).

4.3. Although suggestive, taxonomies of this sort probably require to be
more elaborated to be really useful. In dealing with the functional labelling
of neural codes, we are clearly faced with two different systems of description : one is that of the experimenter-observer who will, for example,
describe metrically the amplitude or the speed of a movement ; the other is
that of an autoreferential system for which the coding of date and peak
frequency change suffices in that instance to specify a muscle shortening of
a given amplitude and at a given speed. Kinematic measures accessible to the
experimenter's tools are, in a sense, only the product of the system's
dynamic parameters. Thus, they cannot be appropriately set in the explicit, a
priori prescriptions of an internal programme. Variables controlled by the
system must certainly be different from such measures and depend in some way
on the system's a priori knowledge of the dynamic properties of its own
instrument. Inbuilt, prewired programmes are the clear expression of this
kind of inherited knowledge. In contrast, newly acquired skills seem to
necessitate a programming process (the contribution of cerebellar and striopallidal loops to this process is discussed by WIESENDANGER and by DELONG in
this symposium).

4.3.1. Programming, as an active process, involves the presetting and
pretuning of conditional loops before the decision to act. This programming
process demands precise, structural prescriptions (including the configuration of muscles to be activated), force requirements (speed and amplitude),
and time specifications (date and sequential ordering). Clearly the labelling
of single-cell activity has to be referred, at this level, to the control of
each of these three classes of variable. In the case of delayed action, this
pretuning can be preserved but, as soon as the decision to act is taken, it
is supposed that the neocerebellar loop is involved in starting, updating
during its execution and stopping this programming process. The paleocerebel-

lar loop, for its part, assists the evolving action with special reference to postural constraints. But pretuning generally presupposes permissive action on specific parts of the circuitry and, with the exception of time specifications, the labelling of activity underlying this process is usually difficult to assess (see REQUIN, 1980, and LECAS et al. this symposium).

4.3.2. Planning is generally considered as a higher level process that precedes and promotes the programming process by the selection of the most suitable strategy in accordance with the intended goal, the initial state of the body, its expected postural changes, and the estimated requirements of the task in intra- and extra-personal space (cf. PAILLARD, 1982). We may therefore expect the language of planning to be rather different from that of programming and of execution. The activity of single cells, supposedly involved in the planning process, would then be related to the movement by its anticipatory timing but would generally be labelled as "task-related" and not as "movement-related" in so far as this activity is not directly correlated with parameters of execution like speed, force, position etc. Such is the case of units recorded in the parietal region and described as "projection" or "manipulation" units for arm movements and also of "saccadic acquisition", "fixation" and "pursuit" units for eye movements. The study of the striopallidal loop enabled the labelling of "sensory units" - "task-related" or "movement-related units - depending on their time of intervention in the chain of operations underlying the planning process (ROLLS et al., 1979 ; and ROLLS, this symposium)). The frontal lobe appears to be chiefly involved in the definition of the goal in accordance with drive and the priorities supplied by limbic information. It is here that the "meaning" of the goal, with reference to a system of biological and psychological values, is appreciated and thus that the attribution of a "meaning-dependency" label could profitably be exploited. The evaluation of the correct achievement of the act, in relation to its initially expected sensory consequences, also seems to be within the province of frontal-lobe operations. The label of "reinforcement-dependency" has been sucessfully used to differentiate frontal from parietal-lobe activity (PERRET et al., 1978).

4.3.3. Finally, attentional processes are required to prepare, initiate, enable and control voluntary action. The label of "attention-dependency" has shown its capacity to map the populations of neurones that are and those that are not under attentional control (BUSHNELL et al., 1981). This brings us closer to the labelling of higher and still mysterious brain functions described as will and conscious control and to the realisation of the hope formulated by the late Hans-Lucas TEUBER twenty years ago when he encouraged neurophysiologists to look for "physiological markers of voluntariness" in the functioning brain.

4.4. These few examples are indeed sufficient to demonstrate new possibilities of exploring the higher functions of the nervous system via the systematic search for the functional labelling of single-cell activity when such activity is temporarily related to well-prescribed behavioural tasks. They illustrate the richness of the universe of meanings engendered by the variety of "the languages of the brain" (PRIBRAM, 1971) and the multiplicity of the codes in which they are expressed.

5 - CONCLUSIONS

Let me conclude with a final comment : we ought not to forget that the concept of coding - to which we allocate a central place at this meeting - belongs to the constructs of information theory, of computer language, and of cybernetic models that may eventually prove to be no more than metaphors when applied to the nervous system (MOORE et al., 1966). There is not the place to discuss the role and significance of metaphors in scientific endeavour but we must be aware of their limitations whatever their local explanatory power. An alternative model to that of information-processing has been advanced to describe the "design logic" of the system only in terms of the physical principles of statistical mechanics (The homeokinetic physics of IBERALL, 1977). Instead of attributing organization and regulation in the system to explicit, a priori coded prescriptions (engrammed or generated by some programing process) coordination and control are described by this theory as a direct a posteriori consequences of the system's dynamic behaviour and of the selective constraints imposed upon it by the related nervous architecture. A recent review by Scott KELSO (1981) deals with an application of such principles to motor control problems. It would appear for instance, that problems of timing specification and of sequential ordering - difficult to handle by the information processing model (but see GALLISTEL, 1980) - receive obvious and simple solutions in this conceptual framework (MOROWITZ, 1979).

Whatever the future of this kind of approach, it is my belief that we are no longer faced with the traditional opposition of the holistic and the analytic approach to the study of living systems - to an either-or dilemma. Instead, we are becoming progressively more sensitive to the fact that the evolutionary status of the nervous system confers upon its internal organization the properties of both an _organized_ and an _organizing_ machine (PAILLARD, 1977).

The former aspect involves a structure of a rather rigid connectivity reasonably well described by the cybernetic properties of its hardware logic ; the latter provides through its architectual component the requisite redundancy, variety and lability for generating its plastic properties. These properties ensure its self-preserving and self-organizing functions and are responsible for the dynamic patterning of its activity and then for the creation of new languages and new codes. Thus organisms reinforce their internal cohesion and autonomy while increasing their complexity and conse-quently enrich the uninterrupted dialogue they entertain with their environ-ment (PAILLARD, in press).

REFERENCES

ADRIAN ED (1928) The basis of sensation. Norton, New-York

ALLEN GI, TSUKAHARA N (1974) Cerebrocerebellar communication systems. Physiol Rev 54:957-1006

ARBIB MA (1982) Perceptual structures and distributed motor control. In: BROOKS VB (ed) Handbook of Physiology. Section on Neurophysiology. Vol III. Motor control. Amer Physiol Soc, Bethesda, p 1449-1480

BENATI M, CAGHIO S, MORASSO P, TAGLIASCO V, ZACCARIA R (1980) Anthropomorphic robotic. I. Representing mechanical complexity. II. Analysis of manipulator dynamics and the output motor impedance. Biol Cybern 38:125-140 and 141-150

BROOKS VB, STONEY Jr. V (1971) Motor mechanisms : the role of the pyramidal system in motor control. Ann Rev Physiol 33:337-392

BUSHNELL MC, GOLDBERG ME, ROBINSON DL (1981) Behavioral enhancement of visual responses in monkey cerebral cortex. I. Modulation in posterior parietal cortex related to selective visual attention. J Neurophysiol 46:755-787

ENGBERG I, LUNDBERG A (1969) An electromyographic analysis of muscular activity in the hindlimbs of the cat during unrestrained locomotion. Acta Physiol Scand 75:614-630

FESSARD A (1969) Les problèmes du code nerveux. In: Theoretical Physics and Biology. North Holland, Amsterdam, p 230-245

FESSARD A (1970) Approche neurophysiologique des problèmes de la mémoire. In: La mémoire. Symposium Assoc Psychol de Langue Française. PUF, Paris, p 59-98

GALLISTEL CR (1980) The organization of action. A new synthesis. John Wiley, New-York

GRILLNER S (1975) Locomotion in vertebrates : central mechanisms and reflex interaction. Physiol Rev 55:247-303

GROSSBERG S (1978) A theory of human memory : self organization and performan-ce of sensory-motor codes, maps and plan. In: ROSEN R, SNELL D (eds) Progress in theoretical biology, vol 5. Academic Press, New- York, p 233-374

HENN V, COHEN B (1976) Coding of information about rapid eye movements in the pontine reticular formation of alert monkeys. Brain Res 108:307-325

18

IBERALL AS (1972) Toward a general science of viable systems. Mc Graw- Hill, New-York

JACKSON H (1932) Selected writings (vol 2). TAYLOR J (ed). Hodder and Stoughton, London

MACKAY WA (1980) The motor program : back to the computer. Trends Neurosc 3:284-287

MOORE GP, PERKEL DH, SEGUNDO JP (1966) Statistical analysis and functional interpretation of neuronal spike data. Am Rev Physiol 28:493-522

MORASSO P (1981) Spatial control of arm movements. Exp Brain Res 42:223-227

MOROWITZ HJ (1979) Energy flow in Biology. Woodbridge Conn, Ox Bow Press

MOUNTCASTLE VB (1978) An organizing principle for cerebral function : the unit module and the distributed system. In: EDELMAN GM, MOUNTCASTLE VB (eds) The mindful brain. MIT Press, Cambridge Mass, p 7-50

MÜLLER J (1833) Handbuch der Physiologie des Menschen, vol I, Coblentz, Holscher

NASHNER LM (1977) Fixed patterns of rapid postural responses among muscles during stance. Exp Brain Res 30:13-24

PAILLARD J (1976) Le codage nerveux des commandes motrices. Rev EEG Neurophysiol Clin 6:453-472

PAILLARD J (1977) La machine organisée et la machine organisante. Revue de l'Education Physique Belge XVII:19-48

PAILLARD J (1982a) Apraxia and the neurophysiology of motor control. Phil Trans R Soc London B298:111-134

PAILLARD J (1982b) Le corps et ses langages d'espace. Nouvelles contributions psychophysiologiques à l'étude du schéma corporel. In: JEDDI E (ed) Le corps en Psychiatrie. Masson, Paris, p 53-69

PAILLARD J (in press) Système nerveux et fonction d'organisation. In: PIAGET J, BRONCKART JP, MOUNOUD P (eds) La Psychologie, Encyclopédie de la Pléïade, Gallimard, Paris

PELLIONISZ A, LLINAS R (1980) Tensorial approach to the geometry of brain function. Cerebellar coordination via a metric tensor. Neuroscience 5:1125-1136

PERKEL DH, BULLOCK TH (1968) Neural coding. NRP Bulletin 6: n°3, 221-248

PERRET D, PUERTO A, ROLLS ET, ROPER-HALL A, THORPE SJ (1978) Area 7 neurones do not respond only to desired objects. J Physiol London 284:82 p

POWER WT (1973) Behavior : the control of perception. Aldine Pub Cy, Chicago

PRIBRAM K (1971) Languages of the brain. Englewood Cliffs, Prentice Hall, New Jersey

REQUIN J (1980) Toward a psychobiology of preparation for action. In: STELMACH GE, REQUIN J (eds) Tutorial in motor behavior. North Holland, Amsterdam, p 243-258

ROLLS ET, THORPE SJ, MADISON S, ROPER-HALL A, PUERTO A, PERRET D (1979) Activity of neurones in the neostriatum and related structures in the alert animal. In: DIVAC I, OBERG RGS (eds) The neostriatum. Pergamon Press, Oxford, p 163-182

SCOTT KELSO JA (1981) Contrasting perspectives on order and regulation in movement. In: LONG J, BADELEY A (eds) Attention and Performance IX, chapter 25, p 437-457

SHIK ML, ORLOVSKY GN (1976) Neurophysiology of locomotor automatism. Physiol Rev 56:465-501

SIGGINS GR, BLOOM FE (1981) Modulation of unit activity by chemically coded neurons. In: POMPEIANO O, AJMONE MARSAN C (eds) Brain mechanisms and perceptual awareness. Raven Press, New-York

SOECHTING JF, LACQUANITI F (1951) Invariant characteristics of a pointing movement in man. J. of Neuroscience 1:710-720

VIVIANI P, TERZUOLO CA (1980) Space time invariance in learned motor skill. In: STELMACH GE, REQUIN J (eds) Tutorial in motor behavior. North Holland, Amsterdam, p 525-533

Neural Systems
in the Context of Coding

Neuronal Activities in Primary Motor Area and Premotor Regions

R. Porter

John Curtin School of Medical Research, The Australian National University,
P.O. Box 334, Canberra City, ACT, 2601, Australia

Even before we can begin to approach the question of coding of aspects of
movement performance by neurons in motor regions of the cerebral cortex, we
need to have some definitions of the terminology which should be applied to
these regions. Some authors would include within the term "motor cortex" the
whole area of cerebral surface from which movement responses can be obtained
upon electrical stimulation. Yet the anatomist can recognize within this
total territory several different cyto-architectonic areas. Evidence is also
rapidly accumulating for functional differences in the neuronal populations
within these separable areas (Table 1). Finally, even within a single
cyto-architectonic area, there may be several levels of organization and
multiple representations, if recent studies using micro-stimulation and recording are confirmed.

So our starting point must be regional geography. Since I have been asked to
speak about neuronal activities in the primary motor and in premotor regions
of the cerebral cortex, I will have to provide some definitions and describe
my version of the map which we are to follow. Those who have examined
cyto-architectonic regions of the cerebral cortex have all separated an area
gigantopyramidalis (area 4) in the precentral gyrus from zones in front of
it, of which the most immediately relevant is area 6. For purposes of this
discussion, I intend to regard these as separable on anatomical grounds. Area
4 may be considered as the primary motor area and area 6, lying in front of
it, is then premotor. The cyto-architectonic zone of area 6 extends medially
to occupy a region of cortex on the medial surface of the hemisphere within
the sagittal sulcus. From this medial zone of cortex, electrical stimulations
produced movement responses when these stimuli were applied by PENFIELD and
his colleagues in studies of the human cerebral cortex. In an anatomical
sense, this zone is also premotor in that its efferent fibres project into
area 4, and it therefore lies upstream of the motor cortex. It was given the
name "supplementary" motor area, and such a zone has been defined in monkeys

Experimental Brain Research, Suppl. 7
© Springer-Verlag Berlin · Heidelberg 1983

as well as in man. We must always remember that WOOLSEY's descriptive illustration of this supplementary motor area is a cartoon and can not be taken to delineate separate zones of representation for the movements of the body parts.

Most of the hints about functions of cortical regions must derive from observations of the movement disorders which follow cortical lesions. Hence lesions of area 4 disturb skill and agility in contralateral movement performance. The most distally-acting muscles are most affected and show least recovery. Fractionation of the use of distally-acting muscles is interfered with and, as a consequence, the precision grip of the monkey's contralateral thumb and index finger is impaired. Using these hints, it should be possible to define questions of relevance to coding in terms such as : How do neurons in area 4 code for skill and precision of use of distal musculature ? Dr. LEMON will contribute more information on this topic later in this symposium.

The results of all experiments addressing coding by neurons in the precentral motor cortex can be interpreted only in terms of the questions asked and the potential codes that are examined. Experimental design factors influence the information that can be obtained. Hence, the now well-known arrangements used by EVARTS (1968) allowed recognition of the fact that some pyramidal tract neurons in area 4 of monkeys showed changes in firing rate which were clearly related to the force generated in identified muscle groups and that changes in firing could not be regarded as coding for the position achieved by the animal's limb. Yet when the position of the limb was purposely disturbed, information about the perturbation was able to influence the same cortical neurons after a very brief latency. In this experiment the same cell could then have been considered to be coding disturbances of limb position, including their timing and direction (EVARTS, 1969 ; 1973 ; PORTER and RACK, 1976). Neither of these experiments addressed the possibility of coding of skill or precision or fractionation of distal muscle action. SMITH et al. (1975) found that precentral cortical neurons did appear to code, in their firing rate, the force and rate of change of force to be generated in contralateral "finger" muscles during a precision grip movement. Other evidence implicates other pyramidal tract neurons in the timing of muscle contraction which could be important in skilled use of the hand, or in use of only a part of a muscle when that muscle is involved in relatively independent finger movements. Is it necessary to invoke a cortical subset of cells concerned with the inhibition of muscle action ?

It is also clear from other experiments that the areas of cortex occupied by cells associated with finger movements are large and that part of the code for the precise control of these muscles may reside in the number of corticospinal neurons making connections with "finger" motoneurons or the power of their cortico-motoneuronal influences (WOOLSEY et al., 1952 ; PHILLIPS and PORTER, 1964 ; CLOUGH et al., 1968). Hence both spatial and temporal aspects of neuronal activity may be elements of a candidate neural code and this will include "the representation and transformation of information in the nervous system" (NRP Bulletin N° 3, 1968). The existence of convergent and divergent neural pathways (cortico-cortical and thalamo-cortical), together with the complex cellular and synaptic arrangements at each link in a neural chain, with both excitatory and inhibitory influences at work, suggests that there is the possibility for considerable editing and integration of the coded information at each level.

Spatial coding of movements or of muscles within the "representation" of movements in the primary motor cortex has been one of the dominant questions in motor physiology for a long period. The search for representation of the body parts in an orderly sequence which occupied WOOLSEY and his colleagues (1952) for so long has recently been dissected into component elements of representation by ASANUMA and others (1975). But the debate remains about whether these component representations are "columnar" or more diffuse and about whether or not there are single or multiple representations of, for example, finger flexion movements. It makes a difference to our theories about the keyboard for execution of movement performance which may be played upon by a variety of other influences concerned with the planning and organization of movement performance.

Part of the coding which must be imposed on area 4 in relation to its functions of imparting skill and precision on movement performance must come from the influences which converge on its pyramidal tract neurons from other areas of cerebral cortex. Immediately "upstream" of the motor cortex lies the premotor cortex (area 6) and its extension on the medial aspect of the hemisphere, the supplementary motor area (SMA). Recordings from neurons in these regions of the monkey's cerebral cortex during natural movement performance reveal significant differences in behavioural associations. BRINKMAN and PORTER (1979) found that many neurons in SMA changed their firing in relation to particular movements (proximal or distal) performed by either limb, but were little influenced, at least at short latencies, by natural stimuli delivered to the relaxed limb. These cells could be coding aspects of the programming of bimanual performance and are found in a zone which operates to feed-forward instructions to the primary motor area (area 4). It is of interest that regional cerebral blood flow in man increased in relation to SMA on both sides in association with the voluntary performance of unilateral finger and thumb opposition (ROLAND et al., 1980) : the increase occurred in these zones without a similar increase over the contralateral primary motor area when the patient thought about the movement but did not produce it. Further evidence for a role of SMA in the planning of movements is found in the bilateral disability in the sequencing of distal movement control which follows a unilateral lesion in this zone (BRINKMAN, 1980).

Behavioural observations which relate to the motor deficits which follow lesions confined to the lateral part of area 6, the premotor cortex, are much less certain in defining a global functional role for this premotor zone and the debate about whether or not lesions in area 6 are involved in the production of spasticity continue. MOLL and KUYPERS (1977) have recently indicated that monkeys with a premotor lesion had no manual deficits but showed deficiencies in visually guiding the arm through a hole to a food target.

Recordings from neurons in area 6 revealed similarities to the findings in SMA. Hence some neurons changed their firing in relation to specific movements of the forelimb musculature and the changes in discharge clearly preceded the occurrence of the movement. A proportion of these cells was active in association with movements of the contralateral and also of the ipsilateral limb (BRINKMAN and PORTER, 1979).

But other cells in area 6 have a complex association with movement performance in which visual effects associated with the position of a target or attention to it were combined with responses in association with movement towards that target (BRINKMAN and PORTER, 1981 ; WISE and WEINRICH, 1981). This and the behavioural information (MOLL and KUYPERS, 1977) suggests that aspects of visuomotor control may be coded in the premotor cortex and then relayed to the primary motor area.

Taken together with the accumulating knowledge about local connectivities within the cerebral cortex and between the thalamus and the cerebral cortex, these findings draw us towards the conclusion that area 4 contains the essential machinery for command of the execution of an appropriate movement response, particularly using the most distally-acting muscles of the contralateral limbs. These same neuronal populations in area 4 are in receipt of a very short latency indicator signal which arises within the peripheral motor territory which is affected by the natural discharge of these same cells. These afferent responses are apparently not essential for normal performance of learned movements. Whether or not the indicator signal operates as a servo-feedback system for control of force development requires further evaluation in experiments designed to test more rigorously the force-feedback control system and to evaluate the role of flexibility and plasticity and learning in relation to these responses. (FETZ and FINOCCHIO, 1971 ; EVARTS and TANJI, 1974 ; CONRAD et al., 1974).

Neurons in the premotor cortex of area 6 seem to be much more involved in the generation of signals which could influence outputs from area 4. These are less subject to short-latency effects from peripheral detectors of movement. Some of them seem to be concerned in specification of movements whether or not these are to be performed by the contralateral or the ipsilateral limb. But many cells in area 6 may be concerned with visuo-motor responses.

Neurons in the supplementary motor area exhibit complex responses in relation to movement performance. They too are little affected at short latency by detectors of movement in the limbs. They too discharge in relation to particular movement performances whether these are performed with the ipsilateral or the contralateral limb. And most of the recent evidence suggests a function for these cells in the planning and programming of the signal which will be directed from area 4 in relation to the execution of movement performance.

REFERENCES

ASANUMA H (1975) Recent developments in the study of the columnar arrangement of neurons within the motor cortex. Physiol Rev 51:143-156

BRINKMAN C, PORTER R (1979) Supplementary motor area in the monkey : activity of neurons during performance of a learned motor task. J Neurophysiol 42:681-709

BRINKMAN J (1980) Effects of supplementary motor area ablation in the monkey. Proc Aust Physiol Pharmacol Soc 11:170P

BRINKMAN J, PORTER R (1979) "Premotor" area of the monkey's cerebral cortex : activity of neurones during performance of a learned motor task. Proc Aust Physiol Pharmacol Soc 10:

BRINKMAN C, PORTER R (1981) Supplementary motor and premotor areas of the cerebral cortex in the monkey : activity of neurons during performance of a learned movement task. In: Motor control mechanisms in man, edited by J.E. DESMEDT, Raven Press, New York, in press.

CLOUGH JFM, KERNELL D, PHILLIPS CG (1968) The distribution of monosynaptic excitation from the pyramidal tract and from primary spindle afferents to motoneurones of the baboons hand and forearm. J Physiol 198: 145-166

CONRAD B, MATSUNAMI K., MEYER-LOHMANN J, WIESENDANGER M., BROOKS VB (1974) Cortical load compensation during voluntary elbow movements. Brain Res 71:507-514

EVARTS EV (1968) Relation of pyramidal tract activity to force exerted during voluntary movement. J Neurophysiol 31:14-27

EVARTS EV (1969) Activity of pyramidal tract neurons during postural fixation. J Neurophysiol 32:375-385

EVARTS EV (1973) Motor cortex reflexes associated with learned movement. Science 179:501-503

EVARTS EV, TANJI J (1974) Gating of motor cortex reflexes by prior instruction. Brain Res 71:479-494

FETZ EE, FINOCCHIO DV (1971) Operant conditioning of specific patterns of neural and muscular activity. Science NY 174:431-435

MOLL L, KUYPERS HGJM (1977) Premotor cortical ablations in monkeys : contralateral changes in visually guided reaching behaviour. Science 198:317-319

PHILLIPS CG, PORTER R (1964) The pyramidal projection to motoneurons of some muscle groups of the baboon's forelimb. In: ECCLES JC, SCHADE JP (eds) Progress in Brain Research : Physiology of spinal neurones. Elsevier, Amsterdam, vol 12, pp 222-242

PORTER R, RACK PMH (1976) Timing of the response in the motor cortex to an unexpected disturbance of the finger position. Brain Res 103:201-213

ROLAND PE, LARSEN B, LASSEN NA, SKINHOJ E (1980) Supplementary motor area and other cortical areas in organization of voluntary movements in man. J Neurophysiol 43:118-136

SMITH AM, HEPP-REYMOND MC, WYSS UR (1975) Relation of activity in precentral cortical neurons to force and rate of change during isometric contractions of finger muscles. Exp Brain Res 23:315-332

WISE SP, WEINRICH M (1981) The monkey's premotor cortex. Soc Neuroscience Abstracts vol 7, p 18

WOOLSEY CN, SETTLAGE PH, MEYERS DR, SENCER W, HAMUY TP, TRAVIS AM (1952) Patterns of localization in precentral and "supplementary" motor areas and their relation to the concept of a premotor area. Res Publs Ass nerv ment Dis 30:238-264

AREA 4 : "PRIMARY" MOTOR AREA	SUPPLEMENTARY MOTOR AREA (S.M.A.) AREA 6 ON MEDIAL SURFACE	AREA 6 : "PREMOTOR" CORTEX : LATERAL SURFACE OF HEMISPHERE
1. Predominantly contralateral relationships to movement. Associations with distal or proximal movements.	1. Many "bilateral" associations usually symmetrical. Associations with distal or proximal movements. Some complex relationships to whole task performance.	1. Some contralateral, some bilateral associations (not usually symmetrical).
2. Short latency responses to natural stimulation of peripheral receptors. Localized "receptive zones" - predominantly deeply situated.	2. No significant short latency responses from detectors of peripheral disturbances. (?Highly processed afferent input from other cortical areas)	2. Many complex relationships dominated by visual "context" of the task.
3. Some neurons code force to be developed or derivatives of force. (Weakness occurs after area 4 lesions).	3. Behavioural evidence for feed forward to motor cortex of plan for movement. Deficit of sharing of work in bimanual task follows unilateral lesion.	3. No significant short latency inputs from detectors of peripheral disturbance.
4. But other aspects of movement must be also coded a) Skill and agility (evidence for coding of timing of contraction). b) Fractionation (?Inhibition direct to some motoneurons or reciprocal effects).		4. Visuomotor responses imposed on motor cortex from premotor cortex.
5. Both "motor" and "sensory" responses of PTN show marked flexibility and plasticity with changes in instructions (?Relationship to learning).		

Cortico-Basal Ganglia Relations and Coding of Motor Performance

M.R. DeLong, A.P. Georgopoulos, and M.D. Crutcher

Departments of Neurology and Neuroscience, Johns Hopkins University, School of Medicine, Baltimore, Maryland 21205, USA

The precise contributions of the basal ganglia to the control of normal movement and the role of these nuclei in pathophysiologic mechanisms of movement disorders are poorly understood. The present paper will consider selected aspects of the functional organization of the basal ganglia, and the neuronal coding of movement parameters in these nuclei. For a more detailed review and discussion of these and related matters, see DELONG and GEORGOPOULOS (1981).

Functional organization

The striatum, the "receptive" portion of the basal ganglia is divided in primates by the internal capsule into the caudate nucleus and the putamen. The sensorimotor and premotor cortices project to the putamen (KÜNZLE, 1975 ; 1978) while the "association" cortices project to the caudate (GOLDMAN and NAUTA, 1977 ; YETERIAN and VAN HOESEN, 1978). These anatomic features indicate a role of the putamen in more strictly "motor" and the caudate in more "complex" behavioral functions. Indeed, it has been shown repeatedly that restricted bilateral lesions of specific areas of the caudate nucleus in the primate can produce an impairment of performance in behavioral tasks similar to those seen after restricted lesions of regions of the prefrontal cortex which project to these areas (see DIVAC (1977) for a review). The most clear-cut impairments have been observed in performance of delayed alternation tasks after lesions of the dorsolateral prefrontal cortex or its projection area in the head of the caudate nucleus (the anterodorsal portion) and in performance of object reversal tasks after lesions of the orbitofrontal cortex or the ventrolateral portion of the caudate nucleus. Neurophysiological evidence for the predominant motor function of the putamen and portions of the pallidum came from early studies of arm-movement related cells in both segments of the globus pallidus (GP) (DELONG, 1971) and the putamen (DELONG, 1973 ; DELONG and STRICK, 1974). More recent studies in our laboratory provided clear evidence for a somatotopically organized grouping of cells related to the leg, arm and face in both the putamen and the ventral two-thirds of each segment of the GP (DELONG and GEORGOPOULOS, 1979 ; 1981), i.e. in those portions of GP which receive projections from the putamen.

The finding that the somatotopic motor representation established in the putamen is subsequently maintained in GP suggested that there exist segregated pathways through the basal ganglia for the control of different body parts. These findings led us to reexamine (DELONG and GEORGOPOULOS, 1981) the evidence for the widely held view that the basal ganglia serve as a "funnel" from association areas to the motor cortex (EVARTS and THACH, 1969 ; KEMP and POWELL, 1971 ; KORNHUBER, 1971). We have reviewed in detail (DELONG and GEORGOPOULOS, 1981) the anatomical evidence which indicates that influences from the association areas are ultimately directed back upon more rostral regions of the frontal lobe while influences from the sensorimotor and premotor cortices are directed largely upon premotor areas (not directly to area 4). This is shown schematically in Figure 1. Just as the arm, leg, and face representations remains segregated throughout the cerebral cortex, basal ganglia and thalamus, so the influences from the cortical association areas appear to be separately routed through these nuclei with no evidence of convergence upon the motor areas of these structures. In an early study JOHNSON and ROSVOLD (1971) showed that the topographical separation of the anterodorsal and the ventrolateral regions of the caudate nucleus is preserved in the projections of these behaviorally defined regions upon the pallidum and substantia nigra. These workers postulated that the dorsolateral frontal system is concerned with the spatial aspects of behavior (where to respond), whereas the orbitofrontal system participates in the control of temporal response tendencies (when to respond), and that the efferent pathways from these two regions remain distinct not only in the striatum, but also in the globus pallidus and the substantia nigra (SN).

The segregation of influences from the "association" and sensorimotor cortices in the caudate and putamen, respectively, is thus preserved at the next stage of processing by virtue of non-overlapping, topographically organized projections from the caudate and putamen to both segments of the GP and the SN (SZABO, 1967 ; 1970). This segregation of "motor" and "complex" functions appears to be maintained as well at the thalamic level by subsequent topographic projections to the thalamus from the inner segment of the GP (GPi) and the pars reticulata of the SN (SNpr) (NAUTA and MEHLER, 1966 ; KUO and CARPENTER, 1973 ; CARPENTER et al., 1976 ; KIM et al., 1976). The efferents from GPi and the SNpr together constitute the major output from the basal ganglia.

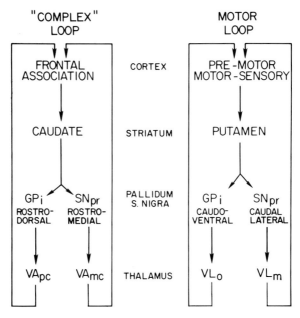

Fig. 1. Schematic depiction of the suggested segregation of pathways from the "association" (complex loop) and the sensorimotor areas (motor loop) through the basal ganglia and thalamus

Although the segregation of influences from association and sensorimotor cortices appears to be maintained throughout the basal ganglia, there is abundant evidence that integration of input from different cortical regions does take place. This was suggested by the studies of KEMP and POWELL (1970), who demonstrated overlapping corticostriate projections to the striatum from adjacent cortical areas. Recent autoradiographic studies (KÜNZLE, 1975 ; GOLDMAN and NAUTA, 1977 ; JONES et al., 1977) further suggest that the overlap may be even more extensive than indicated by degeneration studies. Recent studies by YETERIAN and VAN HOESEN (1978) indicate, however, that the overlapping of corticostriate projections is based not simply on proximity of cortical regions, but on whether or not cortical regions are interconnected. A theoretical outcome of the application of this organizing principle to the "arm" representation at cortical and putaminal levels is shown in Figure 2. This hypothetical scheme depicts integration within the putamen of cortical inputs from the "arm" areas in cortical areas 6, 4, 3, 1, 2 and 5. In a recent study, JONES et al. (1977) in fact demonstrated overlapping projections in the putamen from hand regions in cortical areas 4, 3, 1, 2 and 5. These studies suggest that, although corticocortical interactions do take

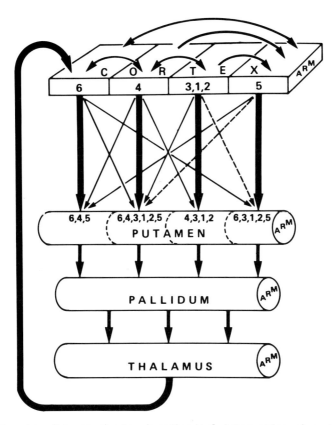

Fig. 2. Schematic diagram showing hypothetical integration of cortical inputs within the putamen. The arm representation is chosen as an example. In the putamen this representation consists of a long anteroposterior cylinder where inputs from "arm" representation in cortical areas 6, 4, 3, 1, 2 and 5 are integrated. This cylindrical representation is maintained in the pallidum and ventrolateral nucleus of the thalamus by virtue of topographically organized connections. Main corticoputaminal projections are shown as heavy lines ; projections from reciprocally interconnected cortical areas are shown as continuous light lines and those from nonreciprocally connected areas as dashed lines. (From DELONG and GEORGOPOULOS (1981) with permission of the American Physiological Society)

place at the cortical level, new interactions may arise in the basal ganglia, leading to novel integration within the striatum or at later stages in the pallidum and thalamus (DELONG and GEORGOPOULOS, 1981). According to this scheme, integration of afferent inputs to the putamen (and more generally the entire striatum) takes place primarily in the rostrocaudal plane. Specifically, motor and sensory inputs to the arm, leg, and face areas within the putamen remain highly segregated whereas inputs related to a single body part (e.g. arm) from a variety of cortical areas appear to converge along a rostrocaudal functional (arm) cylinder. This organizational scheme, which indicates a flow of information from the cerebral cortex (arm areas) → putamen (arm) → pallidum (arm), clearly suggests that one could study the function of the basal ganglia and the operations of each structure by characterizing the activity of neurons along the pathway from input (cortex) to output (GPi) in a behavioral task in which sensory inputs and motor responses can be identified and characterized.

Although major emphasis has been given to the pathway from the cortex to the striatum, recent anatomic studies (HARTMANN-VON MONAKOW et al., 1978) have revealed a topographically organized projection from the motor and premotor cortices to the subthalamic neurons (STN) in primates. In recent studies of the activity of neurons in the STN we have observed a somatotopic organization of the movement-related neurons similar to that suggested by the anatomical studies. The STN projects topographically to both segments of the GP and to the SN (CARPENTER and STROMINGER, 1967 ; NAUTA and COLE, 1978) and, thus, can influence directly the output from the basal ganglia. Lesions of the STN in man and primates result in involuntary movements of the contralateral limbs (hemiballismus) (WHITTIER, 1947 ; CARPENTER et al., 1950 ; WHITTIER and METTLER, 1949). Since these movements can be abolished by subsequent lesions of GPi or its efferent projections (CARPENTER et al., 1950), it has been postulated that loss of the modulating influences of the STN on GPi leads to involuntary movements because of the abnormal output from GPi. It is possible, however, that it is the disconnection of the GP from the cortico-subthalamic input which is responsible for this disorder which appears to be unique to primates.

Encoding of movement parameters

In earlier studies (DELONG, 1971) a relation of basal ganglia neurons to specific aspects of limb movement was demonstrated in single cell experiments in monkeys. It was found that the activity of many neurons in GP was related to arm or leg movements during performance of a motor task and, moreover, to movements of the arm in a particular direction (e.g., push or pull or side to side). In a later study, it was found that cell discharge in the putamen was influenced by the speed of internally generated non-pursuit arm movements (DELONG, 1973 ; DELONG and STRICK, 1974). In this study the animals had to generate either a fast or a slow movement in response to a red or green light, respectively. The activity of a large percentage of cells in the putamen and a smaller percentage in the pallidum was preferentially related to the slow movements in that task.

Those studies formed the starting point of further investigations (DELONG and GEORGOPOULOS, 1979 ; 1981) of the relation of neuronal discharge to movement parameters. We studied neuronal activity in STN and SN as well as GPe and GPi. Animals were trained on both step and pursuit tracking tasks in which the amplitude, speed and direction of movement were varied. All cells in these studies were related to arm movements during examination of the animal outside the behavioral task. Eighty three neurons in GPe, 35 in GPi and 36 in STN were studied in the step tracking task ; of these, 66 in GPe, 26 in GPi and 13 in STN were also studied in the pursuit tracking task.

Many cells in GPe, GPi and STN discharged at different frequencies with opposite directions of movement. This difference in discharge was achieved through different combinations of increase or decrease in activity in different cells. Significant relations to the direction to movement were observed during both the movement time (MT) and the initial premovement time (IPT, i.e., the 100 msec prior to the onset of movement), during which most of the changes in EMG began to occur.

A high proportion of cells in GPe, GPi and STN showed a significant relation to the amplitude of movement. An example is shown in Figure 3. In general, the frequency of cell discharge was a linear function of the amplitude of movement. The incidence of significant amplitude effects was highest in the MT, but the effects were also present in the IPT. The effects of movement amplitude became apparent when a wide range of amplitudes was used (25mm to 100mm). These effects were not marked in initial experiments probably because of the small range of movement amplitudes used.

The relations between cell discharge and peak velocity of movement in the step tracking task were similar to those described above for the amplitude of movement. This was expected since amplitude and peak velocity were highly correlated. No significant relations to ramp velocity in the pursuit task were observed, however.

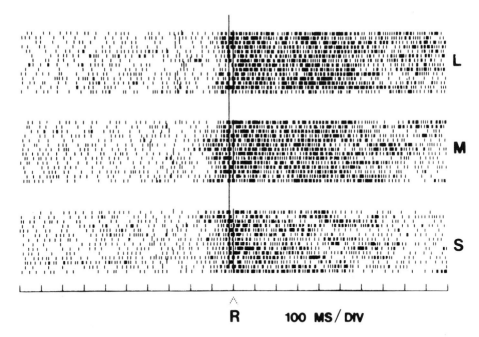

Fig. 3. Activity of a cell in monkey subthalamic nucleus during arm flexion movements of different amplitudes : S (small = 25 mm), M (medium = 62.5 mm), and L (large = 100 mm). Trials for each class are aligned on the response (R), the first detectable change in velocity. A clear relationship of cell discharge to amplitude of movement can be seen. (From DELONG and GEORGOPOULOS (1981) with permission of the American Physiological Society)

Studies of the relations between neuronal activity and movement in the SN indicated that the discharge of most cells in the pars compacta (SNpc) was unrelated to movement of specific body parts and most movement-related cells in the pars reticulata (SNpr) were related to orofacial movements. The observed lack of phasic modulation of SNpc neurons during movement suggested a more tonic or "gating" rather than a phasic role of the nigrostriatal dopamine system in movement (DELONG and GEORGOPOULOS, 1979).

The finding of significant directional effects in GP is not surprising since neurons in both the putamen (CRUTCHER and DELONG, 1981) and the STN, which project to GP, show a strong relation to the direction of movement. The presence of directional relations in the putamen and STN can, in turn, be accounted for by the input to these structures from the cerebral cortex, since both precentral and parietal cortical cells show significant relations to the direction of movement (EVARTS, 1966 ; SCHMIDT et al., 1975 ; GEORGOPOULOS et al., 1980 ; KALASKA et al., 1981).

Monkeys were studied in a behavioral paradigm which was designed to determine whether the activity of neurons in the putamen is related to the direction of movement, per se, or to the underlying pattern of muscular activity (CRUTCHER and DELONG, 1981). The animals were trained to perform a visuomotor tracking task which required elbow flexion/extension movements with assisting and opposing loads. Thus the direction of arm movement was dissociated from the pattern of muscular activity. The activity of 91% of neurons (n=120) was related to the arm movements in the step portion of the task : 58% of neurons were best related to the direction of arm movement irrespective of the muscles used, whereas 13% showed a pattern of activity "like muscle". These results indicate that neurons in the putamen are predominantly related to the direction of arm movement rather than to the activity of individual muscles, and that the basal ganglia may play a role in the specification of parameters of movement independent of the pattern of activity of specific muscles.

Relations of basal ganglia neurons to static force have been observed in both the GP (BRANCH et al., 1980) and the putamen (CRUTCHER and DELONG, 1981). Neurons in both structures exhibited sustained changes in discharge in association with maintained loads. Of 120 arm cells in the putamen, 23% had a significant linear relation to the level of static load.

The finding of significant neural relations to the amplitude of movement may be relevant to the observation that patients with diseases of the basal ganglia frequently have difficulty in controlling the amplitude of their limb movements. For example, in patients with Parkinson's disease, single-step large amplitude movements are impaired : these movements fall short of the target (FLOWERS, 1978), which is then reached by a series of small-amplitude movements (DRAPER and JOHNS 1964 ; FLOWERS, 1978). The mechanism of this phenomenon was partially elucidated recently by HALLETT and KHOSHBIN (1980) who observed that Parkinsonian patients were unable to increase the amplitude of the agonist burst in step-tracking movements. Thus, large amplitude movements were achieved by several small-amplitude steps. Loss or derangement of pallidal influence in the control of movement amplitude might account on the one hand for the hypometric movements and overall bradykinesia of Parkinsonian patients and on the other hand for the wild, large amplitude movements of patients with chorea and hemiballismus.

In conclusion, it appears on the basis of recent anatomical and physiological studies that previous concepts of the functional organization of the basal

ganglia and their relations with the cerebral cortex must be revised. While
the striatum receives input from the entire neocortex, this input appears to
remain segregated along the lines established at the cortical level. Rather
than a "funneling" of input from different cortical areas through the
pallidum to the thalamus and motor cortex, there appears to be, in the
broadest sense, a maintained segregation of information relevant to motor and
"complex" functions and within each of these two divisions, a finer grain for
movements of individual body parts (leg, arm, face, etc.) and for complex
behaviors (e.g., delayed alternation, delayed response, object reversal). The
concept of segregated parallel subcortical loops subserving "motor" and
"complex" functions is proposed. On the output side, it should be emphasized
that the output from the "motor loop" terminates in those regions of the
thalamus which project to premotor areas (area 6), rather than to area 4, and
that at the thalamic level there is no evidence for significant integration
of basal ganglia and cerebellar output. Single cell studies in the basal
ganglia of behaving animals have revealed specific relations of neuronal
activity to movements of individual body parts and a relation to specific
parameters of movement, particularly direction, amplitude, and force. Therefore, the basal ganglia may play a specific role in integration of information from related cortical areas and in the determination of specific
parameters of movement. Some evidence suggests that such relations to
movement parameters may be coded independently of the pattern of muscular
activity.

REFERENCES

ALLEN GI, TSUKAHARA N (1974) Cerebrocerebellar communication systems. Physiol
Rev 54:957-1006

BRANCH MH, CRUTCHER MD, DELONG MR (1980) Globus pallidus : neuronal responses
to arm loading. Soc Neurosci Abstr 6:272

CARPENTER MB, WHITTIER JR, METTLER FA (1950) Analysis of choreoid hyperkinesia in the rhesus monkey : surgical and pharmacological analysis of
hyperkinesia resulting from lesions in the subthalamic nucleus of Luys. J
comp Neurol 92:293-331

CARPENTER MB, STROMINGER NL (1967) Efferent fibers of the subthalamic nucleus
in monkey. Am J Anat 121:47-72

CARPENTER MB, NAKANO K, KIM R (1976) Nigrothalamic projections in the monkey
demonstrated by autoradiographic technics. J comp Neurol 165:401-416

CRUTCHER MD, DELONG MR (1981) Relation of putamen neuronal discharge to
direction of movement or pattern of muscular activity. Soc Neurosci Abstr
7:778

DELONG MR (1971) Activity of pallidal neurons during movement. J Neurophysiol
34:414-427

DELONG MR (1973) Putamen : activity of single units during slow and rapid arm movements. Science 179:1240-1242

DELONG MR, STRICK PL (1974) Relation of basal ganglia, cerebellum, and motor cortex units to ramp and ballistic limb movements. Brain Res 71:327-335

DELONG MR, GEORGOPOULOS AP (1979) Motor functions of the basal ganglia as revealed by studies of single cell activity in the behaving primate In:

POIRIER LJ, SOURKES TL, BEDARD PJ (eds) Advances in neurology. Raven Press, New York, pp 13⊦-140

DELONG MR, GEORGOPOULOS AP (1981) Motor functions of the basal ganglia. In: Handbook of Physiology. American Physiological Society, pp 1017-1061

DEVITO J, SMITH OJ (1964) Subcortical projections of the prefrontal lobe in the monkey. J comp Neurol 123:413-424

DIVAC I (1977) Does the neostriatum operate as a functional entity ? In: COOLS AR, LOHMANN AHM, VAN DEN BERCKEN JHL (eds) Psychobiology of the striatum. Elsevier, Amsterdam, pp 21-30

DRAPER IT, JOHNS RJ (1964) The disordered movement in parkinsonism and the effect of drug treatment. Bull John Hopkins Hosp 115:465-480

EVARTS EV (1966) Pyramidal tract activity associated with a conditioned hand movement in the monkey. J Neurophysiol 29:1011-1927

EVARTS EV, THACH WT (1969) Motor mechanisms of the CNS : cerebrocerebellar interrelations. Ann Rev Physiol 31:451-498

FLOWERS K (1978) Some frequency response characteristics of parkinsonism on pursuit tracking. Brain 101:19-34

GEORGOPOULOS AP, DELONG MR (1979) Quantitative studies of neuronal activity in basal ganglia during limb movements. Can J Neurol Sci 6:79

GEORGOPOULOS AP, KALASKA JF, MASSEY JT (1980) Cortical mechanisms of two-dimensional aiming arm movements. I. Aiming at different target locations. Soc Neurosci Abstr 6:156

GOLDMAN PS, NAUTA WJH (1977) An intricately patterned prefronto-caudate projection in the rhesus monkey. J comp Neurol 171:369-386

HALLETT M, KHOSHBIN S (1980) A physiological mechanism of bradykinesia. Brain 103:301-314

HARTMANN-VON-MONAKOW K, AKERT K, KUNZLE H (1978) Projections of the precentral motor cortex and other cortical areas of the frontal lobe to the subthalamic nucleus in the monkey. Exp Brain Res 33:395-403

JOHNSON TN, ROSVOLD HE (1971) Topographic projections on the globus pallidus and the substantia nigra of selectivity placed lesions in the precommissural caudate nucleus and putamen in the monkey. Exp Neurol 33:584-596

JONES EG, COULTER JD, BURTON H, PORTER R (1977) Cells of origin and terminal distribution of corticostriatal fibers arising in the sensory- motor cortex of monkeys. J comp Neurol 173:53-80

KALASKA JF, CAMINITI R., GEORGOPOULOS AP (1981) Cortical mechanisms of two-dimensional aimed arm movements. III. Relations of parietal (areas 5 and

2) neuronal activity to direction of movement and change in target location. Soc Neurosci Abstr 7:563

KEMP JM, POWELL TPS (1970) The corticostriate projection in the monkey. Brain 93:525-546

KEMP JM, POWELL TPS (1971) The connexions of the striatum and globus pallidus : synthesis and speculation. Phil Trans R Soc Lond B 262:441-457

KIM R, NAKANO K, JAYARAMAN A, CARPENTER MB (1976) Projections of the globus pallidus and adjacent structures : an autoradiographic study in the monkey. J comp Neurol 169:263-290

KORNHUBER HH (1971) Motor functions of cerebellum and basal ganglia :the cerebellocortical saccadic (ballistic) clock, the cerebellonuclear hold regulator, and the basal ganglia ramp (voluntary speed smooth movement) generator. Kybernetik 8:157-162

KUNZLE H (1975) Bilateral projections from precentral motor cortex to the putamen and other parts of the basal ganglia. An autoradiographic study in Macaca fascicularis. Brain Res 88:195-209

KUNZLE H (1978) An autoradiographic analysis of the efferent connections from premotor and adjacent prefrontal regions (areas 6 and 9) in Macaca fascicularis. Brain Behav Evol 105:185-234

KUO JS, CARPENTER MB (1973) Organization of pallidothalamic projections in the rhesus monkey. J comp Neurol 151:201-236

LILES SL (1978) Unit activity in the putamen associated with conditioned arm movements : topographic organization. Federation Proc 37:396

NAUTA HJW, COLE M (1978) Efferent projections of the subthalamic nucleus : an autoradiographic study in monkey and cat. J comp Neurol 180:1-16

NAUTA WJH, MEHLER WR (1966) Projections of the lentiform nucleus in the monkey. Brain Res 1:3-42

SCHMIDT EM, JOST RG, DAVIS KK (1975) Reexamination of the force relationship of cortical cell discharge patterns with conditioned wrist movements. Brain Res 83:213-223

SZABO J (1967) The efferent projections of the putamen in the monkey. Exp Neurol 19:463-476

SZABO J (1970) Projections from the body of the caudate nucleus in the rhesus monkey. Exp Neurol 27:1-15

WHITTIER JR (1947) Ballism and subthalamic nucleus. Arch Neurol Psychiatry 58:672-692

WHITTIER JR, METTLER FA (1949) Studies of the subthalamic of the rhesus monkey. II. Hyperkinesia and other physiologic effects of subthalamic lesions with special references to the subthalamic nucleus of Luys. J comp Neurol 90:319-372

YETERIAN EH, VAN HOESEN GW (1978) Cortico-striate projections in the rhesus monkey : the organization of certain cortico-caudate connections. Brain Res 139:43-63

Cortico-Cerebellar Loops

M. Wiesendanger

Institut de Physiologie, Université de Fribourg, CH-1700 Fribourg, Switzerland

1. INTRODUCTION

The aim of this presentation is to provide an overview on the main corti-co-cerebellar circuits and to discuss current views about the function of these loops in motor control, i.e. in execution of, as well as in programming motor tasks. The cerebellar input-output systems are commonly separated into medial, intermediate and lateral components which is in accord with hodology and, to some extent, also reflects a functional division : the vermal and paramedian zones of the cerebellum are considered to be involved in the updating of ongoing movements, the hemispheres (neocerebellum) with the planning of movements (e.g. ALLEN and TSUKAHARA, 1974). It should be noted, however, that the anatomical interrelations between cerebral cortex and cerebellum cannot be filled strictly into these medio-lateral divisions.

I have deliberately omitted the discussion of the olivary circuit because it would have considerably enlarged and complicated the present account. It should be remembered, though, that the climbing fibre system does also transmit feedforward signals from "higher" motor centres including the cere-bral cortex, most probably via polysynaptic routes (cf. recent review by BLOEDEL and COURVILLE, 1981).

2. LOOPS CONSIDERED TO BE IMPLICATED IN UPDATING ONGOING MOVEMENTS

The main classical deficits caused by lesions of the medial-intermediate zones of the cerebellum concern the difficulties in stance, gait, limb movements, and in ocular motility (see GILMAN et al. (1981) for recent review). It has been proposed that these zones continuously update the descending control signals in response to the incoming feedback signals in the course of evolving movements, "...like the controlling system of a target-finding missile" (ECCLES, 1979). In the following are brief accounts

Experimental Brain Research, Suppl. 7
© Springer-Verlag Berlin · Heidelberg 1983

about the structures which might be implicated in this "dynamic loop of movement control". Anatomically identified mossy fibre inputs from these precerebellar nuclei are chiefly (but not exclusively) distributed to the vermis, flocculus and nodulus, to the paramedian lobe and to the respective underlying intracerebellar nuclei. The cortical inputs to these relays originate mainly (but not exclusively) from the sensorimotor cortex.

2.1. The lateral reticular nucleus (LRN)

Figure 1 is a summarizing diagram of the known afferent and efferent connections (for details see also BLOEDEL and COURVILLE, 1981). As most precerebellar nuclei, the LRN receives descending, ascending spinal and cerebellar return signals. In a single unit study from our laboratory (BRUCKMOSER et al., 1970b), it was found that a subset of LRN neurons received rubral, but not fastigial short-latency inputs ; another subset of LRN neurones conversely received short-latency fastigial, but not rubral inputs. Many LRN neurones could be activated from the sensorimotor cortex at relatively long latencies (suggesting multisynaptic links or reflecting the need of much temporal summation), but a subset of LRN neurones was excited from the cortex at short (probably monosynaptic) latencies with great synaptic efficacy (BRUCKMOSER et al., 1970a). Anatomical data indicated that the connections are via collaterals from the bulbar pyramid (KUNZLE and WIESENDANGER, 1974) and electrophysiological observations (ZANGGER and WIESENDANGER, 1973) suggested that part of the cortical impulses are mediated via collaterals of corticospinal fibres (see, however, recent investigation by ALSTERMARK and LUNDBERG, 1980).

Degeneration studies in cats (P. BRODAL et al., 1967) revealed a non-topographic cortical projection, principally from the anterior sigmoid gyrus. In an autoradiographic study in monkeys, we have addressed the question of the cortical origin and of somatotopy (R. WIESENDANGER and M. WIESENDANGER, unpublished observations). Labelled amino acids were injected into various areas of the frontal and parietal cortex. In all positive cases, the labelling in the LRN was weak or moderate. So far an unambiguous projection was seen only in area 4 cases. The precentral arm and hindlimb cortex had overlapping projections with the forelimb projection occupying more medial and the hindlimb projection more lateral zones. A single unit study in monkeys (WIESENDANGER and MARINI, unpublished) likewise revealed excitatory inputs from precentral areas only. The rather strong effects also obtained by stimulations in area 6 were considered to be mediated indirectly via the red nucleus.

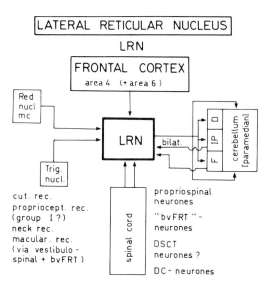

Fig. 1. Connections of the lateral reticular nucleus (LRN). On the lower left type of afferent information transmitted, on the lower right types of neurones projecting to the LRN. See text. (bvFRT = bilateral ventral flexor reflex tract ; DSCT = dorsal spino-cerebellar tract ; DC = dorsal columns)

It is known since long that the LRN receives a massive spinal input, partly via the so-called bilateral ventral flexor-reflex tract (GRANT et al., 1966). In line with LUNDBERG's hypothesis that ascending pathways monitor the activity of spinal interneurones rather than peripheral events (cf. BALDISSERA et al., 1981 ; for recent discussion), it was postulated that LRN neurones may "compare" feedforward signals from higher motor centres with internal feedback signals from lower (spinal) motor centres (OSCARSSON, 1973 ; ZANGGER and WIESENDANGER, 1973). In recent years, our knowledge of the wiring diagram of spinal afferent fibres to the LRN has greatly increased. Thus, it appears that the cord segments have somatotopically organized projections to the LRN (KUNZLE, 1973), and that a particularly important input is derived from collaterals of high cervical propriospinal cells which integrate signals from various descending pathways and which project monosynaptically to motoneurones. This circuit seems ideally suited for the monitoring of activity in spinal motor centres as proposed in LUNDBERG's hypothesis.

Generally, the receptive fields of LRN neurones were large and relatively strong electrical stimuli had to be used to activate LRN neurones (OSCARSSON, 1973). However, small receptive fields, the involvement of group I afferents, and responses to muscle stretch have also been described (see BLOEDEL and COURVILLE, 1981).

Functionally, the LRN appears to be involved in a number of motor activities. First, it was discovered that LRN neurones participate in the control of locomotion and rhythmic scratching (ARSHAVSKY et al., 1978). Since modulation of LRN cell-discharges persisted during fictive locomotion one may conclude that this modulation was caused by internal feedback signals and/or descending signals. As yet it is unknwon whether LRN neurones are also implicated in movements other than locomotion and scratching. However, there is now accumulating evidence that the LRN may also play an important role in tonic postural mechanisms as evidenced by lesion studies (CORVAJA et al., 1977) and by the findings that macular and neck afferents influence LRN neurones to a remarkable degree (KUBIN et al., 1981a, b).

2.2. The paramedian reticular nucleus (PRN)

Figure 2 summarizes the connectivity of this precerebellar nucleus (cf. BLOEDEL and COURVILLE, 1981, for references). The functional implication of these anatomically identified connections are so far unknown ; the hodological similarities with the LRN suggest that it subserves perhaps also similar functions.

2.3. The nucleus reticularis tegmenti pontis of Bechterew (NRTP)

As illustrated in Figure 3, this is the only precerebellar relay nucleus for which no spinal input has been found. The NRTP is included somewhat arbitrarily in this section, inspite of its close relation with the pontine nuclei proper, because its efferent fibres project mainly to the median and paramedian zones of the cerebellum and because its major cortical input originates from the motor cortex (P. BRODAL, 1980a, b). The inflow from the intracerebellar nuclei (mainly interpositus and dentate) appears to be very powerful, and it has been suggested that this nucleus might more appropriately be considered as a relay in a cerebello-cerebellar (reverberating) circuit. Degeneration studies in the monkey by BRODAL (1980c) had revealed a relatively diffuse pattern of cortical projection which contrasted with the cortical projection to the pontine nuclei proper. A renewed analysis with autoradiographic methods disclosed, however, a somewhat more distinct topographical relationship (HARTMANN VON MONAKOW et al., 1981).

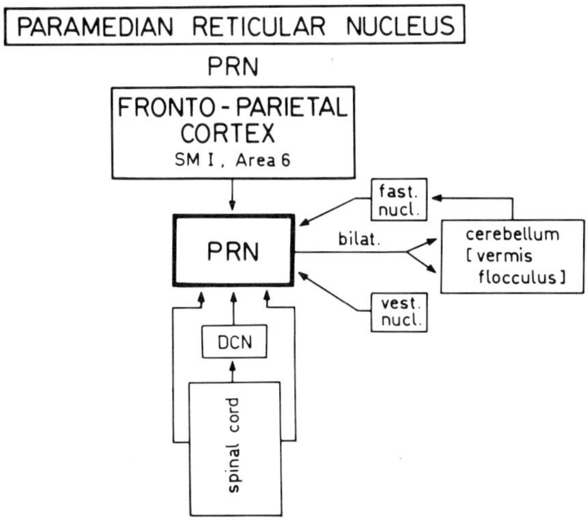

PARAMEDIAN RETICULAR NUCLEUS

PRN

FRONTO - PARIETAL CORTEX

SM I, Area 6

PRN

fast. nucl.

bilat.

cerebellum [vermis flocculus]

vest. nucl.

DCN

spinal cord

Fig. 2. Connections of the paramedian reticular nucleus (PRN). See text for description. (DCN = dorsal column nuclei)

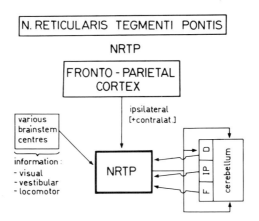

N. RETICULARIS TEGMENTI PONTIS

NRTP

FRONTO - PARIETAL CORTEX

various brainstem centres

ipsilateral [+contralat.]

information :
- visual
- vestibular
- locomotor

NRTP

D

IP

F

cerebellum

Fig. 3. Connections of the N. reticularis tegmenti pontis (NRTP). On the lower left are indicated the types of information transmitted via brainstem centres to the NRTP. See text

New insights on the function of the NRTP have been obtained recently in electrophysiological and lesion studies in cats. Thus, PRECHT and STRATA (1980) addressed the problem of the pathway by which optokinetic information reaches the vestibular nuclei (known to integrate information from the horizontal canal system and horizontal optokinetic information). Rather surprisingly, it was found that lesions involving the NRTP in cats critically interfered with both the optokinetic response properties of the vestibular neurones and also with the elaboration of the optokinetic nystagmus. These results suggested that signals from visual centres are mediated to the vestibular nuclei via the NRTP. Single unit studies on NRTP neurones in rats confirmed this conclusion (CAZIN et al., 1980). Moreover, MAEKAWA et al. (1981) found NRTP cells in rabbits which could be activated orthodromically from the optic tract and antidromically from the flocculus (known to receive NRTP afferents). Optokinetic signals may thus also reach the vestibular nuclear neurones via a cerebellar loop. These important new results then suggest that the NRTP contributes to the control of eye movements.

In other studies on decorticate cats, it was found that about two-thirds of the NRTP neurones investigated changed their activity during induced locomotion ; these were either tonic changes or rhythmic modulations (ZANGGER and SCHULTZ, 1978). Since the NRTP receives no spinal afferents it is likely that these changes in cell discharge were induced either via the cerebellar afferents or by the mesencephalic locomotor area shown to project to the NRTP (EDWARDS, 1975). It was previously proposed by BOYLLS (1975) that the NRTP could mediate a powerful reticulocerebellar recurrent excitation during locomotion.

3. LOOPS CONSIDERED TO BE IMPLICATED IN THE PLANNING AND PROGRAMMING OF MOVEMENTS

Gordon HOLMES' (1917) documentation that hemi-cerebellar patients are delayed in releasing a grasp on the affected side has been influential in current considerations about the role of the cerebellum in movement initiation (cf. BROOKS, 1979). The pioneering anatomical work on the corticopontine projection by NYBY and JANSEN (1951) seemed to fit with the concept that the pontocerebellum is upstream to the motor cortex as expected from the proposed role of the cerebellum in movement initiation and programming. ALLEN and TSUKAHARA (1974) emphasized this functional aspect of the neocerebellum by the well-known diagram displaying the flow of information from cortical association cortex via the neocerebellum and the ventrolateral thalamus to the motor cortex. This open loop was considered to be one of the candidates subserving the "long-range planning of movements". In man, there are more than 20 million cells in the pontine nuclei (PN) and they give rise to the dominant mossy fibre input to the cerebellum, especially to its lateral zones. Newer results about the cortico-pontocerebellar system will be summarized below.

3.1. The cortico-pontocerebellar system in monkeys

Figure 4 displays diagrammatically the connections of the PN in monkeys as revealed in studies by P. BRODAL (1978), VILENSKY and VAN HOESEN (1981), HARTMANN-v. MONAKOW et al. (1981) and in our own investigations (DHANARAJAN et al., 1977 ; WIESENDANGER et al., 1979a). Much of this work has already been reviewed (WIESENDANGER et al., 1979b) and I will therefore point only to a few features which seem important in the context of the present review. All investigators seem to agree that the peri-Rolandic areas including MI, premotor cortex, SMA, SI, SII and area 5 as well as the visual cortex provide the bulk of cortical afferents to the PN. Area 24 of the anterior cingulate gyrus may be considered as another premotor area as discussed elsewhere (MacPHERSON et al., 1982). Contrary to expectation, however, the contribution from high-order association cortex appears to be sparse or even lacking. The other result which became strikingly apparent in autoradiographic studies was the widely distributed "patchy" projection from small cortical areas (espe-

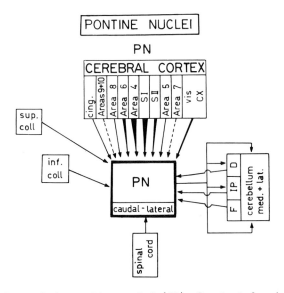

Fig. 4. Connections of the pontine nuclei (PN). See text for description

A

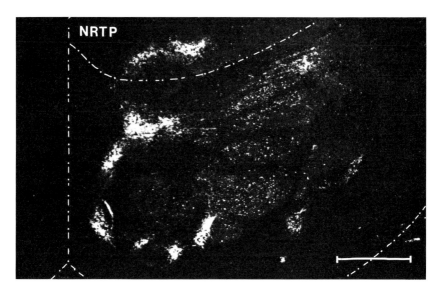

B

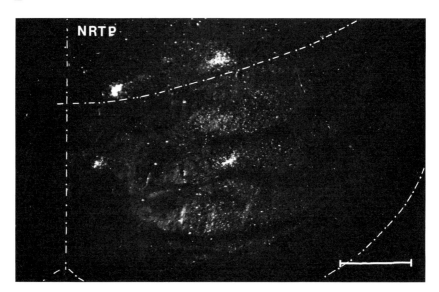

Fig. 5. A : Autoradiograph showing multiple patches of silvergrains in the PN and the NRTP following an injection of labeled aminoacids in area 4. B : Case of a SMA injection with two patches in the PN and in the NRTP. Calibration : 1 mm. Unpublished observations from experiments by R. and M. WIESENDANGER

cially of the motor cortex, see Fig. 5). Retrograde HRP studies (P. BRODAL, 1979) also revealed the complex pattern of divergence and convergence of the pontocerebellar projection. Furthermore, a remarkable convergence pattern from subdivisions of peri-Rolandic areas to identified pontocerebellar neurones was found in microelectrophysiological investigations by RUEGG et al. (1977).

From these anatomical and physiological results, taken together, it can be concluded that the "pontocerebellum" is mostly interested in information from cortical motor, somatosensory and visual areas. The sensory information transmitted from the cortex (and also from tectal relays) is therefore not as highly processed as would be the case if high-order association cortex was the chief source of inputs to the PN. The intricate "patchy" organization within PN neurones, the presence of interneurones and recurrent collaterals would, however, allow for integrative processes to take place at the pontine level.

3.2. Theoretical implications

That part of the loop which originates from the motor cortex and which feeds back, via the dentate nucleus and the ventrolateral thalamus, to the motor cortex can be considered as a closed loop and might share functions similar to those attributed to the other loops described in section 2. In fact, anatomical data have shown that the PN project not only to the lateral, but also to the medial zones. BLOMFIELD and MARR (1970) conjectured that this fast excitatory loop might function as a reinforcing mechanism for generation of rapid movements. We (WIESENDANGER et al., 1979b) and others (BROOKS and THACH, 1981) have considered alternative propositions which take into account also the sensory inputs to the PN. Anatomical, physiological, behavioural and clinical data were discussed which were taken to favour the role played by the cerebellum in triggering movement programs by sensory signals, or in re-structuring on-going movement programs. Such a role is perhaps in better agreement with clinical symptomatology than the proposed role of "long-range planning" of movements.

4. CONCLUDING REMARKS

In this short overview on corticocerebellar loops I discussed the multitude of afferents from peripheral and central sources which may influence the relays of the loops. The medial and paramedian zones of the cerebellum, including the flocculus, have traditionally been considered to be implicated mainly in the immediate co-ordination of on-going movements and in the control of posture. However, it is clear that one cannot attribute one particular function to each of the relays. For instance there are at least two relays concerned with the control of locomotion (the NRTP and the LRN). Eye, head and posture co-ordination by means of vestibular and/or visual signals implicate the NRTP, the LRN and the PRN. Some electrophysiological evidence is available indicating that each relay encodes different aspects of motor behavior in distinct subsets of neurones. We do not know as yet whether a given cell population is specialized for a given task (e.g. locomotion), or whether it integrates multiple aspects of motor behaviour (e.g. locomotion and head position).

With respect to the proposed role of the lateral cerebellum in planning and programming movements, there are a number of difficulties which may partly be caused by the loose definitions of the terms "planning" and "programming". If "long-range planning" is viewed as a process of higher-order preparation of movement, i.e. selection of movement strategies, then it is unlikely that the neocerebellum fulfills this function (see also BROOKS, 1979, on this subject). Cerebellar lesions do not interfere with cognitive aspects of motor behaviour. If "programming" is viewed as a process tightly associated with the immediate execution, i.e. with the detailed instructions (direction, speed, force etc.), then such a role of the neocerebellum appears at least compatible with clinical observations. Few people would doubt that high-order association areas are of great importance in the "planning" of movements. Since these areas have little or no access to the cerebellum, it might be more profitable to study the role of cortico-striate or cortico-cortical loops in this respect. Several "premotor" areas, including the supplementary motor area, have powerful links with the motor cortex and evidence is accumulating that these areas indeed play an important role in movement initiation (cf. WIESENDANGER, 1981).

ACKNOWLEDGEMENT

The research work of the author was supported by the Swiss National Science Foundation (grant n° 3-752-80).

REFERENCES

ALLEN GI, TSUKAHARA N (1974) Cerebrocerebellar communication systems. Physiol Rev 54:957-1006

ALSTERMARK B, LUNDBERG A (1980) Do corticospinal fibers send collaterals to the lateral reticular nucleus ? Acta Physiol Scand 108:4A

ARSHAVSKY YI, GELFAND IM, ORLOVSKY GN, PAVLOVA GA (1977) Messages conveyed by spinocerebellar pathways during scratching in the cat. I Activity of neurons of the lateral reticular nucleus. Brain Res 151:479-491

BALDISSERA F, HULTBORN H, ILLERT M (1981) Integration in spinal neuronal systems. In: BROOKS VB (ed) Handbook of Physiology, section I, The Nervous System, vol II, Motor Control, part I. Am Physiol Soc, Bethesda, pp 509-595

BLOEDEL JR, COURVILLE J (1981) Cerebellar afferent systems. In: BROOKS VB (ed) Handbook of Physiology, section I, The Nervous System, vol II, Motor Control, part 2. Am Physiol Soc, Bethesda, pp 735-829

BLOMFIELD S, MARR D (1970) How the cerebellum may be used. Nature (London) 227:1224-1228

BOYLLS CC (1975) A theory of cerebellar function with applications to locomotion. I. The physiological role of climbing fiber inputs in anterior lobe operation, Technical Report, Dept of Computer and Information Sciences, Univ Mass Amherst, p 18

BRODAL P (1978) The corticopontine projection in the rhesus monkey. Origin and principles of organization. Brain 101:251-283

BRODAL P (1979) The pontocerebellar projection in the rhesus monkey :an experimental study with retrograde axonal transport of horseradish peroxidase. Neuroscience 4:193-208

BRODAL P (1980a) The cortical projection to the nucleus reticularis tegmenti pontis in the rhesus monkey. Exp Brain Res 30:19-27

BRODAL P (1980b) The projection from the nucleus reticularis tegmenti pontis to the cerebellum in the rhesus monkey. Exp Brain Res 38:29-36

BRODAL P, MARSALA J, BRODAL A (1967) The cerebral cortical projection to the lateral reticular nucleus in the cat, with special reference to the sensorimotor cortical areas. Brain Res 6:252-274

BROOKS VB (1979) Control of intended limb movements by the lateral and intermediate cerebellum. In: ASANUMA H, WILSON VJ (eds) Integration in the nervous system. Igaku-Shoin, Tokyo New-York

BROOKS VB, THACH WT (1981) Cerebellar motor of posture and movement. In: BROOKS VB (ed) Handbook of Physiology, section I, The Nervous System, vol II, Motor Control, part 2. Am Physiol Soc, Bethesda, pp 877-946

BRUCKMOSER P, HEPP-REYMOND MC, WIESENDANGER M (1970a) Cortical influence on single neurons of the lateral reticular nucleus of the cat. Exp Neurol 26:239-252

BRUCKMOSER P, HEPP MC, WIESENDANGER M (1970b) Effects of peripheral, rubral and fastigial stimulation on neurons of the lateral reticular nucleus of the cat. Exp Neurol 27:388-398

CAZIN L, PRECHT W, LANNOU J (1980) Firing characteristics of neurons mediating optokinetic responses to rat's vestibular neurons. Pflügers Arch 386:221-230

CORVAJA N, GROFOVA I, POMPEIANO O, WALBERG F (1977) The lateral reticular nucleus in the cat. II Effects of lateral reticular lesions on posture and reflex movements. Neuroscience 2:929-943

DHANARAJAN R, RUEGG DG, WIESENDANGER M (1977) An anatomical investigation of the corticopontine projection in the primate (Saimiri sciureus). The projection from motor and somatosensory areas. Neuroscience 2:913-922

ECCLES JC (1979) Introductory remarks. In: MASSION J, SASAKI K (eds) Cerebro-cerebellar interactions. Elsevier-North Holland Biomedical Press, Amsterdam New-York Oxford, pp 1-18

EDWARD SB (1975) Autoradiographic studies of the projections of the midbrain reticular formation : descending projections of nucleus cuneiformis. J Comp Neurol 161:341-358

GILMAN S, BLOEDEL JR, LECHTENBERG R (1981) Disorders of the cerebellum. Davis Comp, Philadelphia, pp 189-221

GRANT G, OSCARSSON O, ROSEN I (1966) Functional organization of the spinoreticuloocerebellar path with identification of its spinal component. Exp Brain Res 1:306-319

HARTMANN-v. MONAKOW K, AKERT K, KUNZLE H (1981) Projection of precentral, premotor and prefrontal cortex to the basilar pontine grey and to nucleus reticularis tegmenti pontis in the monkey (Macaca fascicularis). Arch Suisses Neurol, Neurochir Psychiat 129:189-208

HOLMES G (1917) The symptoms of acute cerebellar injuries due to gunshot injuries. Brain 40:461-535

KUBIN L, MAGHERINI PC, MANZONI D, POMPEIANO O (1981a) Responses of lateral reticular neurons to sinusoidal rotation of the neck in the decerebrate cat. Neuroscience 6:1277-1290

KUBIN L, MANZONI D, POMPEIANO O (1981b) Responses of lateral reticular neurons to convergent neck and macular inputs. J Neurophysiol 46:48-64

KUNZLE H (1973) The topographic organization of spinal afferents to the lateral reticular nucleus of the cat. J Comp Neurol 149:103-116

KUNZLE H, WIESENDANGER M (1974) Pyramidal connections to the lateral reticular nucleus in the cat : a degeneration study. Acta Anat Basel 88:105-114

MACPHERSON J, WIESENDANGER M, MARANGOZ C, MILES TC (1982) Corticospinal neurones of the supplementary motor area of monkeys. A single unit study. Exp Brain Res (in press)

MAEKAWA K, TAKEDA T, KIMURA M (1981) Neural activity of nucleus reticularis tegmenti pontis - the origin of visual mossy fiber afferents to the cerebellar flocculus of rabbits. Brain Res 210:17-30

NYBY O, JANSEN J (1951) An experimental investigation of the cortico-pontine projection in Macaca mulatta. Skr Nor Vidensk Akad 3:1-47

OSCARSSON O (1973) Functional organization of spinocerebellar paths. In: IGGO A (ed) Somatosensory system. Springer, Berlin (Handbook of sensory physiology, vol 2 pp 339-380)

PRECHT W, STRATA P (1980) On the pathway mediating optokinetic responses in vestibular nuclear neurons. Neuroscience 5:777-787

RUEGG DG, SEGUIN JJ, WIESENDANGER M (1977) Effects of electrical stimulation of somatosensory and motor areas of the cerebral cortex on neurones of the pontine nuclei in squirrel monkeys. Neuroscience 2:923-927

VILENSKY JA, VAN HOESEN GW (1981) Corticopontine projections from the cingulate cortex in the rhesus monkey. Brain Res 205:391-395

WIESENDANGER M (1981) Organization of secondary motor areas of cerebral
cortex. In: BROOKS VB (ed) Handbook of Physiologyy, section I, The Nervous
System, vol II, Motor Control, part 2. Am Physiol Soc, Bethesda pp 1121-1147

WIESENDANGER M, RUEGG DG, WIESENDANGER R (1979) The corticopontine system in
primates : anatomical and functional considerations. In: MASSION J, SASAKI K
(eds) Cerebrocerebellar interactions. Elsevier-North Holland Biomedical
Press, Amsterdam New York Oxford, pp 45-65

WIESENDANGER R, WIESENDANGER M, RUEGG DG (1979) An anatomical investigation
of the corticopontine projection in the primate (Macaca fascicularis and
Saimiri sciureus). II The projection from frontal and parietal association
areas. Neuroscience 4:747-765

ZANGGER P, SCHULTZ W (1978) The activity of cells of nucleus reticularis
tegmenti pontis during spontaneous locomotion in the decorticate cat. Neuroscience Letters 7:95-99

ZANGGER P, WIESENDANGER M (1973) Excitation of lateral reticular neurones by
collaterals of the pyramidal tract. Exp Brain Res 17:144-151

Presynaptic Controls in the Neostriatum: Reciprocal Interactions Between the Nigro-Striatal Dopaminergic Neurons and the Cortico-Striatal Glutamatergic Pathway

A. Nieoullon, L. Kerkerian, and N. Dusticier

Département de Neurophysiologie Générale - INP - CNRS - B.P. 71 - 13277 Marseille Cedex 9 France

Until the initial report on presynaptic inhibition by FRANK and FUORTES (1957) neurophysiological investigations emphasized the exclusive role of nerve impulses in coding the transmission of information in the brain by the frequency of their firing. Presynaptic inhibitory fibres were shown to make synapses on excitatory fibres and it was suggested that by the action of a chemical transmitter the excitatory nerve terminal is depolarized. As a result of this a spike potential in this nerve ending is diminished and the release of the excitatory substance is decreased leading to a reduction in excitation of the effect produced by this synapse. Presynaptic inhibition was described for primary afferents in the spinal cord but electrophysiological studies have found no evidence for such a mechanism at higher levels of the mammalian central nervous system where postsynaptic inhibition is prevalent (see Mc GEER, ECCLES and Mc GEER, 1980).

During the last decade neurochemical and neuropharmacological studies have introduced the idea of presynaptic receptors. It has been suggested that neuronal information is subjected to complex integration processes which are not only due to spatial and temporal summation mechanisms on the cell's membrane but also to the intervention of synaptic properties producing complex changes of the afferent message with presynaptic mechanisms.

The receptors localized on nerve endings are thought to contribute to the modification of the coding of neuronal information mainly by acting on the release of the neurotransmitters. They seem to be involved in at least three types of mechanisms. First, such receptors are thought to exert a coupling in the activity of afferent pathways to a given structure suggesting axo-axonic interactions. Second, presynaptic receptors could also be involved in the regulation of the activity of a given nerve ending by its own neurotransmitter ; in that case the presynaptic receptors are called autoreceptors. Finally, the presynaptic receptors have also been suggested to be implicated

Experimental Brain Research, Suppl. 7
© Springer-Verlag Berlin · Heidelberg 1983

in coupling the activity of a postsynaptic neuron and its afferent pathways. In this situation the neurotransmitter is supposed to be released from the dendrites of the postsynaptic neuron and to act on receptor sites presynaptically localized on fibres afferent to the neuron as suggested for dopamine in the substantia nigra (NIEOULLON et al., 1977).

The presynaptic regulation occurring between the activity of afferent fibres to a given structure could have a reciprocal nature. This short review describes such interactions occurring in the basal ganglia at the level of the neostriatum between the nigro-striatal dopaminergic pathway and the cortico-striatal glutamatergic neurons and illustrates the possible intervention of both inhibitory and excitatory presynaptic mechanisms in the integration of neuronal information. The interactions are discussed as a model of modulation of the cortical output by a monoaminergic afferent pathway at a subcortical level. However, if in the case of the primary afferent fibers in the spinal cord axo-axonic synapses have been seen in electron micrographs, so far in basal ganglia there is no evidence for such a morphological substrate of these presynaptic mechanisms.

THE STRIATAL MODEL OF PRESYNAPTIC INTERACTIONS

The neostriatum is known to receive two main afferent pathways originating in the substantia nigra and the cerebral cortex. The nigro-striatal dopaminergic system has been for many years extensively investigated. The monoaminergic neurons arise from the substantia nigra pars compacta and exert an inhibitory influence on cholinergic interneurons in the striatum. Cortico-striatal fibres have been more recently shown to contain glutamate. This cortical input, excitatory in nature, also influences the striatal interneurons which have been demonstrated to receive convergent afferents from substantia nigra, cerebral cortex and in some cases also from the thalamic nuclei (KOCSIS et al., 1977).

Biochemical studies of receptor sites to neurotransmitters in association with lesion experiments have contributed to define the localization of these receptor sites in the striatum. Results have shown that some of the receptor sites for dopamine, glutamate or GABA are localized at presynaptic levels on striatal afferent fibres. Indeed, nigral 6-hydroxydopamine (6-OHDA) lesions which delete dopaminergic terminals in the neostriatum revealed that the density of high affinity ^{3}H-dopamine and ^{3}H-apomorphine binding sites was reduced by 40 to 47% in the rat striatum (NAGY et al., 1978 ; SEEMAN, 1980). These results suggest that about half of the high affinity sites for these ligands were located on presynaptic terminals of nigral dopaminergic neurons and therefore could be considered as autoreceptors. The same lesion also revealed a 40% decrease in the number of glutamate binding sites presumably reflecting loss of glutamatergic receptors presynaptically located on dopaminergic nerve terminals (ROBERTS et al., 1982).

Kainic or ibotenic acid lesions of the neostriatum which are thought to destroy the cell bodies of neurons and spare the axons and nerve endings induced a complete elimination of some particular dopaminergic receptors linked to an adenylate cyclase mechanism (DA_1 receptors) and of about 50% of the high affinity ^{3}H-neuroleptic binding sites (DA_2-like receptors ; see SEEMAN, 1980). The same type of lesion is followed by a 35% reduction of specific glutamate binding (ROBERTS et al., 1982) showing a postsynaptic location of these dopaminergic and glutamatergic receptors. Similar experiments apparently failed to cause a reduction in GABA receptor binding suggesting that these receptors have a large presynaptic localization particularly on striatal afferent fibres (CAMPOCHIARO et al., 1977).

Finally hemidecortication has also been used to specify the location of neurotransmitter receptor sites in the striatum. Lesions of a large part of the cerebral cortex induced a 30 to 40% decrease in the number of dopaminergic receptors not linked to the adenylate cyclase suggesting these dopaminergic receptors are situated on corticofugal nerve terminals (SCHWARCZ et al., 1978). Decortication experiments also suggested the presence of GABA receptors on cortical afferents to the striatum (CAMPOCHIARO et al., 1977). However, the number of glutamatergic receptor sites is unchanged or increased after lesions of the cerebral cortex (BIZIERE et al., 1980 ; ROBERTS et al., 1982) suggesting they are not situated on corticofugal fibres.

The localization of the cholinergic receptors in the striatum has not yet been identified but pharmacological experiments suggest that they exist at a presynaptic level on dopaminergic nerve endings (GIORGUIEFF et al., 1977a).

Results from the above experiments show that neuronal processes can exhibit receptor sites for neurotransmitters at presynaptic level. Studies on the nigro-striatal dopaminergic nerve endings have shown that these presynaptic receptors could be the substrate for multiple functional interactions. The dopaminergic nerve endings have been shown to have dopaminergic, glutamatergic, and cholinergic presynaptic receptors and were more recently proposed to also exhibit opiate receptor sites. This suggests a higher level of complexity in presynaptic interactions. Such presynaptic mechanisms have also been described in other structures of the brain : in the substantia nigra between dopaminergic and GABA-ergic systems and at the spinal cord level between substance P and enkephalin peptidergic nerve terminals suggesting the presynaptic interactions could be involved in synaptic transmission of neuronal information.

NATURE OF PRESYNAPTIC CONTROLS IN THE STRIATUM

The first evidence that cortico-striatal neurons may regulate dopamine mediated functions in the striatum was obtained from electrical stimulation of the motor cortex which enhanced the release of newly synthesized ^{3}H-dopamine in the cat caudate nucleus in vivo (NIEOULLON et al., 1978). The application of glutamate or kainic acid to rat striatal slices was also shown to stimulate the release of ^{3}H-dopamine by a tetrodotoxin-resistant process suggesting a direct action of glutamate on the dopaminergic terminals (GIORGUIEFF et al., 1977b ; ROBERTS and SHARIFF, 1978 ; ROBERTS et al., 1979). These results suggest glutamate in the striatum exerts a facilitatory control on the dopaminergic nerve terminals by acting on the presynaptic receptors located on these nerve endings (ROBERTS et al., 1982).

More recent experiments on glutamate release provided evidence that dopamine could modulate the activity of the cortico-striatal nerve endings. Dopamine and dopaminergic agonists were found to decrease the K^+-evoked endogenous glutamate release from rat striatal tissue in vitro (MITCHELL and DOGGETT, 1980 ; ROWLANDS and ROBERTS, 1980) and this effect was shown to be enhanced after 6-OHDA lesions suggesting for the first time a supersensitivity of dopaminergic presynaptic receptors localized on the cortico-striatal nerve endings (ROBERTS et al., 1982). In the same way since high affinity glutamate transport as well as glutamate release can be activated by depolarisation, we have investigated the effects of dopamine on the glutamate uptake taken as an index of glutamatergic neuronal activity in vitro. Incubation of the tissue in the presence of dopamine, apomorphine and bromocriptine produced marked inhibition of ^{3}H-glutamate transport from rat striatal homogenates. Dopaminergic inhibition was shown to be reversed in the presence of haloperidol or domperidone which act by blocking dopaminergic neuronal activity in the striatum by the nigro-striatal dopaminergic input. The effect would be due to the activation of the DA_2-like receptors located at presynaptic levels on cortico-striatal nerve endings (NIEOULLON et al., 1982).

Finally acetylcholine was known to exert a facilitatory action on dopamine release by means of both muscarinic and nicotinic presynaptic receptors directly located on nigro-striatal dopaminergic nerve terminals (GIORGUIEFF et al., 1977a). GABA was thought not to directly influence dopamine release (GIORGUIEFF et al., 1978) but was recently shown to activate glutamate release (MITCHELL, 1980) suggesting the activation of the presynaptic GABA receptors located on cortico-striatal nerve terminals as indicated from binding experiments (CAMPOCHIARO et al., 1977). Using the measurement of the high affinity glutamate uptake as an index of the activity of cortico-stria-tal glutamatergic neurons we have recently shown that acetylcholine exerts an inhibitory action on this glutamate transport (Fig. 1). Acetylcholine and cholinergic agonists added to an incubation medium from the rat striatum indu-ced a marked inhibition of glutamate uptake. This effect is no longer detected in the presence of atropine. To avoid a possible indirect action of acetylcholine on the glutamatergic nerve endings by means of the activation of dopamine release, we have also verified that the inhibitory effects of acetylcholine are still present when the dopaminergic receptors are blocked by haloperidol (KERKERIAN and NIEOULLON, submitted). Therefore, these results suggest a possible control of cortico-striatal glutamatergic nerve endings by means of presynaptic cholinergic receptors. This effect of acetylcholine seems to involve both muscarinic and nicotinic receptors and is similar to the action of acetylcholine on the dopaminergic nerve terminals. One interes-ting result is that acetylcholine exerts opposite effects on two different nerve terminals. This compound facilitates dopamine release while it reduces glutamatergic activity. Thus the response of nerve endings to a given neurotransmitter could be excitatory or inhibitory. This would indicate that the properties of the effector linked to the receptor, inducing the physiolo-gical response, are different. Although the neurotransmitter and the receptor sites are similar, the response of the neuron to the receptor activation is apparently dependant on the properties of the individual neuron.

In summary, dopaminergic neurons which inhibit cholinergic interneurons in the striatum seem to be controlled by glutamatergic and cholinergic nerve terminals by mean of presynaptic receptors which activate dopamine release when stimulated. Glutamatergic activity, mainly linked to the cortico-stria-tal pathway, exerts a facilitatory action on striatal cholinergic interneu-rons as shown by the decreased acetylcholine turn-over measured after corti-cal ablation (WOOD et al., 1979) and the enhanced ^{3}H-acetylcholine release in rat striatal slices preloaded by ^{3}H-choline induced by glutamate (see SCATTON et al., 1982). At the presynaptic level, glutamatergic activity is submitted to the double inhibitory action of dopamine and acetylcholine while GABA seems to exert a facilitatory action on this glutamatergic transmission. The main results concerning acetylcholine, dopamine and glutamate interactions in the striatum are summarized in Figure 2.

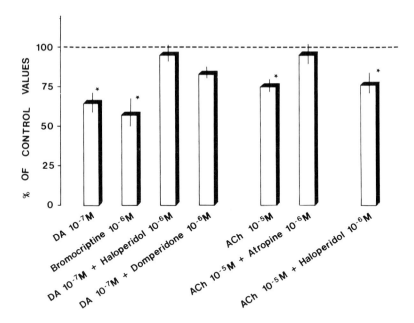

Fig. 1. Effects of dopamine (DA), bromocriptine and acetylcholine (ACh) on the sodium-dependant high affinity glutamate uptake in homogenates from rat striatum. DA, bromocriptine or ACh were incubated (3 min at 25°C) with homogenates from rat striatum in the presence of L-^{3}H-glutamate (specific activity 35 Ci.mmole) 1 M. For the details of the assay, see NIEOULLON et al. (1982). In some experiments, haloperidol, domperidone or atropine were added to the incubation medium to test the reversal of DA or ACh induced inhibition of high affinity glutamate uptake. Control values correspond to 110 nmoles of ^{3}H-glutamate incorporated per minute incubation and per gramme proteines. Experiments were performed in 6 to 12 animals. * : P < 0.02 when compared to control values (Student's t-test)

POSSIBLE FUNCTIONAL IMPLICATIONS

Results of biochemical experiments indicate that the cerebral cortex influences the neostriatum by a mechanism which is antagonistic to dopamine mediated events. The cortico-striatal glutamatergic pathway exerts a facilitatory action on the striatal cholinergic interneurons while the nigro-striatal dopaminergic pathway inhibits their activity. These two striatal afferent systems seem to be reciprocally linked at the presynaptic level.

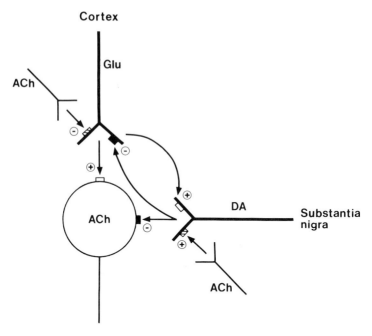

Fig. 2. Proposed model of functional interactions occurring in the striatum between the nigro-striatal dopaminergic system, the cortico-striatal glutamatergic pathway and the striatal cholinergic interneurons. + : excitatory effect ; - : inhibitory influences ; Glu : glutamate ; DA : dopamine ; ACh : acetylcholine

An increased dopaminergic transmission which induces a direct decrease in cholinergic activity could also reduce the excitatory cortical input to these cholinergic neurons by acting presynaptically on cortico-striatal glutamatergic nerve endings. The resulting action is to augment the reduction of the striatal cholinergic activity. Therefore, the nigro-striatal dopaminergic system could prevent the excitatory action of the cortico-striatal glutamatergic pathway on the cholinergic interneurons. Similarly, a decreased dopaminergic activity leads to an increase of the excitability of cholinergic neurons both by a reduced direct inhibitory input and by decreasing the inhibitory control at the presynaptic level on cortico-striatal glutamatergic nerve endings. In this situation the cortical input would have a more powerful effect on cholinergic activity in the striatum.

When there is an increase in the activity of cortico-striatal glutamatergic neurons, the resulting changes can not be explained simply by reversal of the above situations. It results in a direct increase in the excitation of striatal cholinergic interneurons and also in activation of dopamine release from the nigro-striatal endings. The resulting action on the striatal cholinergic interneuronal activity is in that case a competition between the excitatory effects of the glutamatergic neurons and the inhibitory action of the dopaminergic afferent pathway presynaptically activated (Fig. 2).

In addition, the interpretation of these situations is probably complicated by the retroaction of acetylcholine on dopaminergic and glutamatergic nerve terminals which could be considered as a negative feed-back response of the striatal interneurons during changes in dopaminergic activity. When there is an increase in the activity of nigro-striatal dopaminergic neurons it is possible that the subsequent reduction in cholinergic activity reduces the excitatory cholinergic influence on dopaminergic nerve endings and consequently leads to a decreased dopaminergic activity. Inhibition of cholinergic interneurons could also decrease cholinergic inhibition exerted at a presynaptic level on cortico-striatal nerve endings. When there is an increase in cortico-striatal glutamatergic activity, changes in cholinergic function in the striatum are probably more transient due to the competition between the effects of the excitatory cortico-striatal and the inhibitory nigro-striatal afferent pathways.

These results are supported by the fact that cortical ablations enhance the amphetamine-induced stereotyped behaviour (IVERSEN et al., 1971) which results from an increased dopaminergic transmission. In the reverse situation where dopaminergic receptor sites are blocked by haloperidol, these lesions prevent its cataleptogenic action (SCATTON et al., 1982). These mechanisms could also explain why lesions of the frontal cortex in the rat fail to alter striatal choline acetyltransferase activity and acetylcholine levels (SCATTON et al., 1982). Similar results on choline acetyltransferase have also been obtained in the cat (NIEOULLON and DUSTICIER, submitted). The cortical lesion leads to decreased excitation of cholinergic neurons by suppression of direct glutamatergic input but also results in an indirect decrease in inhibitory dopaminergic action on these interneurons which counteracts the decreased excitation.

Our proposed organization of the striatal network suggests that a decreased dopaminergic input could result in an increased cortico-striatal glutamatergic neurotransmission. This situation occurs in Parkinson's disease where dopaminergic neurons are likely to have been destroyed. Biochemical measurements reveal in that case the number of DA_2 receptor sites in the striatum is

62

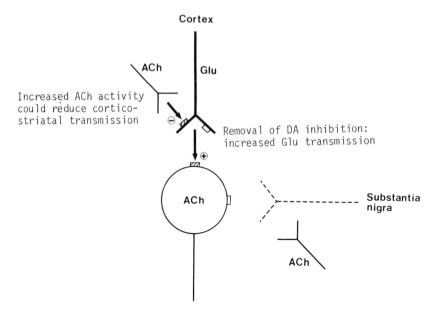

Increased ACh activity
could reduce cortico-
striatal transmission

Removal of DA inhibition:
increased Glu transmission

Cortex

ACh   Glu

ACh

Substantia
nigra

ACh

PARKINSONISM

Fig. 3. Proposed model of modification of presynaptic interactions in the
striatum between cortico-striatal glutamatergic pathway and cholinergic interneurons after disappearance of nigro-striatal dopaminergic nerve terminals
such as in Parkinson's disease. + : excitatory effects ; - : inhibitory
influences ; Glu : glutamate ; DA : dopamine ; ACh : acetylcholine

increased (LEE et al., 1978) corresponding to denervation hypersensitivity
mechanisms. Therefore, the lack of stimulation of these receptors sites
probably located on cortico-striatal nerve terminals could result in an
hyperactivity of the cortico-striatal glutamatergic neurons which could be
responsible for the major symptoms of the disease and particularly of
akinesia. Possibly the ergot-derivative bromocriptine and lisuride effects
against akinesia can be attributed to the action of these drugs on the DA_2
receptors (SCHACHTER et al., 1980). The effect of their activation could be
to reduce the cortico-striatal glutamatergic transmission (Fig. 3).

In conclusion, in this short review we have discussed the evidence to support
the idea that a monoaminergic pathway could exert a modulatory effect of
cortical output in subcortical structures by means of mechanisms involving
receptors presynaptically localized on nerve terminals. In the case of the
nigro-striatal dopaminergic system this monoaminergic pathway could contribu-

te by presynaptic mechanisms to tonically modulate the activity in the striatum. The effects of the other inputs to this structure may be modulated as a function of the level of dopamine release. A similar hypothesis has been developped to explain the hyporeactivity of rats treated with 6-OHDA in the substantia nigra to sensory stimuli (see BJORKLUND et al., 1981). The sensory neglect could be reversed in these animals by arousing stimuli which have been shown to increase the release of dopamine, probably from the remaining intact dopaminergic nerve terminals (see NIEOULLON and DUSTICIER, 1982). This could contribute to presynaptically decrease the cortico-striatal glutamatergic transmission.

SUMMARY

The neostriatum is known to receive two main afferent pathways, the nigro-striatal dopaminergic system and the cortico-striatal glutamatergic projection. These two neuronal systems exert opposite influences on cholinergic interneurons. Biochemical experiments have shown interactions occurring between the dopaminergic and the glutamatergic nerve terminals at the presynaptic level mediated by presynaptic receptors. Glutamate as well as acetylcholine were shown to directly activate dopamine release. In a series of experiments we have measured in vitro, an index of the activity of the glutamatergic system, the sodium-dependant high affinity glutamate uptake, from rat striatal samples in the presence of dopamine or acetylcholine. Both neurotransmitters were shown to decrease glutamate uptake and the effects were demonstrated to be related to dopaminergic and cholinergic receptor activation.

The results are discussed in terms of reciprocal interactions occurring at the presynaptic level in the neostriatum between the nigro-striatal dopaminergic system and the cortico-striatal glutamatergic neurons. It is suggested that the dopaminergic system can act in the neostriatum as a neuromodulator of cortico-striatal transmission. These mechanisms are finally considered in the situation where the dopaminergic nerve terminals disappear such as in Parkinson's disease.

ACKNOWLEDGEMENTS

This work was supported by grant n° 816020 from the "Institut National de la Santé et de la Recherche Médicale". The authors are grateful to Dr. J.P. TASSIN for his advice on uptake assay and to Dr. C. PALMER who kindly revised the English. Drugs were generously provided by JANSSEN PHARMACEUTICA (neuroleptics) and by Laboratoires SANDOZ (bromocriptine).

REFERENCES

BIZIERE K, THOMPSON H, COYLE JT (1980) Characterisation of specific, high-affinity binding sites for L-^{3}H-glutamic acid in rat brain membranes. Brain Res 183:421-433

BJORKLUND A, STEVENI U, DUNNETT S, IVERSEN SD (1981) Functional reactivation of the deafferented neostriatum by nigral transplants. Nature 289:497-499

CAMPOCHIARO PR, SCHWARCZ R, COYLE JT (1977) GABA receptor binding in rat striatum, localisation and effects of denervation. Brain Res 136:501-511

FRANK K, FUORTES MGF (1957) Presynaptic and postsynaptic inhibition of monosynaptic reflexes. Fed Proc 16:39-40

GIORGUIEFF MF, LE FLOCH ML, GLOWINSKI J, BESSON MJ (1977a) Involvement of cholinergic presynaptic receptors of nicotinic and muscarinic types in the control of the spontaneous release of dopamine from striatal dopaminergic terminals in the rat. J Pharmacol Exp Ther 200:535-540

GIORGUIEFF MF, KEMEL ML, GLOWINSKI J (1977b) Presynaptic effect of L-glutamic acid on dopamine release in rat striatal slices. Neurosci Lett 6:73-78

GIORGUIEFF MF, KEMEL ML, GLOWINSKI J, BESSON MJ (1978) Stimulation of dopamine release by GABA in rat striatal slices. Brain Res 139:115-130

IVERSEN SD, WILKINSON S, SIMPSON B (1971) Enhanced amphetamine responses after frontal cortex lesions in the rat. Europ J Pharmacol 13:387-390

KERKERIAN L, NIEOULLON A (submitted) Effects of acetylcholine on sodium-dependant high affinity glutamate transport in rat striatal homogenates

KOCSIS JD, SUGIMORI M, KITAI ST (1977) Convergence of excitatory synaptic inputs to caudate spiny neurons. Brain Res 124:403-413

LEE T, SEEMAN P, RAJPUT A, FARLEY IJ, HORNYKIEWICZ O (1978) Receptor basis for dopaminergic supersensitivity in Parkinson's disease. Nature (Lond) 278:59-61

Mc GEER PL, ECCLES JC, Mc GEER EG (1980) Molecular neurobiology of the mammalian brain. Plenum Press, New York, pp 643

MITCHELL R (1980) A novel GABA receptor modulates stimulus-induced glutamate release from cortico-striatal terminals. Europ J Pharmacol 67:119-122

MITCHELL PR, DOGGETT NS (1980) Modulation of striatal (^{3}H)-glutamic acid release by dopaminergic drugs. Life Sci 26:2073-2081

NAGY JI, LEE T, SEEMAN P, FIBIGER HC (1978) Direct evidence for presynaptic and post-synaptic dopamine receptors in brain. Nature (Lond) 274:278-281

NIEOULLON A, CHERAMY A, GLOWINSKI J (1977) Release of dopamine in vivo from cat substantia nigra. Nature (Lond) 266:375-377

NIEOULLON A, CHERAMY A, GLOWINSKI J (1978) Release of dopamine evoked by electrical stimulation of the motor and visual areas of the cerebral cortex in both caudate nuclei and in the substantia nigra in the cat. Brain Res 145:69-83

NIEOULLON A, DUSTICIER N (1982) Effect of superficial radial nerve stimulation on the activity of nigro-striatal dopaminergic neurons in the cat : role of cutaneous sensory input. J Neural Trans 53:133-146

NIEOULLON A, DUSTICIER N (submitted) Changes in glutamate uptake, glutamate decarboxylase and choline acetyltransferase in subcortical areas after sensorimotor cortical ablations in the cat.

NIEOULLON A, KERKERIAN L, DUSTICIER N (1982) Inhibitory effects of dopamine on high affinity glutamate uptake from rat striatum. Life Sci 30:1165-1172

ROBERTS PJ, ANDERSON SD (1979) Stimulatory effect of L-glutamate and related amino acids on ^{3}H-dopamine release from rat striatum : an in vitro model for glutamate actions J Neurochem 32:1539-1545

ROBERTS PJ, Mc BEAN GJ, SHARIF NA, THOMAS EM (1982) Striatal glutamatergic function : modifications following specific lesions. Brain Res 235:83-91

ROBERTS PJ, SHARIF NA (1978) Effects of L-glutamate and related amino acids upon the release of ^{3}H-dopamine from rat striatal slices. Brain Res 157:391-395

ROWLANDS GJ, ROBERTS PJ (1980) Activation of dopamine receptors inhibits calcium-dependent glutamate release from cortico-striatal terminals in vitro. Europ J Pharmacol 62:239-242

SCATTON B, WORMS P, LLOYD KG, BARTHOLINI G (1982) Cortical modulation of striatal functions. Brain Res 232:331-343

SCHACHTER M, BEDARD P, DEBOND AG, JENNER P, MARSDEN CD, PRICE P, PARKES JD, KEENAN J, SMITH B, ROSENTHALER J, HOROWSKI R, DOROW R (1980) The role of D-1 and D-2 receptors. Nature (Lond) 286:157-159

SCHWARCZ R, CREESE I, COYLE JT, SNYDER SH (1978) Dopamine receptors localized on cerebral cortical afferents to rat corpus striatum. Nature (Lond) 271:766-768

SEEMAN P (1980) Brain dopamine receptors. Pharmacol Rev 32:229-313

WOOD PL, MORONI F, CHENEY DL, COSTA E (1979) Cortical lesion modulate turnover rates of acetylcholine and gamma-aminobutyric acid. Neurosci Lett 12:349-354

From Immobility to Motion

Patterns of Activities in the Ventrobasal Thalamus and Somatic Cortex SI During Behavioral Immobility in the Awake Cat: Focal Waking Rhythms

A. Rougeul-Buser, J.J. Bouyer, M.F. Montaron, and P. Buser

Laboratoire de Neurophysiologie Comparée, Université Pierre et Marie Curie, 75005 Paris, France.

INTRODUCTION

Many species may display sudden states of bodily immobility during waking, possibly accompanied by a high degree of vigilance. These episodes which belong to the behavioral repertoire of each species, can occur e.g. during hunting, prior to attack ("arrest" attitude while expecting prey to appear, or while watching an already visible prey), or as a defense reaction (at the sight of a frightening stimulus). Such attitudes have been considered by some authors as part of the "orienting" reaction, although only very few investigators or theorists have actually insisted very much on this particular behavioral feature, i.e. that of body immobility (see e.g. BERLYNE, 1960 , 1970). In our study on cats, we have tried to characterize certain electrophysiological correlates of such alert immobility states, at the cortical and thalamic levels, while placing the animal in situations that could be considered as mimicking those of "hunting". In looking for such correlations, we then endeavoured to identify some of the neuronal events which take place at the thalamic level in connection with the development of at least one of these behavioral immobility states. Finally, the question was raised whether these particular neuronal activities, observed at some CNS sites, only represent consequences of immobility or if some more complex link can be established between the two phenomenological categories, behavioral and electrophysiological, implying some kind of circular causality.

About fifty cats were used in these studies. The animals were first prepared under fluothane anaesthesia for two stages of investigations : (i) for focal electrocorticographic (ECoG) exploration, to localise the characteristic waking immobility rhythms, an array of 15 electrodes, 2 mm apart, was implanted over the sensorimotor and proximal parietal cortices. Each such electrode was made of a fine wire slightly penetrating into the cortex ; an indifferent electrode was fixed into the frontal bone. All ECoG recordings

Experimental Brain Research, Suppl. 7
© Springer-Verlag Berlin · Heidelberg 1983

were later performed with a "monopolar" montage, i.e. against the frontal (quasi-silent) reference.

(ii) for microelectrode exploration of the thalamus, two horizontal bars oriented in the frontal plane were secured to the skull, after adequately removing the skin and tissues and covering the skull itself with dental acrylic. This system, which is now widely used in a large number of laboratories, allowed exploration of the animal in painless fixation in the standard Horsley-Clarke position, in a fully alert condition.

To investigate the behavioral correlates of the ECoG activity, the animal was placed in a relatively sound-proof chamber. It was left alone with no specific target or source of interest or, on the contrary, it was placed in either one of two situations which, as expected, could draw its attention : a) a mouse hidden behind a wall with a hole that the cat would watch, to wait for the prey to come out ; b) a mouse placed in a perspex box, that the cat could see but could not catch. The cat's behavior in its chamber was constantly followed on the screen of a close circuit video TV system.

During these behavioral investigations, the ECoG activity was recorded on a multichannel inkwriter for visual inspection and also processed (on or off line) with a PDP computer to evaluate the spectral power in the 0-50 Hz band, using the Fast Fourier Transform algorithm (for details see BOUYER et al., 1981). The data was displayed in successive periods of one min as "evolutive spectra", to follow changes in spectral content throughout a whole session (90 min).

The single unit study *per se* took place only one or two weeks after implantation. For this investigation, the animal was fixed into the stereotaxic frame and the latter was then oriented to give the animal its preferred position, generally sitting on the table in a "sphinx-like" position. A hole was drilled through the acrylic layer and underlying skull at the appropriate antero-posterior (AP) and lateral (L) positions to reach the ventrobasal thalamus (nucleus ventralis posterior, VP) and its vicinity. The dura was then gently opened and a 2M K citrate filled microelectrode was introduced into the brain. Before beginning the exploration, the microelectrode impedance was measured ; only those electrodes displaying a value between 5 and 15 Mohms were used.

For cortical stimulation, single shocks were delivered from a conventional device, as rectangular pulses of 0.3 msec, 0.1 to 1/sec, 10 to 20 V, between the two adjacent electrodes that had been selected in a preliminary ECoG recording (see below). To investigate by means of the collision test the stimulator could, as is usual, be triggered by spontaneous thalamic spikes, the cortical stimulus itself being delivered at a variable delay after the trigger time.

In each penetration, when the electrode had reached its maximal depth, histological marking was performed by passing a high frequency current (500 KHz, 15 μA) for 10 min. With this technique, the complete descent was usually well marked as a fine line on post-mortem histological sections made in the appropriate plane. After completion of the descent, the microelectrode was removed and the skull hole closed with a drop of cement. As a rule, a variable number of such penetrations were made on one side within one session, the latter lasting from 3 to 5 h, during which the animal remained generally quiet, as long as no intercurrent, unexpected stimulation occurred in the room. The same animal was then taken for a second, similar exploration of the contralateral side on the next day. After this second session, it was immediately sacrificed with an overdose of barbiturate, and carefully perfused with Ringer and formalin, to provide optimal conditions for histological identification of the penetration tracks.

In particular, the time relationships between thalamic spikes and ECoG were investigated through either superimposing the successive cortical waves and comparing the resulting time distribution of the spikes or, instead, using specific spikes as trigger signals and estimating the superposition of the corresponding waves. More details are given in legends.

RESULTS

We shall briefly summarize the two main steps of our present research : (i) behavioral-electrocortical correlates ; (ii) electrocortical-single thalamic unit relationships.

1) Stages of vigilance and somatosensory rhythms

Let us first consider some of the salient points of our previous data on somatosensory ECoG and waking immobility.

a) It was observed that rhythmic synchronized activities develop in the sensorimotor cat cortex whenever the awake animal becomes motionless, the only remaining movements occasionally involving tail and eyes. While these anterior rhythms develop, the rest of the cortex is usually in an activated state ("desynchronized"). Therefore, if no particular care was taken to place the electrodes upon adequate loci, no such activities could be recorded. Thus with only one or two pairs of electrodes in position on the suprasylvian cortex to monitor the state of alertness of the animal, as is so often used, the conclusion would unavoidably be that the animal only displays desynchronized cortical activity. It is especially remarkable that when synchronized rhythms developed in the anterior foci, the posterior cortical areas did not necessarily show any "alpha" type activity.

b) Sensorimotor rhythms are of several distinct types. When exploring the motor cortex, area somatic I and area SII, as well as the most anterior part of the "associative" parietal cortex, known to coincide with area 5a (HASSLER and MUHS-CLEMENT, 1964), where another somatic territory has in fact been characterized (area S III, DARIAN-SMITH et al., 1966 ; TANJI et al., 1978), we could isolate two main sets of such rhythms. Both developed when the animal was behaviorally alert. The two sets were distinguished by their frequency (14 Hz and 36 Hz) and their precise localization within the anterior cortex. Moreover, and this is an essential point, they could be shown to accompany two distinct behavioral situations with different overt signs of attention by the animal.
(i) when the cat was in a position of expectancy, waiting for the unseen mouse to come out through the hole, rhythms were at about 14 Hz ; they were localized precisely over the wrist and hand zone of area S I (Fig. 1, A2).
(ii) when the animal was watching the visible (but unseizable) mouse, rhythms were surprisingly and distinctly at a higher frequency (about 36 Hz) ; they were this time located within two foci, one in the "associative" parietal area, i.e. clearly behind S I, the other one in the pericruciate motor cortex (Fig. 1, B2).

c) The spatial extent of these foci has always appeared to be rather restricted, in the order of 4 to 10 mm^2. This size is compatible with data that has led to the concept of "macrocolumn", as recently developed (MOUNTCASTLE, 1978).

Evolutive spectra could well illustrate the difference between these two situations (Fig. 1). As can be seen, expectancy, when the animal was waiting for the mouse to come out of its hole, was quasi-permanently accompanied by a frequency peak at 14 Hz, for as long as 60 minutes. On the other hand, when the cat was watching its potential "prey", displaying an overt focused attention on it, 36 Hz activities were this time highly dominant, for as long as 90 minutes of recording.

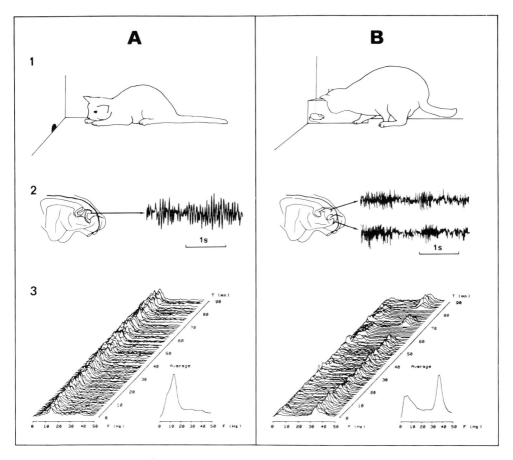

Fig. 1. Waking immobility rhythms on cat cortex.
A, expectancy or quiet waking (mean frequency, 14 Hz) ; B, focused attention (mean frequency, 36 Hz).
1 : illustrate the animal's most common attitudes in the used experimental set ups.
2 : types of rhythmic patterns and their localization : one focus in SI in A and two foci, one motor and one parietal in B.
3 : evolutive spectra taken during the 90 min recording time. Each spectrum was computed from 1 min recording. Heights of peaks indicate spectral power (in μV^2) in the frequency band 0-50 Hz (resolution $\Delta f = 0.2$ Hz). Added to each set of evolutive spectra is the average spectrum computed over the 90 min recording time

These two sets of rhythms may evidently also develop in other environmental situations (see discussion). But in none of these cases have we been able to record intermediate frequencies over the cortical areas studied. It is thus clear that we are dealing with two distinct rhythmic systems, each developing in correlation with a specific type of situation requiring immobility and that, with our experimental set up, either one or the other may dominate.

d) A systematic macroelectrode exploration of the thalamus, including different approaches such as focal destruction of thalamic areas, and above all
computation of the coherence function between activities simultaneously recorded at the two sites, cortical and thalamic, has led us to the conclusions
(which we only briefly summarize herein) that : (i) the cortical rhythms are
governed by thalamic "pace-makers" i.e. that the cortex is secondarily
entrained by the thalamus ; this conclusion has been reached by several
investigators before (see discussion) ; no indication exists as yet of a
participation of the descending cortico-thalamic neurons in the generation of
these rhythms ; (ii) in our experimental conditions (animal awake, vigilant
and immobile), each set of rhythms is highly correlated with the activity of
a distinct thalamic area : the hand area of n.VP for the 14 Hz "expectancy"
patterns and a zone belonging to the posterior group (POm) for the parietal
36 Hz high vigilance patterns. On the other hand, we have not been able as
yet to localize the thalamic area involved in the anterior motor cortex 36 Hz
focus (possibly ventralis lateralis or dorsalis medialis).

e) Finally, these focal rhythms seem to be homologous to activities described
in human EEG investigations under the designation of "mu" and "beta" rhythms
respectively. However, no observation is available (to our knowledge) on
functional differences between the two, which would parallel our animal

Table 1. Somatosensory rhythms during waking immobility

Frequency (Hz)	14	36
Localisation	SI hand area	- Motor cortex (M I) - "Associative" parietal cortex (area 5a)
Conditions for occurrence	"expectancy" ; quiet waking	Watching prey ; focused attention ; "hypervigilance"
Thalamic source	VP (hand area)	Unknown for motor cortex POm for associative parietal

studies here (JASPER and PENFIELD, 1949 ; GASTAUT et al., 1957 ; PFURTSCHELLER, 1981). Table 1 summarizes the above data.

2) Microelectrode explorations of the thalamus (VP nucleus and vicinity)

As a next step in our study, we tried to explore the thalamic neuronal events accompanying the development of synchronized waking immobility rhythms. The preliminary question was obviously whether the animal, being held in painless stereotaxic fixation, would display at least one type of such rhythms, with the same temporal and spatial characteristics as the normal behaving cat. This turned out to be true for both activities : cats under fixation, while waking, developed 36 Hz rhythms chiefly at the beginning of the experiment, then later preferentially 14 Hz; at times the animal could even become drowsy, with slower rhythms (about 8 Hz ; the latter are not mentioned elsewhere in the present study).

From then on, a microelectrode exploration of the thalamic pacemaker of the immobility rhythms became technically much simpler than in the freely beha-ving cat. Considering the relative importance of "expectancy" 14 Hz activi-ties in such preparations, our thalamic exploration was oriented toward the VP forelimb area. Our aim was of course to detect cells that would modify, in one or other way, their firing pattern at each occurrence of a train of cortical rhythms at 14 Hz. The latter usually developed as sequences of variable duration, but were very often sufficient (2 sec) to enable us to search for possible correlation with the simultaneously recorded unit activi-ty.

Whenever possible, we tested all encountered cells for their responsiveness : (i) to various peripheral somatic stimulations such as light touch, hair bending, tapping, passive joint movement, etc... (ii) to cortical electrical stimulation, using as stimulating electrodes the pair of recording leads that displayed the largest and most characteristic 14 Hz activity ; this method allowed us to use the classical collision test to determine whether the studied cell could be activated antidromically (and thus represent a thala-mo-cortical neuron) or not (see discussion).

To summarize our results :

a) A first striking fact was that in our explorations, only a very limited proportion of cells encountered in the VP area altered their discharge in connection with the 14 Hz rhythms. About 600 cells could be followed for sufficient time to allow for a systematic search for correspondance. Only 75 units could be isolated that correlated in any way with the cortical synchrony state.

b) Among the 75 cells of our sample, not all units displayed the same pattern of changes during the cortical 14 Hz rhythm. A major distinction could be made between :

(i) cells that became rhythmically active during the cortical rhythm ("R" cells) ;

(ii) other cells, that showed a sustained change, lasting throughout the whole rhythmic sequence ; we called these "tonic" ("T") cells ;

(iii) seventeen other cells behaved in a much more complex way. They were all "tonic" but never changed their firing during the development of the 14 Hz VP-S I system alone. On the other hand, they altered their discharge during phases of drowsiness, which are electrophysiologically more complex (BOUYER et al., 1974), since they are characterized by the simultaneous development of 14 Hz and of another set of rhythms, at 8 Hz, that does not originate from VP nor from the PO nucleus. These cells will not be considered here.

c) Going further into details, not all R cells (39 in total) behaved in the same way. Twenty five fired randomly during the cortical "desynchronized" state and displayed one or two spikes at each cortical wave of the 14 Hz episode, with a fairly constant time relationship (Fig. 2A) between spike and wave ("spiking" cells, R_S). The antidromic invasion test indicated that these units were thalamo-cortical neurons. Fourteen units behaved somewhat differently ; they were almost totally silent during all episodes other than the 14 Hz ones, during which they discharged with rhythmic, high frequency bursts (intraburst frequency, 200-300 Hz). Here again, the superposition of the tracings indicated that these "bursting" cells (R_B) fired with a fairly constant time relationship to the cortical waves (Fig. 2B). On the other hand, at variance with R_S cells, R_B units did not display collision between spontaneous firing (the latter being, as indicated above, of very low frequency) and that elicited through cortical stimulation. Their latency of response to single cortical shock was rather variable, in the order of 15 to 20 msec for the same cell.

d) T cells were also of two distinct types. The ones called here T(+) showed a low spontaneous activity during cortical desynchronisation and suddenly increased their firing rate while a 14 Hz sequence was developing on the cortex (Fig. 2D). Others cells, designated as T(-), fired under all conditions except during the 14 Hz episodes, during which they became completely

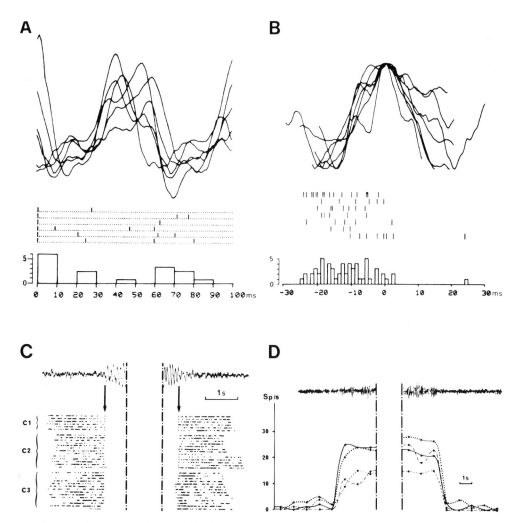

Fig. 2. Patterns of unit discharges in nucleus VP and vicinity in relation to the 14 Hz cortical rhythms recorded from cortex SI.
A. R_S type cell. The computer was set to obtain successive triggering of the scope sweep through spikes during a rhythmic 14 Hz sequence. Six successive sweeps were superimposed and the positions of the subsequent spikes is marked by vertical lines. At bottom, sequential histogram of number of spikes ; bin width 10 msec.
B. R_B type cell. Seven successive waves of a cortical 14 Hz rhythmic sequence were superimposed by the computer (top traces). All spikes of each burst were then plotted as short vertical lines on the middle traces, for the 7 successive sweeps. Spike number vs time histogram at bottom.
C. T(-) type cell. During 33 successive 14 Hz trains (sample visible on top) the cell suddenly ceased firing throughout the rhythmic sequence and returned back to the initial discharge level at the end of the cortical rhythm. The 33 cortical sequences were graphically lined up for their beginning and ending, since they were of different lengths.
D. T(+) type cell. During 4 successive trains of rhythms, the cell suddenly increased its firing rate (spikes/sec in ordinates). Same graphical lining up of start and stop as in C

silent (Fig. 2C). Only a few T cells could be tested for their antidromic activation from the cortex. None of them displayed any response to cortical stimulation.

e) An interesting but somewhat unexpected feature was that none of the encountered cells, R_S, R_B, T(+) and T(-) could ever be activated through one of the tested somatic stimuli (cutaneous or joint). R cells appeared to be scattered among other units that were encountered during the same penetration of the microelectrode and could be typically activated especially through light tactile stimulus ; these displayed a well circumscribed peripheral, contralateral field and very little fatigue to repetition of the natural adequate stimulus. Such cells, which also clearly fulfilled the criterion of antidromic activation from the cortex, could be classified as thalamo-cortical relay (TCR) cells as is usually understood by this term (POGGIO and MOUNTCASTLE, 1963 ; ANDERSEN et al., 1964). On the other hand (and this was also a surprise), these cells never displayed any rhythmic firing or any other type of modification of firing during the 14 Hz sequences.

f) Let us finally consider the localisations of these various units as determined from the post-mortem histological control, combined with micrometer reading data during recording itself.

All R cells, either spiking or bursting, were encountered within the VP nucleus itself ; more precisely in its middle part, in the zone of projection of the anterior limb. As was mentioned earlier, R cells were intermingled with typical TCR units activated through tactile wrist and hand stimulation.

T cells were found either in the VP itself, or its immediate vicinity (fringe of nucleus lateralis posterior LP, and nucleus suprageniculatus, SG).
Table 2 summarizes these single unit data.

DISCUSSION

1) In the first part of our presentation, we briefly recalled some of our previous findings (BOUYER et al., 1974) emphasizing the existence of two subclasses of rhythms that can be recorded over the sensorimotor cortical areas. These subsets differ in frequency (14 and 36 Hz, respectively) and develop in connection with distinct environmental conditions. They have in common occurrence only when the animal is waking and immobile and both display a very restricted spatial extent, as small foci located either on cortical area SI (14 Hz) or on the motor cortex and associative parietal cortex (36 Hz).

Table 2. Types of units found in VP

Class	R cells (39)		T cells (19)	
Subclass	R_S	R_B	T(+)	T(-)
Number	25	14	9	10
Behavior during 14 Hz	1-2 spikes per wave	one burst per wave	accelerated	silent
Behavior to cortex stimulation	antidromic response	orthodromic response	?	?
Localisation	VP hand area		VP or vicinity (LP, SG)	

The behavioural correlates of the beta rhythms, i.e. "focused attention", are relatively easy to establish, because of the typical attitude of the animal. Our experimental set up provided a favourable condition for their development. Another situation that has also been appropriate is the exploratory behaviour at an unfamiliar place : while exploring, the animal stands still from time to time and then simultaneously develops trains of 36 Hz activities.

On the other hand, the conditions for obtaining mu rhythms seem at first less precise and somewhat less specific. When a cat is progressively passing from active wakefulness into sleep, with no overt source of "expectancy", it usually displays episodes characterized as "quiet waking", with eyes open, which are also accompanied by mu activity ; the same holds true in the even more artificial conditions of painless stereotaxic fixation. The difference with our experimental situation implying "expectancy" is essential, though : during quiet waking, the 14 Hz is as a rule very labile, only transient and quickly replaced by drowsiness rhythms (at about 8 Hz), while the significant feature of a situation presumed to involve expectancy is the existence of prolonged episodes of mu rhythms, without any interspersed drowsiness-type ECoG. Another interesting case for development of 14 Hz rhythms was that during operant conditioning : in this situation, such an activity regularly appeared while the animal was waiting for the go-signal to press the lever to be rewarded (ROUGEUL et al., 1972).

Focal rhythms accompanying immobility have been noted before by other groups (ROTH et al., 1967 ; STERMAN and WYRWICKA, 1967) but, to our knowledge, only those belonging to *one* of our subclasses (14 Hz) have been described. Data has also been gathered showing that the subsets are generated by a distinct thalamic zone : a restricted area of VP for the 14 Hz rhythms (HOWE and STERMAN, 1972 ; BOUYER et al., 1974) ; an area belonging to the PO group for the parietal 36 Hz ; an (as yet) not well identified thalamic zone for the motor cortex 36 Hz. The more general, but indeed still provisional, hypothesis may thus be proposed, that some specific thalamocortical "sectors" undergo a given change in their pattern of activity ("synchronization"), in relation to a particular environmental and behavioral situation. Such sectors may be restricted precisely in their spatial extent, which would explain why these focal rhythms were often overlooked, and can in fact only be observed and followed with the use of a high spatial density of recording electrodes. This limited spatial distribution may perhaps also explain why the "mu" and "beta" activities, that were described in human EEG to occur in conditions that are, roughly speaking, those of body immobility, were claimed to be only recordable in a limited number of subjects. The possibility should be considered that their presence over the scalp is conditioned by the individual spatial topography of the cortical sources of rhythms. But it could also be that the tested subjects were not confronted with adequate psychological situations that would favor the development of one or the other type of central rhythms.

The sensori-motor rhythms should be clearly distinguished from the "alpha-like" rhythms that develop over the occipital cortex, in animals as well as in humans, as a consequence of particular (sometimes complex) situations of visual environment (eyes closed ; eyes open on an unpatterned uniform visual field etc...), quite distinct from those favoring the anterior rhythms. Also, they are in no way similar to the sleep "spindles" so often described in numerous species as occurring in part of the sleep states. Spindles are morphologically quite different and their spatial distribution is also not identical to those of the frontal waking rhythms. In the cat, 14 Hz sleep spindles are particularly conspicuous very near to the midline in the frontal cortex, where 36 Hz rhythms are recorded during hypervigilance ; on the contrary, they seldom appear in SI, where 14 Hz rhythms are recorded during the quiet waking state.

Finally, deep barbiturate narcosis is also well known for eliciting spindles with a very wide cortical distribution. Briefly then, it thus appears that none of the studies performed, either on non-anaesthetized drowsy or sleepy animals, or on deeply barbiturized preparations, can be compared to our model (ROUGEUL et al., 1972).

2) Regarding the second part of our data, let us first briefly stress three points in our findings (see also BOUYER et al., 1982) : (i) VP and its vicinity contains two categories of cells that distinctly alter their firing rate during sequences of 14 Hz somatosensory rhythms, "rhythmic" and "tonic" cells. (ii) None of the neurons that were shown to react during the rhythms clearly appeared as classical thalamo-cortical relay cells (TCRs) carrying specific sensory messages to the cortex. (iii) Conversely none of the TCR cells, characterized through light tactile stimulation, seemed to change its spontaneous firing during a rhythmic sequence.

Our data deserves the following remarks :

a) A striking result is the small proportion of cells in the VP and its vicinity that underwent changes during the studied rhythms (13%). This contrasts with the relatively high number of cells, found in the VP of preparation under nembutal anaesthesia, that fired in relation to the "barbiturate" spindles. No doubt the two conditions are fairly distinct : barbiturate spindles extend over a large part of the cortex, and therefore involve a much higher number of cortical as well as thalamic cells, including typical TCRs (ANDERSEN et al., 1964 ; ANDERSEN and ANDERSSON, 1968 ; GANES and ANDERSEN, 1975). On the other hand, 14 Hz somatosensory rhythms are confined within a very restricted cortical surface (order of magnitude of 3-10 mm^2), representing a forepaw and wrist subarea ; therefore it was not unexpected that the corresponding thalamic area be, in this case, also of very limited extent. It is striking that the thalamic "center" seems to be composed of cells interspersed among the TCR cells. The finding that the long axon thalamocortical cells which participate in the rhythms do not obey the criterion of "relay cell", of the kind that carries somatic information to the cortex, awaits further confirmation on a larger sample. It would obviously be interesting to be able to generalize and consider that thalamocortical cells responsible for any type of focalized cortical rhythm never carry peripheral information.

However, these conclusions could be completely altered if, for the thalamic relay cells that do not display an overt rhythmicity during 14 Hz ECoG, some kind of statistical rhythmicity could be revealed as the result of a more sophisticated processing of their spike trains, as was performed e.g. for the hippocampal theta (GARCIA-SANCHEZ et al., 1978) or for cells in the respiratory brain-stem centre (BERTRAND and HUGELIN, 1971).

b) One may then speculate about the type of circuitry that could account for the observed effects. The distinction between two subsets of rhythmic R cells, spike cells and burst cells has often been made by others (ANDERSEN et al., 1964 ; BURKE and SEFTON, 1966 ; STERIADE et al., 1971 ; STERIADE, 1978).

From data with the collision test, we could conclude that R_S cells were long thalamo-cortical axon neurons. On the other hand, the R_B cells, that were quasi-silent during "desynchronization" episodes, displayed a response with variable and longer latency to cortex stimulation, with no visible collision. Their activation from the cortex could in this case be considered as transsynaptic. The alternative test which is currently employed to further confirm the antidromic versus transsynaptic character, is resistance to high frequency stimulation. Since we wanted to keep the cortex in its best possible shape, we did not perform such repetitive stimulation (over 100/sec). Despite this, one is tempted to consider R_B cells as short axon interneurons (but this may not be the only possible interpretation ; further tests are needed). The way these bursting cells are transsynaptically activated also remains a matter of speculation. It could be through a descending cortico-thalamic long axon neuron (whose existence is amply documented by the anatomists but whose physiological impact or functional importance remains incompletely known) ; or it could be through the recurrent collaterals of neighbouring thalamo-cortical cells activated by the cortical shock.

That such collaterals exist is of course also well-known ; most existing interpretations of the thalamic rhythm generator are in fact based upon this latter type of organization, whatever the complexity of the hypothetized circuitry.

Another point of interest is the existence of cells in the vicinity of the VP and even within the VP, that displayed sustained alterations of their firing during a sequence of 14 Hz rhythms. The role of these tonic cells remains obscure. Our present hypothesis is that they contribute to the development of the rhythms through acting as "enabling" cells, one type (T+) firing, the other type (T-) becoming silent during the same period. The way these two cell categories are connected both to each other and to the rhythm generator itself should be elucidated in the future. One may suggest that the enabling (+) cells (those which are accelerated) initiate the process, inhibiting the enabling (-) cells, those which are silenced and are normally inhibitory to the rhythms. This is for the moment only speculative. A somewhat similar hypothesis was put forward for the occurrence of sleep spindles in the encéphale isolé cat ; in the latter case, however, neurones belonging to nucleus reticularis thalami were implicated (LAMARRE et al., 1971 ; SCHLAG and WASZAK, 1971 ; WASZAK, 1974).

3) As a third point in this discussion, one may finally speculate on the functional meaning of the observed rhythms in relation to motor behavior considered in general.

The states of non-motion as observed here, of expectancy of a prey, or of focused attention on a desired prey, do not represent a non-specific kind of immobility. Some authors would consider them as part of the orienting reaction ; this we shall not discuss here. Whatever their relation to orienting, the described immobilities may represent "premotion postures", i.e. an active attitude of behavioral arrest preceding an adjusted intentional and directed motor behavior.

Whether synchronisation in one or other thalamocortical sector (depending on the specific situation) is purely a consequence of immobility may be discussed. The simplest (and most conservative) hypothesis would indeed be that synchrony is determined by the sudden occurrence of a time invariance of the afferent message : phasic somatic receptors are silenced while tonic receptors (cutaneous, joint, muscles) send a message pattern invariant in time. The mechanism thus postulated for such local synchrony, based on what could be called a "dynamic deafferentation" (ROUGEUL-BUSER et al., 1978) is in a way at variance with the classical views on the genesis of "synchronized" activities, essentially based upon withdrawal of activating influences. Local synchronisations could well be common processes in the higher centers, whereby the function of one or other discrete thalamo-cortical sector involved in a specific task (perceptive, elaborative, etc...) could be influenced, without necessarily implying a shift into drowsiness or even more into sleep. This brings up the next, obvious question, i.e. whether immobility rhythms that are elicited because the animal is motionless, in turn have an influence upon further processing mechanisms. In other words, are rhythms a simple consequence of immobility or do they themselves represent some causal link in some CNS mechanism ?

Rather surprisingly, we still do not know if and how the message processing is altered in a given sensory afferent channel during the development of synchronized rhythms. We mentioned above that the spontaneous activity was apparently not modified in typical TCR neurones during such rhythms. This however did not provide any information on the possible bearing of thalamocortical synchrony on the transfer of specific sensory messages through the VP and/or their processing at the cortical level. As yet only some isolated observations have been performed, showing how orthodromic impulse transmission through the VP was disturbed during spontaneous - in this case barbiturate - spindles (ANDERSEN and ANDERSSON, 1968).

If we assume that a directed movement requires for its adjustment somatic controls that may originate from either area SI, or from the more posterior parietal sectors, possibly through direct or indirect cortico-cortical pathways to the motor cortex (see e.g. JONES and POWELL, 1968), it is conceivable that synchrony could in this case cause a loss of adequate somatic control (or an inhibition of such control) upon the motor cortex and hence, a no-movement episode. Rhythms may in turn reinforce immobility, and this positive feed-back process would last until an external or internal drive overtakes the synchronizing influence. Teleologically one could even suggest that synchrony in the somatic sphere, with immobility, could facilitate attention processing in the visual sphere to prepare the movement i.e. a mechanism which is probably governed by area 7 (MOUNCASTLE et al., 1975) and possibly 19.

As a final remark, we wish to emphasize that the mechanisms which we have hypothesized herein are - in our opinion - different from those which have emerged in the past from experiments with electrical stimulation of some central structures like medial thalamus (HUNTER and JASPER, 1949 ; ROUGEUL et al., 1967), or caudate nucleus (BUCHWALD, et al., 1961 ; ROUGEUL, 1965) as producing states of generalized "arrest" or "freezing" ; the latter attitudes are probably quite distinct from the natural behavioral immobilizations that we have described in the present paper. The relation between the two sets of findings remains to be discovered.

SUMMARY

1) Electrocorticographic studies performed in waking cats have demonstrated the existence of two sets of "rhythmic" patterns that may develop in the sensorimotor and parietal cortex when the animal is displaying attentive behavior. One set (at 14 Hz), on the somatic I cortex, characterizes "expectancy" and quiet waking ; the second (36 Hz), on two areas, motor cortex and parietal cortex behind SI, develop while the cat is focusing attention, e.g., on prey. The thalamic structures likely to constitute the pace-makers of these rhythms are respectively the hand and wrist area of n. ventralis posterior for the 14 Hz and a part of the posterior group (POm) for the parietal 36 Hz activities.

2) A microelectrode study was then performed in n. ventralis posterior (VP) of the fully alert cat, to study the correlation between thalamic unit activity and the cortical synchronized 14 Hz rhythms. (i) Only a small proportion of VP cells underwent changes during the studied cortical rhythms. (ii) None of these cells were typical thalamo-cortical relay cells carrying tactile messages to the cortex. (iii) Cells altering their discharge were of two types, rhythmic (R) cells, discharging at the frequency of the cortical rhythms, and tonic (T) cells, displaying an overall, sustained change during the whole sequence of cortical 14 c/sec. (iv) Among R cells, some were long axon thalamo-cortical cells and others were likely to be interneurones. (v) Some T cells increased their firing rate during rhythmic trains, other were silent during the same period.

The possible functional meaning of these synchronized activities in relation to control of a "pre-motion immobility" is discussed.

ACKNOWLEDGEMENT

This work was supported in part by the following grants : C.N.R.S. (E.R.A. 411), D.E.S., D.G.R.S.T., D.R.E.T., I.N.S.E.R.M., Fondation pour la Recherche Médicale.

REFERENCES

ANDERSEN P, ANDERSSON SA (1968) Physiological basis of the alpha rhythm. Appleton Century Crofts, 235P

ANDERSEN P, ECCLES JC, SEARS TA (1964) The ventro-basal complex of the thalamus : types of cells, their responses and their functional organisation. J Physiol (Lond) 174:370-399

BERLYNE DE (1960) Conflict, arousal and curiosity. Mc Graw-Hill, N.Y., 350P

BERLYNE DE (1970) Attention as a problem in behavior theory. In: MOSTOFSKY DI (ed) Attention : Contemporary theory and analysis. Appleton Century Crofts, N.Y., 447P

BERTRAND F, HUGELIN A (1971) Respiratory synchronizing function of nucleus parabrachialis medialis : pneumotaxic mechanisms. J Neurophysiol 34:189-207

BOUYER JJ, DEDET L, KONYA A, ROUGEUL A (1974) Convergence de trois systèmes rythmiques thalamo-corticaux sur l'aire somesthésique du chat et du babouin normaux. Rev EEG Neurophysiol 4:397-406

BOUYER JJ, MONTARON MF, ROUGEUL A (1981) Fast fronto-parietal rhythms during combined focused attentive behaviour and immobility in cat : cortical and thalamic localizations. Electroenceph Clin Neurophysiol 51:244-252

BOUYER JJ, ROUGEUL A, BUSER P (1982) Somatosensory rhythms in the awake cat. A single unit exploration of its thalamic concomitant in nucleus ventralis and vicinity. Arch Ital Biol 120:95-110

BUCHWALD NA, WYERS EJ, LAUPRECHT EW, HEUSER G (1961) The "caudate spindle". IV. A behavioral index of caudate-induced inhibition. Electroenceph Clin Neurophysiol 13:531-537

BURKE W, SEFTON AJ (1966) Discharge patterns of principal cells and interneurones in lateral geniculate nucleus of rat. J Physiol (Lond) 187:201-212

DARIAN-SMITH I, ISBISTER J, MOK H, YOKOTA T (1966) Somatic sensory cortical projection areas excited by tactile stimulation of the cat. J Physiol (Lond) 182:671

GANES T, ANDERSEN P (1975) Barbiturate spindle activity in functionnally corresponding thalamic and cortical somatosensory areas in the cat. Brain Res 98:457-472

GARCIA-SANCHEZ JL, BUNO W Jr, FUENTES J, GARCIA-AUSTT E (1978) Non rhythmical hippocampal units, theta rhythm and afferent stimulation. Brain Res Bull 3:213-219

GASTAUT H, JUS A, JUS C, MORRELL F, STORM VAN LEEUWEN W, DONGIER S, NAQUET R, REGIS H, ROGER A., BEKKERING D, KAMP A, WERRE J (1957) Etude topographique des réactions électroencéphalographiques conditionnées chez l'homme. Electroenceph Clin Neurophysiol 9:1-34

HASSLER R, MUHS-CLEMENT K (1964) Architectonischer Aufbau des sensomotorischen und parietalen Cortex der Katze. J Hirnforsch 6:377-420

HOWE PC, STERMAN MB (1972) Cortical-subcortical EEG correlates of suppressed motor behavior during sleep and waking in the cat. Electroenceph Clin Neurophysiol 32:681-695

HUNTER J, JASPER H (1949) Effects of thalamic stimulation in unanaesthetized animals. The arrest reaction and petit-mal like seizures, activation patterns and generalized convulsions. Electroenceph Clin Neurophysiol 1:305-324

JASPER H, PENFIELD W (1949) Electrocorticograms in man : effect of voluntary movement upon the electrical activity of the precentral gyrus. Arch Psychiat Z Neurol 183:163-174

JONES EG, POWELL TPS (1968) The ipsilateral cortical connections of the somatic sensory areas in the cat. Brain Res 9:71-94

LAMARRE Y, FILION M, CORDEAU JP (1971) Neuronal discharges of the ventrolateral nucleus of the thalamus during sleep and wakefulness in the cat. I. Spontaneous activity. Exp Brain Res 12:480-498

MOUNTCASTLE VB (1978) An organizing principle for cerebral function : the unit module and the distributed system. In: EDELMAN GM and MOUNTCASTLE VB (eds) The Mindful Brain : cortical organization and the group-selective theory of higher function. MIT Press, Cambridge, 7-50

MOUNTCASTLE VB, LYNCH JC, GEORGOPOULOS A, SAKATA H, ACUNA C (1975) Posterior parietal association cortex of the monkey : command functions for operations within extrapersonal space. J Neurophyiol 39:871-908

PFURTSCHELLER G (1981) Central beta rhythm during sensorimotor activities in man. Electroenceph Clin Neurophysiol 51:253-264

POGGIO GF, MOUNTCASTLE VB (1963) The functional properties of ventrobasal thalamic neurons studied in unanaesthetized monkeys. J Neurophysiol 26:775-806

ROTH SR, STERMAN MB, CLEMENTE CD (1967) Comparison of EEG correlates of reinforcement, internal inhibition and sleep. Electroenceph Clin Neurophysiol 23:509-520

ROUGEUL A (1965) Inhibition de l'activité motrice par stimulation centrale chez l'animal libre. Actualités Neurophysiologiques 6:183-200

ROUGEUL-BUSER A, BOUYER JJ, BUSER P (1978) Transitional states of awareness and short term fluctuations of selective attention : neurophysiological corre-lates and hypotheses. In: BUSER P, BUSER A (eds) Symp Cerebral Correlates of Conscious Experience. Elsevier, Amsterdam, 215-232

ROUGEUL A, LETALLE A, CORVISIER J (1972) Activité rythmique du cortex somesthésique primaire en relation avec l'immobilité chez le chat libre éveillé. Electroenceph Clin Neurophysiol 33:23-39

ROUGEUL A, PERRET C, BUSER P (1967) Effets comportementaux et électro-graphiques de stimulations électriques du thalamus chez le chat libre. Electroenceph Clin Neurophysiol 23:410-428

SCHLAG J, WASZAK M (1971) Electrophysiological properties of units of the thalamic reticular complex. Exp Neurol 32:79-97

STERIADE M (1978) Cortical long axoned cells and putative interneurons during the sleep waking cycle. Behav Brain Sci 1:465-485

STERIADE M, APOSTOL V, OAKSON G (1971) Control of unitary activities in cerebellothalamic pathway during wakefulness and synchronized sleep. J Neuro-physiol 34:389-413

STERMAN MB, WYRWICKA W (1967) EEG correlates of sleep : evidence for separate substrates. Brain Res 6:143-163

TANJI DG, WISE SP, DYKES RW, JONES EC (1978) Cytoarchitecture and thalamic connectivity of third somatosensory area of the cat cerebral cortex. J Neurophysiol 41:268-284

WASZAK M (1974) Firing pattern of neurons in the rostral and ventral part of nucleus reticularis thalami during EEG spindles. Exp Neurol 43:38-59

Premovement Cortical Potentials Associated With Self-Paced and Reaction Time Movements

K. Sasaki and H. Gemba

Department of Physiology, Institute for Brain Research, Faculty of Medicine, Kyoto University, 606 Kyoto, Japan

CEREBRO-CEREBELLAR INTERCONNECTIONS AND PREMOVEMENT CORTICAL FIELD POTENTIALS RECORDED WITH CHRONICALLY IMPLANTED ELECTRODES IN MONKEYS

Neuronal circuits connecting reciprocally the cerebral cortex and the cerebellum have been studied in cats and monkeys and those of monkeys are diagrammatically drawn as in Figure 1 upper schemata (SASAKI, 1979). Using laminar field potential analysis, three kinds of inputs to the cerebral cortex have been distinguished, i.e., two thalamo-cortical (T-C) projections (deep and superficial) and a cortico-cortical projection (association or commissural) as diagrammatically shown in lower part of Figure 1 (cf. SASAKI, 1979 ; SASAKI et al., 1981b). Under such circumstances, cortical field potentials associated with hand movements have been recorded with electrodes implanted chronically on the surface and in the depth of various cortical areas of unanesthetized monkeys. Our intent was to investigate not only movement related characteristics of neuronal circuits causing field potentials but also to study changes in their characteristics during motor learning and the compensation processes. This report will briefly review some of the results.

Silver needle electrodes insulated except for their pointed tips were implanted on the surface and in the depth (2.5-3.0 mm from the surface S and D in the lower left part of Fig.1) of respectively 8-20 different cortical areas on both sides in a monkey. Potentials were measured with respect to two reference electrodes implanted in the bone just behind each ear and connected together (INDIF). The elctrooculogram (EOG) was picked up by an electrode placed in the rostrolateral edge of the frontal bone above the orbit. INDIF served as reference for the EOG. The amplifiers used for cortical potentials and EOGs had time constants of 2.0 s. Electromyograms (EMG) were recorded bipolarly by electrodes on the skin over the wrist extensor muscles of the operant hand, amplified, rectified and taped.

Experimental Brain Research, Suppl. 7
© Springer-Verlag Berlin · Heidelberg 1983

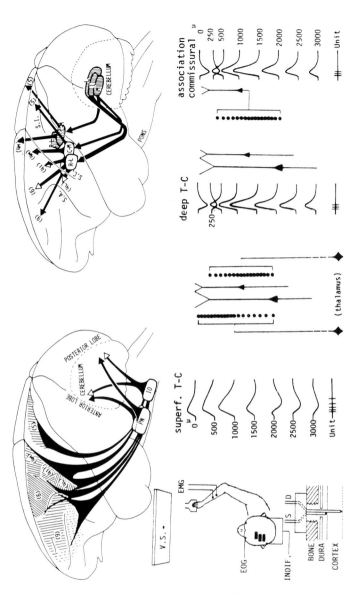

Fig. 1. Schemata of cerebro-cerebellar interconnections in monkeys (upper diagrams) and those of laminar field potentials of two thalamo-cortical (superficial and deep T-C) and cortico-cortical (association or commissural) inputs (lower major part), and diagrams for methods of chronic experiments (lower left). Upper diagrams : numerals indicate area numbers of the cortex. PN : pontine nuclei. IO : inferior olive. S.A. : arcuate sulcus. S.C. : central sulcus. S.I. : intra-parietal sulcus. M, I, L : medial, interpositus and lateral nucleus. R-L, C-M : two nuclear complexes of the thalamus. Lower diagrams : numerals indicate depths from the cortical surface in μm. Unit : schematical pattern of firing of cortical pyramidal neuron. Presumed excitatory synaptic terminals on apical dendrites of cortical pyramidal neurons in layer III and V are schematically shown by dots for three afferent inputs. Laminar field potentials are due to electrical dipoles generated in pyramidal neurons by the EPSPs. See text for lower left diagrams. Modified from SASAKI (1979)

Monkeys (Macaca fuscata) were trained to lift a lever by wrist extension either at their self-paced rate at intervals of more than 2 s or within the duration of a light stimulus lasting for 510-900 ms which was delivered in front of the monkey with a small green light emitting diode (V.S. in Fig. 1) at a random time interval of 2.5-6.0 s. Correct movements were rewarded with a small amount of fruit juice about 600 ms after every movement. Timing pulses indicating the onset of the light stimulus and of the movement (lever elevation) were recorded on FM tape. Cortical potentials, EOGs and EMGs were averaged 100 times using either the stimulus or the movement pulse as the trigger signal. For visually initiated movements, reaction time measured from onset of the stimulus to lever elevation was plotted in a histogram of 16 ms bins for the same 100 movements as those for the potentials. Recording sites in the cortex of all cases and the extent of the cerebellar hemispherectomy in five monkeys (next section) were morphologically verified later.

Self-paced hand movements are preceded by slowly increasing field potentials, surface-negative, deep-positive, in the bilateral premotor, the contralateral forelimb motor and somatosensory cortices for the operant hand. These potentials start at about 1 s and reach the summit at 50-100 ms prior to the movement (HASHIMOTO et al., 1979 ; GEMBA et al., 1980). They are interpreted as being composed mainly of superficial T-C responses (SASAKI et al., 1981b) and are probably the same as "readiness potentials" in human subjects (GILDEN et al., 1966 ; DEECKE et al., 1969). There is a considerable difference between the potential configurations and the distribution in both hemispheres for the premovement potentials of self-paced ("voluntary") movements on the one hand and the visually initiated (conditioned) movements on the other hand (GEMBA et al., 1980 ; 1981). Such different premovement potentials could be elicited in the same monkey when it was sufficiently trained for reacting with both kinds of movements in sequence (SASAKI and GEMBA, 1981 ; GEMBA et al., 1982). This suggests that different central programs are established in the monkey and manifested as the different premovement potentials for the two kinds of movements having the same motor performances.

PREMOVEMENT POTENTIALS WITH VISUALLY INITIATED HAND MOVEMENT AND THE CEREBELLUM

Visually initiated hand movements are preceded by characteristic field potentials in various cortical areas. Potentials in premotor (A) and forelimb motor (B) cortices contralateral to the moving hand are illustrated in Figure 2 left column (PREOP.). When averaged from the pulse of stimulus onset (triangle), bilateral surface-positive, depth-negative potentials appeared at about

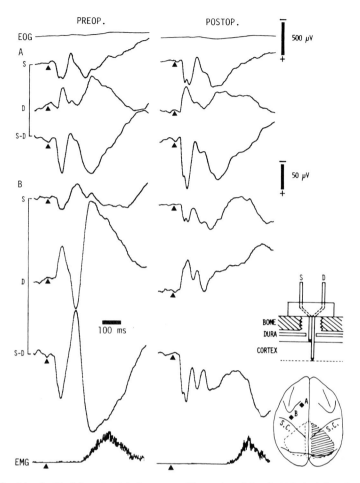

Fig. 2. Cortical field potentials preceding visually initiated hand movements in the premotor (A) and forelimb motor (B) cortices contralateral to the moving hand (see inset). The potentials before (PREOP., left column) and four days after (POSTOP., right column) unilateral cerebellar hemispherectomy (shaded in the lower inset diagram) are recorded from the same monkey. S and D rows present field potentials on the surface (S) and in the depth (D) (2.5-3.0 mm from the surface) respectively as in the upper inset diagram. S-D row gives surface minus depth potentials. 100 ms for all records. 500 μV for EOG and 50 μV for cortical potentials. S.C. : central sulcus. From SASAKI et al. (1981a)

40 ms after the pulse in premotor and motor cortices (A and B). Surface-negative, depth-positive premovement potentials emerged at about 120 ms latency only in the forelimb motor cortex contralateral to the hand. The early surface-positive, depth-negative potentials were found more intimately related to visually evoked impulses than to motor execution, whereas the late surface-negative, depth-positive potentials were connected more closely with

motor execution than to the visual inputs. Thus the early potentials remained almost unchanged but the late potentials in the forelimb motor cortex disappeared entirely when an experimenter lifted the lever for the monkey so that the monkey just watched the light and drank juice without any forelimb movements (GEMBA et al., 1981). The late potentials are considered superficial T-C responses because of their depth profiles and such responses in the forelimb motor cortex will possibly be mediated by the neo-cerebellum (Fig.1 ; SASAKI, 1979), as substantiated in Figure 2 right column.

After the monkey had been trained enough to reveal steady premovement potentials as presented in Figure 2 left column (PREOP.), the cerebellar hemisphere ipsilateral to the moving hand (shaded by oblique lines in the inset figure) was extirpated. Several days after the operation, such monkeys could usually lift the lever but the movement was slow and unstable with a latency of less than 700 or 900 ms after the light stimulus instead of less than 510 ms before the operation, as may be seen in EMG records in Figure 2. As clearly noted in Figure 2 right column, the late surface-negative, depth-positive potentials in the motor cortex were completely eliminated without much change of the early surface-positive, depth-negative potentials in the premotor and motor cortices. When the cerebellar hemispherectomy included both dentate and interpositus nuclei, repeated observations after the operation disclosed the elimination of the late premovement potentials and the delay of movement (90-250 ms in the five monkeys) persisted throughout the whole postoperative period of more than several months. On the contrary, when the operation involved the dentate nucleus but saved the interpositus (SASAKI et al., 1982), the eliminated late premovement potentials and the prolonged reaction times started to recover at several days after the operation and attained improved levels within several weeks. These results indicate that fast and skillful reaction time movements are initiated by the impulses impinging upon the motor cortex through the neo-cerebellum and superficial T-C neurons. Without the cerebellar hemisphere only slow and unstable movements can be performed and are not improved by further training (see next section). In normal situations, the impulses would be conveyed mainly via the dentate nucleus and the thalamus to the forelimb motor cortex, but the interpositus nucleus might substitute for the removed dentate nucleus, at least in early weeks after the operation, according to the mode of innervation of motor cortical areas by the cerebellar nuclei (SASAKI et al., 1976).

DEVELOPMENT AND CHANGE OF PREMOVEMENT POTENTIALS DURING LEARNING PROCESSES OF
VISUALLY INITIATED HAND MOVEMENTS

Premovement field potentials in various cortical areas were successively
recorded during learning processes of the visually initiated hand movement.
Recording loci covered the dorsolateral aspects of both hemispheres except
the temporal lobes, but only five areas are illustrated in Figure 3 A-E. All
training sessions from the commencement to the final steady stages were
recorded for more than several months. They are represented at stages I-VI
for convenience of description. There were differences of the onset times for
the successive stages in the 14 monkeys tested, but sequential events in the
cortical areas were consistently in the same order in all the monkeys. The
S-D potentials averaged from the pulse of the stimulus onset (triangle) and
histograms of reaction times of the same 100 samples are presented for 2nd
day of training (I), 21 days after I (II), 3 days after II (III) and 35 days
after III (IV), training being carried out on 2-5 days per week. Those
movements that occurred within the duration of the stimulus were taken into
the averaged data and histograms. The duration was 900 ms for I-III and 510
ms for IV, and later parts of the 900 ms traces were curtailed in traces of
I-III.

Movements at stages I and II were self-paced as noted in the reaction time
histograms (V.S.-L.E.). Already at stage I, evoked responses were observed in
part of prefrontal (A), and the prestriate (D) cortices, and also in the
premotor (B) and the striate (E) cortices. In the prefrontal cortex, early
surface-positive, depth-negative and late surface-negative, depth-positive
potentials were marked in the caudal part of infraprincipal and ventral
arcuate areas on both sides. Similar potentials were recorded bilaterally in
the prestriate gyri. Stages I and II were not so clearly distinguished but
the potentials in these association cortices, especially the late components
increased considerably at stage II, when the monkey might recognize the light
stimulus to be "meaningful". Then, the monkey suddenly became able to respond
to the stimulus with lever lifting at the reaction times shown in the
histogram of stage III, and surface-positive, depth-negative potentials emerged in the forelimb motor cortex at about 40 ms latency (III C). Potentials
in A and D increased and reached their maximal levels, which were sustained.
The premotor potentials increased often at stage III. The monkey must have
learned at stage III the way to perform the conditioned movement. However,
the movement was still slow and unstable as seen in the histogram and to
encourage the monkey the stimulus had to last for 900 ms. After stage III,
repeated trainings made the movement gradually faster and more skillful and

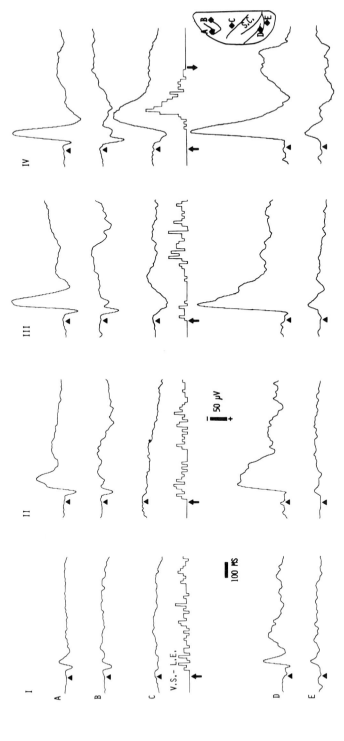

Fig. 3. Changes of S-D (surface minus depth) potentials associated with visually initiated hand movement in learning processes of the movement. Four learning stages (I-IV) are exemplified from observations of eight months. Recording sites are illustrated in the inset diagram by common alphabetical symbols with A-E rows. Reaction times are plotted in 16 ms bins in the V.S.-L.E. row. Upward and downward (only in IV) arrows indicate onset and cessation of the light stimulus. Triangles are the onset times. See text. 100 ms for all traces and 500 μV for all potentials

the monkey attained the final steady accomplished state in motor performance as exemplified in IV, in which early (about 40 ms latency) surface-positive, depth-negative potentials were followed by late (about 120 ms latency) surface-negative, depth-positive potentials in the forelimb motor cortex (Fig. 3, IV C). These potentials are the same as those in Figure 2 left column B. This will indicate that the neocerebellum-superficial T-C projection system is gradually recruited in stages III to IV in order to make the movement faster and more skillful. The consequence of cerebellar hemispherectomy in the well trained monkey appears to correspond to degradation from stage IV to III in respect of motor learning processes.

Much the same (about 40 ms) latencies of premovement potentials in primary visual, prefrontal and occipital association, premotor and motor cortices would suggest that visual information is mostly conveyed not by cortico-cortical serial pathways but in parallel to these cortices via some subcortical structures, presumably thalamic nuclei and their closely related structures. Along stage I to III, such structures under intimate interactions with the cortical areas might distribute the information sequentially and additionally to the cortices and eventually to the motor cortex to initiate the movement, with a kind of "switching" mechanism.

SUMMARY AND CONCLUSION

Field potential analysis with electrodes chronically implanted on the surface and in the depth of various cortical areas in monkeys has demonstrated the following : 1. Different central programs are organized respectively for self-paced ("voluntary") and visually initiated (conditioned) hand movements as revealed by different premovement cortical field potentials in a monkey. 2. Impulses mediated by the neocerebellum and superficial thalamo-cortical projections excite the forelimb motor cortex to initiate the conditioned movement fast and skillfully. Unilateral cerebellar hemispherectomy delays the movement on the ipsilateral side by 90-250 ms. 3. Four stages of the learning processes of the conditioned movement are assumed ; at stage I, visual information arrives bilaterally at striate, prefrontal association, prestriate and often premotor cortices ; at stage II, activities of the prefrontal and occipital association areas increase and the monkey might recognize the light stimulus "meaningful" ; at stage III, impulses arrive at the motor cortex as the monkey has learned the conditioned movement but it is slow and unstable in motor performance ; at stage IV, the movement becomes fast and skillful as the cerebro-cerebellar interactions are recruited.

ACKNOWLEDGEMENTS

We express our gratitude to Prof. Sir John C. ECCLES for valuable advice on
the manuscript.

REFERENCES

DEECKE L, SCHEID P, KORNHUBER HH (1969) Distribution of readiness potential,
pre-motion positivity, and motor potential of the human cerebral cortex
preceding voluntary finger movements. Exp Brain Res 7:158-168

GEMBA H, HASHIMOTO S, SASAKI K (1981) Cortical field potentials preceding
visually initiated hand movements in the monkey. Exp Brain Res 42:435-441

GEMBA H, SASAKI K, HASHIMOTO S (1980) Distribution of premovement slow
cortical potentials associated with self-paced hand movements in monkeys.
Neurosci Lett 20:159-163

GEMBA H, SASAKI K, ITO J (1982) Different cortical potentials preceding
self-paced and visually initiated hand movemnts and their reciprocal transition in the same monkey. Exp Neurol 76:111-120

GILDEN L, VAUGHAN HG Jr, COSTA LD (1966) Summated human EEG potentials with
voluntary movement. Electroencephalogr clin Neurophysiol 20:433-438

HASHIMOTO S, GEMBA H, SASAKI K (1979) Analysis of slow cortical potentials
preceding self-paced hand movement in the monkey. Exp Neurol 65:218-229

SASAKI K (1979) Cerebro-cerebellar interconnections in cats and monkeys. In:
MASSION J, SASAKI K (eds) Cerebro-cerebellar interactions. Elsevier/North
Holland, Amsterdam, pp 105-124

SASAKI K, GEMBA H (1981) Cortical field potentials preceding self-paced and
visually initiated hand movemnts in one and the same monkey and influences of
cerebellar hemispherectomy upon the potentials. Neurosci Lett 25:287-292

SASAKI K, GEMBA H, HASHIMOTO S (1981a) Influences of cerebellar hemispherectomy upon cortical potentials preceding visually initiated hand movements in the monkey. Brain Res 210:425-430

SASAKI K, GEMBA H, HASHIMOTO S (1981b) Premovement slow cortical potentials
on self-paced hand movements and thalamocortical and corticocortical responses in the monkey. Exp Neurol 72:41-50

SASAKI K, GEMBA H, MIZUNO N (1982) Cortical field potentials preceding
visually initiated hand movements and cerebellar actions in the monkey. Exp
Brain Res 46:29-36

SASAKI K, KAWAGUCHI S, OKA H, SAKAI M, MIZUNO N (1976) Electrophysiological
studies on the cerebello-cerebral projections in monkeys. Exp Brain Res
24:495-507

The Initiation of Movements

E.T. Rolls

Oxford University, Department of Experimental Psychology, South Parks Road, Oxford, England

It is the purpose of this paper to consider current concepts on how movements are initiated, and then to introduce evidence leading to a newer formulation according to which the particular functional pathways used in the initiation of a response depend on the nature of the input and output processing required to compute that response.

CURRENT CONCEPTS AND REVISIONS

When considering how movements are initiated, reference is frequently made to a diagram of KEMP and POWELL (1971, see Fig. 1) which draws attention to some similarities of the anatomy of the basal ganglia and the cerebellum. On the right of the diagram, it is shown that many cortical regions, including assocation cortex, project to the striatum, which in turn projects via the globus pallidus and ventrolateral thalamic nuclei to the motor cortex. On the left of the diagram, it is shown that the cerebral cortex projects via the pontine nuclei to the cerebellar cortex, which projects via the cerebellar nuclei (dentate and interpositus) and the ventrolateral thalamic nuclei to the motor cortex. Thus these are two sets of pathways by which information from many regions of the cortex can gain access to the motor cortex, and both could be involved in the initiation of movement. In a similar type of diagram, ALLEN and TSUKAHARA (1974) propose that movements are initiated through connections from the association cortex to the motor cortex via 1) the basal ganglia 2) cortico-cortical connections and/or 3) the lateral cerebellum and dentate nuclei.

Some revision of these hypotheses is required in the light of newer evidence in the primate. First, the striatal and cerebellar systems are not equivalent in the cerebral cortical areas from which they receive inputs, nor in the region of cortex to which their output is directed. The caudate nuclei receive inputs from many areas of the cortex, including connections from

Experimental Brain Research, Suppl. 7
© Springer-Verlag Berlin · Heidelberg 1983

frontal, parietal and temporal lobe association cortex, and send projections via the globus pallidus and the ventroanterior nuclei (VA) of the thalamus to premotor cortex, area 6. The other main part of the neostriatum, the putamen, receives inputs primarily from sensorimotor cortex (areas 6,4,3,1,2 and 5), and sends connections via the globus pallidus and parts of the ventrolateral nuclei of the thalamus (VLo and VLm) to premotor cortex, area 6 (see DELONG, 1982). In contrast, the pontine nuclei and thus the cerebellum receive their heaviest cortical inputs from primary motor and somatosensory areas, followed by secondary motor and visual areas, with only a sparse input from higher order association areas; and the corresponding output of the cerebellum is via the dentate nuclei and parts of the ventrolateral nuclei of the thalamus (VL) to the motor cortex, area 4 (see WIESENDANGER, 1982). Evidence consistent with this is that the activity of dentate neurons tends to slightly precede that of motor cortical neurons (THACH, 1978).

Second, although cooling the dentate nuclei of the cerebellum prolongs the reaction time for an arm movement to a visual signal (MEYER-LOHMANN, HORE and BROOKS, 1977), cooling the VL nuclei of the thalamus did not alter the reaction time (MILLER and BROOKS, 1982). Thus, although the lateral cerebellum may be involved in triggering prompt arm movements (see BROOKS, 1979) (as well as in the execution of the movement once it is initiated, see BROOKS, 1979), this triggering of movements does not appear to require the projection indicated in Figure 1 from the cerebellum via the thalamus to the motor cortex (MILLER and BROOKS, 1982). One reason why this thalamo-cortical pathway was not required for this prompt movement may be that the response was simple elbow movement, and it is known that the motor cortex is required in particular for control of the distal extremities, in for example independent movements of the fingers and thumb (see PHILLIPS and PORTER, 1977 ; PORTER, 1982). It may be that in so far as the cerebello-thalamo-cortical pathway may be involved in the generation of prompt movements, these movements are of the distal extremities, so that only if MILLER and BROOKS had used such a movement, would a prolongation of reaction time have resulted from cooling of the thalamic relay. A second reason may be that this thalamo-cortical pathway is particularly important when a movement is being learned. This is suggested by the finding that VL lesions in the cat impaired the learning of but not the performance of a preoperatively acquired complex limb response made to a moving visual stimulus (FABRE and BUSER, 1980).

This anatomical and functional evidence indicates that not only must the functions of the cerebellum and striatum in the initiation of movement be different, in that their inputs and outputs are different, but also that the

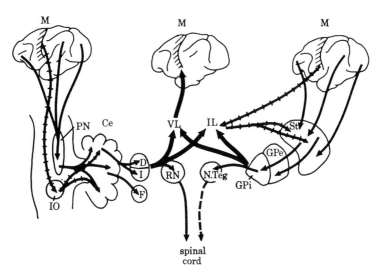

Fig. 1. This figure illustrates similarities in the organization of the cerebral connections of the cerebellum and basal ganglia (from KEMP and POWELL, 1971). Ce, cerebellar cortex ; D, dentate nucleus ; F, fastigial nucleus ; GPe, globus pallidus, external segment ; GPi, globus pallidus, internal segment ; I, interpositus nucleus ; IL, intralaminar nuclei of the thalamus ; IO, inferior olive ; M, motor cortex ; N.Teg., tegmental nucleis ; PN, pontine nuclei ; RN, red nucleus ; St, striatum ; VL, ventrolateral nucleus of the thalamus

type of movement initiated, and whether it has been learned previously, are also important when considering the pathways through which movements are initiated. It will be shown in the following sections that the degree and type of decoding of the stimulus required for the initiation of movement influence the pathways involved in the initiation of movements. The importance of these other pathways in the initiation of movements becomes particularly evident when tasks other than simple reaction time tasks such as the initiation of an elbow movement to a light flash are considered. Examples of the other tasks include choice reaction time tasks, in which on each trial a decision has to be made on whether a response should be made, or on the type of response which should be made. Initiation of movements under these conditions when a choice must be made is common when an animal is in more natural situations. It occurs for example when an animal decides whether to initiate a movement to obtain food when he sees an object which may or may not be food. Investigations of pathways involved in the initiation of feeding are considered next, because they provide information on the pathways involved in the initiation of movement in a situation in which a choice must be made on each trial of whether to initiate a movement, and in which analysis of a patterned visual stimulus is required. Then other pathways involved in different ways in whether movements are initiated are considered. These considerations lead to the view, developed in the synthesis, that for an understanding of the initiation of movement, it is important to determine for the particular type of stimulus analysis required and the particular type of movement, the processing systems which may need to be functionally interconnected for the initiation of that movement.

THE INITIATION OF FEEDING

There is evidence that neurons in the lateral hypothalamus and substantia innominata are involved in the initiation of feeding. Thus damage to the lateral hypothalamus can lead to aphagia, that is to a failure to initiate feeding, even when damage to fibres of passage is minimized with the use of the kainic acid technique, and approximately 13.4% in one sample of 764 neurons in the lateral hypothalamus and substantia innominata had responses to the sight and/or taste of food (see ROLLS, 1981a,b ; ROLLS, BURTON and MORA, 1976). These neurons only responded to the sight of food if the monkey was hungry (BURTON, ROLLS and MORA, 1976), and came through learning to respond to the sight of food as opposed to non-food visual stimuli (MORA, ROLLS and BURTON, 1976). When the monkey had to choose whether to initiate feeding in a visual discrimination task, it was found that the responses of these neurons occurred to the visual stimulus which signified that a lick response could be initiated to obtain food, but not to the visual stimulus which indicated that the monkey should not lick or he would obtain aversive hypertonic saline. The latency of the discriminative responses of these neurons was 140-200 ms, compared to 250-350 ms for the EMG responses associated with licks made at 350-450 ms (ROLLS, SANGHERA and ROPER-HALL, 1979), so that the responses of these neurons preceded and predicted the initiation of feeding responses by the monkey (ROLLS, SANGHERA and ROPER-HALL, 1979). (The neurons did not respond simply in relation to licking movements.) It should be emphasized that this Go/Nogo task requires a visual discrimination, and is not a simple reaction time task.

Motivational specificity. The responses of these neurons in the hypothalamus and substantia innominata thus suggested that they could provide information on which a decision to initiate feeding could be based. To determine whether the responses of these neurons might be involved specifically in the initiation of feeding, or more generally in response initiation, the activity of these neurons was recorded while the monkey performed a visual discrimination in which one stimulus indicated that a lick could be initiated to obtain food, a different stimulus indicated that the same lick could be made to obtain water from the same tube, and a third stimulus that aversive saline would be obtained if a lick was made. The monkey was hungry and thirsty. It was found that although some of these neurons responded to both the food and water related stimuli, others responded either to the food or to the water related stimulus, but not to both. This type of experiment provides evidence that the responses of some of these neurons are related to the initiation of motivationally specific types of response, such as feeding as opposed to drinking.

Output connections. Given that the responses of these neurons in the hypothalamus and substantia innominata suggest that they are involved in the initiation of responses to food, it must next be considered whether they are involved in the initiation of feeding responses to the sight of food, or of autonomic and endocrine responses. To investigate the function of these neurons, their output connections are being investigated by testing for antidromic activation from the different sites to which hypothalamic neurons are known to project. It has so far been shown that some of these feeding-related neurons can be antidromically activated by electrical stimulation of such cortical areas as the prefrontal cortex, the supplementary motor cortex, and the motor cortex (experiments of E.T. ROLLS, E. MURZI and C. GRIFFITHS). This makes it likely that some of these neurons belong to the basal magnocellular forebrain nuclei of Meynert, which send projections directly to the cerebral cortex (KIEVIT and KUYPERS, 1975 ; DIVAC, 1975). Thus through these neurons, a signal reaches the cortex on which a decision to initiate a feeding movement could be based, and this is one way in which these neurons could be involved in the initiation of feeding. A subcortical origin from the ventral forebrain for such a signal is reasonable in that the signal must be modulated by the motivational state of the animal, which is dependent on factors such as stomach distension, plasma nutrient status, etc (see ROLLS, 1982a).

The role of reward in the initiation of movements. These ventral forebrain neurons which respond to the sight of food have responses at a stage of processing at which the signal indicates the availability of food, and that hunger is present. It thus represents a stimulus for which the animal should work, that is a reward-related stimulus. Evidence that the responses of these neurons do signify reward availability, so that the animal will initiate responses in order to activate these neurons, is that the monkeys will work to obtain electrical stimulation delivered in the region of these neurons (ROLLS, BURTON and MORA, 1980 ; ROLLS, 1982a). This evidence is thus consistent with the hypothesis that for the initiation of some types of movements, such as movements made to obtain food, there is decoding of the stimulus to the level at which the signal indicates food reward (i.e. that the stimulus is food and that hunger is present), that this signal is then projected to wide areas of the neocortex, and that on the basis of this signal movements are initiated in order to approach and obtain the food (see further ROLLS, 1982a). The advantage of such a system for the initiation of feeding is that once the stimulus has been decoded to the level of food reward, any movement appropriate to maximize the signal can be made. This allows for flexibility of the initiated behavioral response. It contrasts with the situation in which a particular stimulus is always associated over many trials with a particular motor response, which may allow more rapid, but less flexible, motor responses to be initiated, perhaps through a system involving the basal ganglia (see below).

Pathways required for analysis of the stimulus, and assessment of its significance. The decoding of complex visual stimuli such as the sight of food as compared to non-food objects appears to require visual processing through the inferior temporal visual cortex and amygdala, since lesions in these regions lead monkeys to select non-food as well as food stimuli, and impair the learning of visual discriminations made to obtain food (see ROLLS, 1981a,c ; 1982a,b). Anatomical evidence indicates that the ventral forebain receives visual inputs from the inferior temporal cortex via the amygdala (HERZOG and VAN HOESEN, 1976). It was therefore of interest to investigate the decoding of visual information through this system, to determine at which stage it became coded to represent a signal appropriate for the initiation of movement, such as food reward. It was found that in the inferior temporal visual cortex the significance of a stimulus in terms of its association with reward and dependence on motivational state was not a factor which determined the responses of the neurons, and in the amygdala only the first signs of dependence of neuronal responses on the significance of the stimuli were found (ROLLS, JUDGE and SANGHERA, 1977 ; SANGHERA, ROLLS and ROPER-HALL, 1979 ; see also synthesis below). This evidence is consistent with the hypothesis that neuronal responses which represent the reward value of the stimulus, and on the basis of which it would be appropriate to initiate feeding movements, are elaborated along this pathway, but are not fully evident until the stage of the ventral forebrain neurons, some of which project this information to the cerebral cortex (see further ROLLS, 1981a ; 1982a,b).

THE ORBITOFRONTAL CORTEX

When a monkey must make a decision whether to initiate a movement or not, as
in a Go/Nogo task of the type described above, then the integrity of the
orbitofrontal cortex is required, in that if it is lesioned, responses are
initiated on the Nogo trials (IVERSEN and MISHKIN, 1970 ; see ROLLS, 1981a ;
1982b). In this way the orbitofrontal cortex is important in whether movements are initiated or not. Following orbitofrontal lesions movements are
also initiated when they should be prevented in extinction and in the
reversal of a visual discrimination (BUTTER, 1969 ; JONES and MISHKIN, 1972 ;
see THORPE, ROLLS and MADDISON, 1983). In these situations movements are
initiated to the previously rewarded but now non-rewarded stimulus. To
investigate neuronal processing in the orbitofrontal cortex which might be
related to whether movements are initiated, recordings have been made from
neurons in the orbitofrontal cortex of macaque monkeys performing Go/Nogo
visual discriminations of the type described above, and during reversal of
the discrimination and in extinction (THORPE, ROLLS and MADDISON, 1983). In
a sample of 463 neurons, it was found that a small proportion (3.8%)
responded in one or several non-reward or punishment conditions, such as when
the monkey initiated a response to a previously rewarded visual stimulus and
did not receive reward (extinction) or received punishment with saline (in
reversal). Another population of neurons (32.4% of the sample) responded to
visual stimuli, in some cases on the basis of whether that visual stimulus
had on preceding trials been associated with reward. A third population of
neurons responded after the delivery of the fruit juice reward (see THORPE et
al., 1983). The response properties of these neurons suggest that some of
them respond to visual stimuli on the basis of whether they have been
previously associated with reward, others detect whether reward is obtained
when a response is initiated, and a third group respond if a mismatch is
obtained between expected and obtained reward. Computations such as these
would be required in order to determine whether or not to initiate a response
to a particular stimulus, and it appears that the orbitofrontal cortex is
involved in this type of function (see THORPE et al., 1983).

STRIATUM

Damage to the dopamine pathways which includes the nigrostriatal bundle leads
to akinesia or a failure to initiate movement in Parkinson's disease in man
and to a comparable akinesia or catalepsy which includes a sensorimotor
deficit in animals (see HORNYKIEWICZ, 1973 ; MARSHALL, RICHARDSON and
TEITELBAUM, 1974). Given that the striatum does thus appear to be involved in

the initiation of movement, neurophysiological evidence on the function of the striatum will be considered. This neurophysiological evidence indicates that there is considerable specialization of function within the striatum, and it will be proposed that different parts of the striatum are involved in different aspects of the initiation of movements.

Before considering neurophysiological investigations of the striatum, its main connections will be briefly considered. First, it is in an appropriate position for a role in the initiation of movement in that the main parts of the neostriatum, the caudate nucleus and putamen, together receive inputs from the whole of the cerebral cortex, and send outputs via the globus pallidus and VA/VL thalamic nuclei to the premotor cortex, which in turn projects to the motor cortex (see KEMP and POWELL, 1970 ; 1971 ; DELONG, 1982). Part of its importance in the initiation of movement may be that it provides one of the few routes through which frontal, temporal and parietal association cortices can influence output regions (KEMP and POWELL, 1971 ; DIVAC and OBERG, 1979 ; OBERG and DIVAC, 1979). Second, there is evidence for anatomical segregation in the striatum. The general rule is that each part of the striatum receives inputs most heavily from the part of the cortex which overlies it (KEMP and POWELL, 1970 ; 1971), although there are also more widespread connections (YETERIAN and VAN HOESEN, 1978). Thus the tail of the caudate nucleus receives primarily from the overlying temporal lobe visual and auditory cortex, and the head of the caudate nucleus receives primarily from the prefrontal cortex (KEMP and POWELL, 1970 ; 1971). Also, the putamen receives mainly from sensorimotor cortex (areas 6,4,3,1,2 and 5), and projects through its own parts of the globus pallidus and VL thalamic nuclei to the premotor cortex, area 6 (see DELONG, 1982 ; GRAYBIEL and RAGSDALE, 1979). There is even evidence for functional segregation within this system, in that for example inputs related to the arm from these different cortical areas may converge into one part of the putamen (DELONG, 1982). Neurophysiological evidence on the functions of the striatum in the initiation of movements will now be considered.

Tail of the caudate nucleus. When recordings were made from single neurons in the tail of the caudate nucleus in the macaque monkey, which receives inputs from inferior temporal visual cortex, a population was found which responded with latencies of 90-140 ms to visual stimuli (see ROLLS, 1981a ; ROLLS, THORPE, PERRETT et al., 1981 ; CAAN, PERRETT and ROLLS, in preparation). The visual responses were selective, often on the basis of physical characteristics of the stimuli such as orientation or color. However, unlike the responses of neurons in the inferior temporal visual cortex, the responses of many of these caudate neurons habituated rapidly to a repeated visual stimulus. The responses were in some cases partially restored by a delay, by intervening stimuli, or by rotation of the stimulus, or by changing its color. Damage to the nigrostriatal bundle results in a sensorimotor impairment in which there is a failure to orient to environmental visual stimuli (MARSHALL et al., 1974). It is suggested that this system in the tail of the caudate nucleus is part of a pattern specific mechanism for orientation to a new or changed environmental stimulus, and subsequent habituation to that stimulus (ROLLS, 1981a). In that this system receives from inferior temporal visual cortex, and the habituation is often to specific features of the initially effective stimuli, this "movement initiation system" is specialized for complex, cortically processed, visual inputs to which orientation and subsequent habituation are appropriate, and different mechanisms are probably involved in habituation to simpler stimuli.

Head of the caudate nucleus. In the head of the caudate nucleus, many neurons were found which responded to environmental events which were cues to the monkey to prepare for the initiation of behavior (see ROLLS, 1981a ; ROLLS, THORPE, MADDISON et al., 1979 ; ROLLS, THORPE, PERRETT et al., 1981 ; ROLLS, THORPE and MADDISON, 1983). For example, some of these neurons responded to a tone cue which preceded and signalled the onset of the visual stimuli in the visual discrimination described above. Others responded to a light cue given at the same time. Some of these neurons only responded to these events when they were cues for the start of a trial in the discrimination. Other neurons were tonically active for the duration of each trial, from the cue period until the monkey had completed his response in the discrimination. It is suggested that these neurons are involved, through their inputs from prefrontal cortex, in utilizing environmental stimuli to enable the animal to prepare for and initiate movements, and that the akinesia which follows nigrostriatal damage is due in part to dysfunction of this system (ROLLS, 1981a ; ROLLS et al., 1979 ; 1981).

Putamen. These neurons in the head of the caudate nucleus did not have responses which were phasically related to identifiable movements, and were thus different from neurons recorded in a third part of the striatum, the putamen, in the same test situation. Many of these neurons responded phasically in relation to for example mouth or arm movements (ROLLS, 1981a ; ROLLS et al., 1979 ; 1981). DELONG, who has made an extensive series of recordings in the putamen, has found that neurons in the putamen may respond in relation to the direction of movement rather than the force required to produce the movement (see DELONG, 1982), so that these neurons may be involved in planning the movement, rather than in the details of the muscle activity required to execute the movement.

Ventral striatum. A fourth part of the striatum, the ventral striatum, which includes the nucleus accumbens, the olfactory tubercle and the islands of Calleja, receives inputs from limbic regions such as the amygdala and hippocampus, and from visual association cortex, and projects to the ventral pallidum, and thus perhaps to the mediodorsal nucleus of the thalamus and prefrontal and cingulate cortex, and thus to the motor cortex (HEIMER and WILSON, 1975 ; HEIMER, SWITZER and VAN HOESEN, 1982). There may also be projections from the ventral pallidum to the midbrain locomotor region (L.W. SWANSON and G.J. MOGENSON, personal communication). Damage to the dopaminergic innervation of the ventral striatum impairs the locomotor response which normally occurs in rats placed in a novel environment or exposed to novel stimuli (FINK and SMITH, 1980). In recordings being made in the ventral striatum, we find that some neurons can be activated by visual stimuli. In some cases these responses occur to novel stimuli, and may show memories which last over at least several intervening different visual stimuli. In other cases, these neurons respond to visual stimuli in relation to the aversiveness of these stimuli, and the degree of emotional response they evoke (ROLLS, ASHTON, WILLIAMS et al., 1982). These neuronal responses suggest that the function of at least part of the ventral striatum is related to the initiation of behavioral responses to stimuli which have been processed in relation to memory and emotion through limbic structures. The behavioral responses which result may include the elicitation by environmental stimuli of locomotor activity and exploration when appropriate as determined by limbic decoding (see e.g. MOGENSON, JONES and YIM, 1980).

A main point it is desired to make in this paper is that an account of the initiation of movement can only be given in terms of the input and output processing required for that movement. This is evident even within the context of striatal function, in that as shown above different parts of the striatum appear to perform processing related to the initiation of different types of response to different stimuli. For example, the tail of the caudate appears to be involved in pattern specific orientation and habituation, the head of the caudate to preparation for movement initiation, the putamen to planning movements, and the ventral striatum to locomotor and exploratory responses to novel and emotion-provoking stimuli.

CORTICO-CORTICAL PROCESSING

In addition to the subcortical loops which provide routes for information to reach the motor and premotor cortex, there are also cortico-cortical connections which appear to be important in the initiation of some types of response. For example occipito-frontal cortico-cortical connections are important in visual guidance of finely controlled hand and finger movements (HAAXMA and KUYPERS, 1974).

OTHER PATHWAYS

There is evidence for the existence of at least several other processing systems used in the initiation of movements in particular situations. For example, there is a population of neurons in the cortex in the fundus of the anterior part of the superior temporal sulcus in the macaque monkey with responses specialized to occur to features or combinations of features present in faces (ROLLS, PERRETT and CAAN, 1979 ; PERRETT, ROLLS and CAAN, 1982). There are projections from this region into the amygdala, and neurons with responses which also occur specifically to faces are found in the amygdala (ROLLS, 1981c). This system may be important in the initiation of responses to faces, for damage to the amygdala produces the Kluver-Bucy syndrome in which there is a failure to initiate fearful responses to faces, and to initiate normal social responses in a dominance hierarchy (see ROLLS, 1981c).

In another system of neurons in a perifornical region at the rostral border of the thalamus, the neurons respond to familiar but not to novel stimuli in a memory task which requires relatively long-term memory (ROLLS, CAAN, PERRETT and WILSON, 1981 ; ROLLS, PERRETT, CAAN and WILSON, 1982). These neurons appear to be involved when behavioral responses have to be initiated on the basis of whether a stimulus is familiar or novel, for damage in the medial thalamus of the monkey leads to a failure in a simpler version of this task, and damage may be found in the medial thalamus of humans with amnesia associated with chronic alcoholism or with encephalitis (see AGGLETON and MISHKIN, 1981 ; ROLLS et al., 1982).

These two systems thus provide two further examples of pathways through which information is processed when movements are initiated in particular situations.

SYNTHESIS

According to the approach taken in this paper, instead of considering "the initiation of movement", and whether this depends on for example cerebro-cerebello-motor cortex pathways or cerebro-striato-premotor cortex pathways, it is more helpful to determine for the particular type of stimulus analysis required and the particular type of movement, the processing subsystems which may need to be functionally interconnected for the initiation of the movement. Thus for example if the sensory analysis required involves only detection of the onset of a light (e.g. SASAKI, GEMBA and MIZUNO, 1982 ; MILLER and BROOKS, 1982), then the response may be initiated even with only early or even subcortical stages of visual processing (see e.g. WEISKRANTZ, COWEY and PASSINGHAM, 1977 ; WEISKRANTZ, 1980). If pattern-specific visual analysis is required, then it is likely that at least primary visual cortex will be on the route. If stereopsis or color pattern analysis are required, then it is likely that prestriate cortical visual areas will be on the route. If constancy across different regions of visual space is required, then inferior temporal cortex will probably be on the route (see e.g. COWEY, 1979 ; GROSS, 1973 ; GROSS and MISHKIN, 1977). It is quite possible than the signal is used after sufficient analysis (and the minimal analysis if speed is important) has been completed for the task being performed, and there are output pathways for each of the cortical stages of analysis to for example frontal regions (see JONES and POWELL, 1970) as well as to the striatum (see KEMP and POWELL, 1970).

Another factor which may influence the processing pathways used for the initiation of a movement is whether the task is a simple reaction time task, or requires a decision about whether to initiate a response to the stimulus (as in a Go/Nogo task), or about which response to initiate (as in a choice reaction time task). For a simple reaction time task, relatively direct pathways from sensory to motor regions may be used. For decision tasks in which a decision has to be made about whether to respond, evidence has already been presented above that special processing may be required in regions such as the primate orbitofrontal cortex if responses are not to be initiated inappropriately. When a choice of the response to make is necessary, less is known of the processing involved, but there is evidence for special processing, in that lesions of the parietal or premotor cortex impaired the ability of monkeys to initiate one movement (pulling a handle) to a blue stimulus, and to initiate a different movement (turning the handle) to a yellow stimulus (in the absence of simple sensory or motor impairments ; HALSBAND and PASSINGHAM, 1982). As described here, if the choice is of whether to initiate a response to obtain food, then analysis of the significance of a visual stimulus, in terms of whether as a result of prior learning it is food or signifies food, and whether hunger is present, must be performed. This evaluation of the significance of visual stimuli appears to involve the inferior temporal visual cortex / amygdala / hypothalamus pathway, as described above (see also ROLLS, 1981a, 1982b).

A third factor which may influence the processing pathways used for the initiation of a movement is the type of movement required. Thus if fine finger movements are required, the primary motor cortex will be on the movement initiation pathway (see PHILLIPS and PORTER, 1977). If visual control of limb or finger movements is required, then area 6 of the premotor cortex may be particularly important. If bimanual dexterity is required for a task, then the supplementary motor area may be particularly important (see PORTER, 1982). If the movement initiated is of a whole limb, then its initiation may not require the motor cortex, and the route may follow instead subcortical pathways, which are available for both the cerebellum and the striatum (see NAUTA and DOMESICK, 1979 ; GRAYBIEL and RAGSDALE, 1979).

Thus, it is suggested that the initiation of movements can be analysed and understood in terms of the processing systems and their interconnections which are required for the particular sensory analysis, decision, and output processes which are involved in each situation. These processing systems and their functional interconnections are likely to be different in different situations, and to be selected as needed according to the type of stimulus, decision and response involved for the particular movement being initiated. When analysing pathways involved in the initiation of movement, it is important to specify the sensory analysis and decision processes involved as well as the motor response required, as all three factors will determine the pathways involved in the initiation of a particular movement.

ACKNOWLEDGEMENT. The author is very grateful to G.J. MOGENSON for helpful comments on a draft of this paper.

REFERENCES

AGGLETON JP, MISHKIN M (1981) Recognition impairment after medial thalamic lesions in monkeys. Soc Neurosci Abstr 8:236

ALLEN GI, TSUKAHARA N (1974) Cerebrocerebellar communication systems. Physiol Rev 54:957-1006

BROOKS VB (1979) Control of intended limb movement by the lateral and intermediate cerebellum. In: ASANUMA H, WILSON VJ (eds) Integration in the nervous system. Igaku-Shoin, Tokyo New York, pp 321-356

BURTON MJ, ROLLS ET, MORA F (1976) Effects of hunger on the responses of neurons in the lateral hypothalamus to the sight and taste of food. Exp Neurol 51:668-677

BUTTER CM (1969) Perseveration in extinction and in discrimination reversal tasks following selective prefrontal ablations in Macaca mulatta. Physiol Behav 4:163-171

COWEY A (1979) Cortical maps and visual perception. Quart J Exp Psychol 31:1-17

DELONG MR (1982) Cortico-basal ganglia loops. In: MASSION J, PAILLARD J, SCHULTZ W, WIESENDANGER M (eds), Neural coding of motor performance. Exp Brain Res, Suppl 7, Springer, Berlin

DIVAC I (1975) Magnocellular nuclei of the basal forebrain project to neocortex, brain stem, and olfactory bulb. Review of some functional correlates. Brain Res 93:385-398

DIVAC I, OBERG RGE (1979) Current conceptions of neostriatal functions. In: DIVAC I, OBERG RGE (eds) The neostriatum. Pergamon, New York and London, pp 215-230

FABRE M, BUSER P (1980) Structures involved in acquisition and performance of visually guided movements. Acta Biol Exp 40:95-116

FINK JS, SMITH GP (1980) Mesolimbicocortical dopamine terminal fields are necessary for normal locomotor and investigatory exploration in rats. Brain Res 199:359-384

GRAYBIEL AM, RAGSDALE CW (1979) Fiber connections of the basal ganglia. Prog Brain Res 51:239-283

GROSS CG (1973) Inferotemporal cortex and vision. Prog Physiol Psychol 5:77-123

GROSS CG, MISHKIN M (1977) The neural basis of stimulus equivalence across retinal translation. In: HARNAD S et al. (eds) Lateralization in the nervous system. Academic Press, New York, pp 109-122

HAAXMA R, KUYPERS HGJM (1974) Role of occipito-frontal cortico-cortical connections in visual guidance of relatively independent hand and finger movements in rhesus monkeys. Brain Res 71:361-366

HALSBAND U, PASSINGHAM R (1982) The role of premotor and parietal cortex in the direction of action. Brain Res 240: 368-372

HEIMER L, WILSON RD (1975) The subcortical projections of the allocortex : similarities in the neural associations of the hippocampus, the pyriform cortex and the neocortex. In: SANTINI M (ed) Golgi Centennial Symposium, Raven Press, New York, pp 177-193

HEIMER L, SWITZER GW, VAN HOESEN GW (1982) Ventral striatum and ventral pallidum. Additional components of the motor system. Trends in Neurosciences, in press

HERZOG AG, VAN HOESEN GW (1976) Temporal neocortical afferent connections to amygdala in the rhesus monkey. Brain Res 115:57-69

HORNYKIEWICZ O (1973) Dopamine in the basal ganglia : its role and therapeutic implications. Brit Med Bull 29:172-178

IVERSEN SD, MISHKIN M (1970) Perseverative interference in monkey following selective lesions of the inferior prefrontal convexity. Exp Brain Res 11: 376-386

JONES B, MISHKIN M (1972) Limbic lesions and the problem of stimulus-reinforcement associations. Exp Neurol 36:362-377

JONES EG, POWELL TPS (1970) An anatomical study of converging sensory pathways within the cerebral cortex of the monkey. Brain 93:793-820

JONES EG, PORTER R (1980) What is area 3a ? Brain Res Rev 2:1-43

KEMP JM, POWELL TPS (1970) The cortico-striate projections in the monkey. Brain 93:525-546

KEMP JM, POWELL TPS (1971) The connections of the striatum and globus pallidus : synthesis and speculation. Phil Trans Roy Soc B, 262:441-457

KLEVIT J, KUYPERS HGJM (1975) Subcortical afferents to the frontal lobe studied by means of retrograde horseradish peroxidase transport. Brain Res 85:262-266

MARSHALL JP, RICHARDSON JS, TEITELBAUM P (1974) Nigrostriatal bundle damage and the lateral hypothalamic syndrome. J Comp Physiol Psychol 87:808-830

MEYER-LOHMANN J, HORE J, BROOKS VB (1977) Cerebellar participation in generation of prompt arm movements. J Neurophysiol 40:1038-1050

MILLER AD, BROOKS VB (1982) Parallel pathways for movement initiation in monkeys. Exp Brain Res 45:328-332

MISHKIN M, AGGLETON J (1981) Multiple functional contributions of the amygdala in the monkey. In: BEN-ARI Y (ed) The amygdaloid complex. Amsterdam, Elsevier, pp 409-420

MOGENSON GJ, JONES DL, YIM CY (1980) From motivation to action : functional interface between the limbic system and the motor system. Prog Neurobiol 14:69-97

MORA F, ROLLS ET, BURTON MJ (1976) Modulation during learning of the responses of neurons in the lateral hypothalamus to the sight of food. Exp Neurol 53:508-519

NAUTA WJH, DOMESICK VB (1979) The anatomy of the extrapyramidal system. In: FUXE K, CALNE DB (eds) Dopaminergic ergot derivatives and motor function. Pergamon, Oxford, pp 3-22

OBERG RGE, DIVAC I (1979) "Cognitive" functions of the neostriatum. In: DIVAC I, OBERG RGE (eds) The neostriatum. Pergamon, New York and London, pp 291-313

PERRETT DI, ROLLS ET, CAAN W (1982) Visual neurons responsive to faces in the monkey temporal cortex. Exp Brain Res, 47:329-342

PHILLIPS CF, PORTER R (1977) Corticospinal neurones. Academic Press, New York

PORTER R (1982) Neuronal activities · in primary motor area and premotor functions. In: MASSION J, PAILLARD J, SCHULTZ W, WIESENDANGER M (eds) Neural coding of motor performance. Exp Brain Res, Suppl 7, Springer, Berlin

ROLLS ET (1981a) Processing beyond the inferior temporal visual cortex related to feeding, learning, and striatal function. In: KATSUKI Y, NORGREN

R, SATO M (eds) Brain mechanisms of sensation. Wiley, New York, Ch 16, pp 241-269

ROLLS ET (1981b) Central nervous mechanisms related to feeding and appetite. Brit Med Bull 37:131-134

ROLLS ET (1981c) Responses of amygdaloid neurons in the primate. In: BEN-ARI Y (ed) The amygdaloid complex. Elsevier, Amsterdam, pp 383-393

ROLLS ET (1982a) Feeding and reward. In: NOVIN D, HOEBEL BG (eds) The neural basis of feeding and reward. Haer Institute for Electrophysiological Research, Brunswick, Maine

ROLLS ET (1982b) Neuronal mechanisms underlying the formation and dis-connection of associations between visual stimuli and reinforcement in prima-tes. In: WOODY CD (ed) Conditioning. Plenum, New York

ROLLS ET, BURTON MJ, MORA F (1976) Hypothalamic neuronal responses associated with the sight of food. Brain Res 111:53-66

ROLLS ET, JUDGE SJ, SANGHERA M (1977) Activity of neurons in the infe-rotemporal cortex of the alert monkey. Brain Res 130:229-238

ROLLS ET, SANGHERA MK, ROPER-HALL A (1979) The latency of activation of neurons in the lateral hypothalamus and substantia innominata during feeding in the monkey. Brain Res 164:121-135

ROLLS ET, THORPE SJ, MADDISON S, ROPER-HALL A, PUERTO A, PERRETT D (1979) Activity of neurones in the neostriatum and related structures in the alert animal. In: DIVAC I, OBERG RGE (eds) The neostriatum, Pergamon, Oxford, pp 163-182

ROLLS ET, BURTON MJ, MORA F (1980) Neurophysiological analysis of brain-sti-mulation reward in the monkey. Brain Res 194:339-357

ROLLS ET, THORPE SJ, PERRETT DI, MADDISON S, CAAN W, WILSON F, RYAN S (1981) Neuronal responses in the striatum of the behaving monkey : implications for understanding striatal function and dysfunction. In: SZENTAGOTHAI J, HAMORI J, PALKOVITS M (eds) Advances in physiological sciences, vol 2, Regulatory functions of the CNS. Pergamon, Oxford, pp 205-209

ROLLS ET, CAAN AW, PERRETT DI, WILSON FAW (1981) Neuronal activity related to long-term memory. Acta Neurologica Scandinavica, 64, suppl 89:121-127

ROLLS ET, PERRETT DI, CAAN AW, WILSON FAW (1982) Neuronal responses related to visual recognition. Brain, 105:611-646

ROLLS ET, ASHTON J, WILLIAMS G, THORPE SJ, MOGENSON GJ, COLPAERT F, PHILLIPS AG (1982) Neuronal activity in the ventral striatum of the behaving monkey. Soc Neurosci Abstr 8

ROLLS ET, THORPE SJ, MADDISON SP (1983) Responses of striatal neurons in the behaving monkey. 1. Head of the caudate nucleus. Behav Brain Res, in press

SANGHERA MK, ROLLS ET, ROPER-HALL A (1979) Visual responses of neurons in the dorsolateral amygdala of the alert monkey. Exp Neurol 63:610-626

SASAKI K, GEMBA H, MIZUNO N (1982) Cortical field potentials preceding visually initiated hand movements and cerebellar actions in the monkey. Exp Brain Res 46:29-36

THACH WT (1978) Correlation of neural discharge with pattern and force of muscular activity, joint position, and direction of the intended movement in motor cortex and cerebellum. J Neurophysiol 41:654-676

THORPE SJ, ROLLS ET, MADDISON SP (1983) Neuronal responses in the orbitofrontal cortex of the behaving monkey. Exp Brain Res, in press

WEISKRANTZ L (1980) Varieties of residual experience. Quart J Exp Psychol 32:365-386

WEISKRANTZ L, COWEY A, PASSINGHAM C (1977) Spatial responses to brief stimuli by monkeys with striate cortex ablations. Brain 100:655-670

WIESENDANGER M (1982) Cortico-cerebellar loops. In: MASSION J, PAILLARD J, SCHULTZ W, WIESENDANGER M (eds) Neural coding of motor performance. Exp Brain Res, Suppl 7, Springer, Berlin

YETERIAN EH, VAN HOESEN GW (1978) Cortico-striate projections in the rhesus monkey : the organization of certain cortico-caudate projections. Brain Res 139:43-63

Involvement of Monkey Premotor Cortex in the Preparation of Arm Movements

M. Godschalk and R.N. Lemon

Department of Anatomy II, HB 13, Erasmus University Rotterdam, P.O. Box 1738, 3000 DR Rotterdam, The Netherlands

Mounting evidence suggests that the peri-arcuate cortex of the monkey's frontal lobe is involved in visuo-motor control. The rostral and caudal banks of the arcuate sulcus receive many projections from parietal and striate cortex (PANDYA and KUYPERS, 1969 ; PANDYA and VIGNOLO, 1971 ; JONES et al., 1978) and neurons in the caudal bank project upon the arm and hand area of the motor cortex (area 4) (PANDYA and KUYPERS, 1969 ; MATSUMURA and KUBOTA, 1979 ; MUAKKASSA and STRICK, 1979). Destruction of the peri-arcuate cortex causes a temporary deficit in the visually guided orientation of hand and fingers (MOLL and KUYPERS, 1977). Further, peri-arcuate neurons are activated by presentation of visual stimuli used to condition subsequent motor behavior in trained monkeys (KUBOTA and HAMADA, 1978 ; SAKAI, 1978). Therefore we have tried to determine whether peri-arcuate neurons modulate their activity during preparation for retrieval of a small food reward and whether this modulation is related to the trajectory of the subsequent arm and hand movements.

A monkey (Macaca nemestrina) was trained to execute a reaching task slightly modified from the one described previously (GODSCHALK et al., 1981). The monkey faced a plexiglass plate, in the centre of which was a round hole. On the other side of the plate were three grooves oriented radially around the hole (positions 1, 2 and 3 ; see Fig. 1B). A food reward was placed in one of the three grooves. The monkey had to pass its hand through the hole to recover the reward. The plexiglass plate was covered with a foil which, dependent upon the ambient illumination, appeared either reflective or transparent to the monkey. With the foil reflective, the grooves behind the plate were invisible. Moreover, an opaque disc covered the central hole, so that the monkey was unable to see food being placed in one or other of the grooves by the experimenter. When the foil was made transparent the food reward became visible.

Experimental Brain Research, Suppl. 7

Each trial began with the monkey pressing on a switch with the right hand
(Fig. 1A). During this HOLD phase the food was invisible. After a randomly
variable period (2-4 s), the ambient illumination was changed and the food
reward became visible. However, the monkey had to continue pressing the
switch until this phase (the VISIBLE phase ; also randomly variable from
1.0-2.5 s) was terminated by a buzzer. At the same moment the cover over the
hole, which was initially locked, was released. The buzzer served as a
GO-signal and indicated that the monkey could now release the switch, press
the cover aside and pass its hand through the hole to retrieve the reward
(MOVEMENT phase) (Fig. 1A). If the monkey released the switch before the
buzzer sounded, the trial was terminated. No time constraints were imposed on
the monkey's speed of switch release after the GO-signal ; in most sessions
the GO-release interval was about 350 ms.

The monkey was trained to perform the task and was then prepared under full
anesthesia for chronic recording. A recording chamber was positioned over the
left hemisphere so as to allow microelectrode penetrations in a plane
perpendicular to the cortical surface of the arcuate region. Pairs of
insulated stainless steel wires were implanted in right biceps, triceps,
deltoid and pectoralis major for EMG recording. After full recovery, extracellular records were made with tungsten microelectrodes.

The activity of well-isolated neurons modulating during the task was recorded
on magnetic tape for a minimum of 40 trials ; the position of the reward was
randomised from trial to trial. With the aid of a PDP 11/03 computer, pairs
of peri-event histograms of cell discharges were constructed, one referenced
to the start of the VISIBLE phase, the other to the GO-signal. Each histogram
represents the accumulated number of cell discharges from 10 different trials
with the food in the same position (1, 2 or 3). The moment of switch release
was displayed on each histogram. For several neurons, a third peri-event
histogram was made, referenced to the release of the switch. When modulation
occurred during the MOVEMENT phase, it was slightly more prominent in
histograms referenced to the switch release than in those referenced to the
GO-signal. Surface EMGs were periodically taken from up to ten limb muscles.
Both intramuscular and surface EMG records indicated that there was no
alteration in muscular activity during either the HOLD or VISIBLE phases.

According to the period in which modulation occurred (almost always an
increase in discharge frequency), the cells were divided into four groups,
following qualitative criteria :

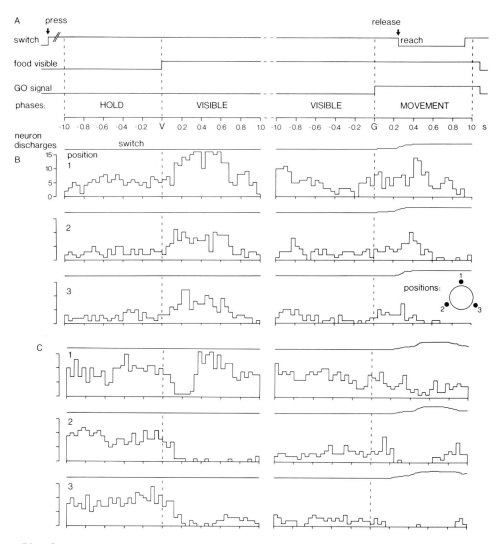

Fig. 1.

A. Schematic representation of the timing of events during a single trial of the task. B,C. Histograms representing the activity of characteristic neurons, accumulated over ten trials. Timing as in A. Thus both histograms in a horizontal row represent the same set of trials, the left one referenced to the start of the VISIBLE phase and the right to the start of the MOVEMENT phase. The histograms are accompanied by a trace indicating the moments at which the monkey released the switch for the 10 sampled trials.

B. Vm-type neuron showing excitation, predominantly for position 1.

C. Vm-type neuron showing inhibition, predominantly for positions 2 and 3

a) V cells altered their discharge frequency in the VISIBLE phase, but showed little or no modulation during the MOVEMENT phase

b) Vm cells began to change their firing rate during the VISIBLE phase, but modulated also during the MOVEMENT phase. Their degree of modulation during VISIBLE phase, however, was greater than that during the MOVEMENT phase

c) vM cells resembled the Vm cells, but the modulation during the MOVEMENT phase was greater than that during the VISIBLE phase

d) M cells altered their activity during the MOVEMENT phase.

About 60% of the neurons in all groups showed different degrees of modulation for each of the three food positions. Thus, V, Vm, vM type neurons usually showed peak modulation during the VISIBLE phase for one preferred position (Fig. 1B). Half of the neurons modulating during both phases showed enhanced modulation for the same position in both the VISIBLE and the MOVEMENT phases (Fig. 1B,C).

As the recording procedure is not yet terminated, no exact number can be given concerning the proportions of neurons in the four groups. Neither is histological verification of the position of recorded neurons available. Preliminary data, however, show a distribution which is similar to that presented in a previous study (GODSCHALK et al., 1981), namely most M and vM neurons were found in the convexity of the precentral gyrus whereas most V and Vm cells were situated close to the arcuate sulcus.

During some recording sessions, the monkey did not retrieve every reward, especially when different rewards were presented alternately, one being preferred to the other (e.g. apple vs. carrot or fresh vs. stale apple). For neurons recorded during these sessions, separate histograms were made for trials in which a food reward presented in a certain position was subsequently retrieved or not retrieved. Analysis of neurons whose activity was modulated during the VISIBLE phase revealed that marked modulation was only present if the monkey subsequently retrieved the food reward. Much less modulation was seen in the VISIBLE phase if no retrieval ensued. Thus the neuron in Figure 2A was strongly inhibited 200 ms after a piece of fresh apple became visible ; this reward was subsequently taken by the monkey. Presentation of stale apple, which was not retrieved, did not elicit this strong inhibitory effect during the VISIBLE phase (Fig. 2B).

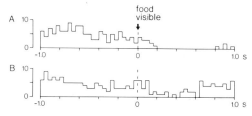

Fig. 2. Histograms from same unit as in fig. 1C, taken from a period during which the monkey was presented randomly with fresh or stale slices of apple in all three positions at random. A. Presentation of fresh apple in position 2, which was subsequently retrieved. B. Presentation of stale apple in position 2, subsequently not retrieved

Since no changes in muscular activity could be detected in the VISIBLE phase, the modulation of neuron activity during this phase cannot be directly related to movement by the monkey. The results therefore suggest that this group of neurons in the peri-arcuate area modulate their activity when visual information is received concerning the position of an object which has to be retrieved. The modulation can not be ascribed to the change in ambient illumination, since it is in general dependent on the position of the object. Neither is the modulation dependent only on the presence of the object in a certain part of the visual field, since a much smaller change in activity was seen when the VISIBLE phase was not followed by food retrieval. It is suggested that these neurons are concerned with the preparation of movements that require specific trajectories, and which are utilised for retrieval of objects in visible space.

REFERENCES

GODSCHALK M, LEMON RN, NIJS HGT, KUYPERS HGJM (1981) Behaviour of neurons in monkey peri-arcuate and precentral cortex before and during visually guided arm and hand movements. Exp Brain Res 44:113-116

JONES EG, COULTER JD, HENDRY SHC (1978) Intracortical connectivity of archi-tectonic fields in the somatic sensory, motor and parietal cortex of monkeys. J Comp Neurol 181:291-348

KUBOTA K, HAMADA I (1978) Visual tracking and neuron activity in the post-arcuate area in monkeys. J Physiol (Paris) 74:297-312

MATSUMURA M, KUBOTA K (1979) Cortical projection to hand-arm motor area from post-arcuate area in macaque monkey. A histological study of retrograde transport of horseradish peroxidase. Neurosci Lett 11: 241-246

MOLL L, KUYPERS HGJM (1977) Premotor cortical ablations in monkeys. Contrala-teral changes in visually guided reaching behavior. Science 198:317-319

MUAKKASSA KF, STRICK PL (1979) Frontal lobe inputs to primate motor cortex. Evidence for four somatotopically organized "premotor" areas. Brain Res 177:176-182

PANDYA DN, KUYPERS HGJM (1969) Cortico-cortical connections in the rhesus monkey. Brain Res 13:13-36

PANDYA DN, VIGNOLO LA (1971) Intra- and interhemispheric projections of the precentral, premotor and arcuate areas in the rhesus monkey. Brain Res 26:217-233

SAKAI M (1978) Single unit activity in a border area between the dorsal prefrontal and premotor regions in the visually conditioned motor task of monkeys. Brain Res 147:377-383

Anticipatory Neuronal Activity in the Monkey Precentral Cortex During Reaction Time Foreperiod: Preliminary Results

J.C.Lecas, J.Requin, and N.Vitton

Department of Experimental Psychobiology, Institute of Neurophysiology and Psychophysiology, National Center for Scientific Research, Marseilles, France

INTRODUCTION

Over the past 10 years, single-cell recordings in awake and freely-moving animals have shown that functional changes can be observed in a number of neuronal systems prior to movement execution, with a delay (from 200 msec to 1 sec) sufficient to exclude that these changes were related to the central command for muscular activation. It was hypothesized that these neural activity changes, found, for instance, in the cerebellar dentate nucleus (STRICK, 1979 ; THACH, 1978), in the motor cortex (EVARTS and TANJI, 1974 ; GANTCHEV, 1978 ; GODSCHALK, LEMON, NIJS and KUYPERS, 1981 ; KUBOTA and HAMADA, 1979 ; NEAFSEY, HULL and BUCHWALD, 1978a ; SCHMIDT, JOST and DAVIS, 1974 ; TANJI and EVARTS, 1976), in the basal ganglia and thalamus (NEAFSEY, HULL and BUCHWALD, 1978b) and in the supplementary motor area (TANJI, TANIGUCHI and SAKA, 1980), reflect the "presetting" of motor processes. As such they may be viewed as the physiological counterparts of the "preparatory" processes referred to by experimental psychologists (REQUIN, 1980). Since the concept of "motor preparation" is mainly employed by psychologists to explain systematic variations in reaction time (RT) as a function of informational parameters, it would therefore seem that the application of neurophysiological techniques in combination with the RT paradigm would be useful in examining how the preparatory processes involved in motor organization are realized in the structure and function of the nervous system.

It must be underlined, that this experimental strategy seems never to have been fully implemented. For instance, in the studies by EVARTS and TANJI (1974) and TANJI and EVARTS (1976), using the methodology which was subsequently employed by a number of authors, a prior instruction provided to the animal about the direction of the wrist movement (extension and flexion) it would have to perform subsequently, resulted in a differential change in the activity of the same neuron of the motor cortex. However, the correlation between those experimentally controlled neuronal changes and the performance level, especially RT, was not reported. On the other hand, such a correlation analysis was undertaken by KUBOTA and HAMADA (1979) in a visual tracking task, but with a procedure in which the anticipatory changes in neuronal activity, and the related changes in RT were not experimentally induced, but were spontaneously observed.

The aim of the present experiment was to study, by means of correlation analysis, the predictive value for performance level of the changes in cortical neuronal activity induced during the preparatory period of a RT paradigm by an experimental manipulation ; the latter was the classical probability effect observed in choice-RT procedures. Here RT is observed to decrease as the probability for the response to be performed increases ; this phenomenon is interpreted as a change in the speed of discovering the correct response in memory and corresponds to an early stage in motor organization preceeding movement parameterization (THEIOS, 1975).

METHOD

Two monkeys were trained to perform a between-hands choice-RT procedure for food reward. In the procedure which was controlled by a PDP 12 computer each trial was started by the animal pressing the left and right-handed levers simultaneously. After a waiting period of variable duration (0.5 to 1.5 seconds), a tone was presented to signal the beginning of a fixed-duration (1 second) preparatory period (PP). At the end of this signalled PP, either the left or the right visual target (each located 15 centimeters above the levers) was illuminated. When this signal occurred, the animal was required to release the lever on the side of the target and to point at the target as quickly as possible while maintaining pressure on the contralateral lever. The pointing movement was performed mainly by biceps activation and each correct response was followed by the delivery of fruit juice. During each session of 256 trials, the probability of one of the targets (either left or right) being illuminated, and hence the response requirement on that side, was randomly modified from .25 to 1.00, in steps of .25 following each block of 64 trials.

After training, a section of the animal's skull 41 mm in the anterior-posterior plane and 12 mm wide, was removed using sterile surgical procedures. The section was located 5 mm lateral to the midline of the animal's skull and on the side contralateral to the best-performing arm according to the reaction-time data. This provided access for recording purposes to an area of cortex that extended from the sulcus principalis to the lunate sulcus. A rectangular plexiglas chamber, the base of which was fitted to the animal's skull was then cemented in place and anchored with stainless steel screws. A horizontal plate about the top of the chamber permitted the animal's head to be held in a fixed position during the placement of two independent tungsten microelectrodes. A specially designed cover permitted the chamber to be maintained in a sealed condition during the manipulation of the electrodes. These were introduced through small apertures in the covers that were sealed with grease. Vertical movements of the electrodes through the holes were controlled by hydraulic systems whereas horizontal movements were achieved by manipulation of the chamber covers which were directly affixed to the horizontal micromanipulators. When a neuron of interest was identified (i.e. one activated during pointing movements and/or during the PP), its activity was recorded continuously throughout the session and stored on magnetic tape. These data were subsequently analyzed, according to behavioral parameters, on a PDP 11 computer.

RESULTS

The behavioral data conform well to the results typically observed in RT studies conducted on human subjects. Following approximately two months of training during which a progressive reduction in reward availability constrains the monkey to perform the task as quickly as possible, a significant effect of probability biases between the two responding arms appears. For a given arm, RT decreases significantly as the probability increases for performing a pointing movement with that arm. The observation that the probability variable does influence the RT but does not influence the movement time indicates that this procedural factor acts by modifying the time taken for selecting the correct response and/or specifying the corresponding motor program, but not the time for executing the movement.

Simultaneous recordings were made from the precentral motor cortex and the posterior parietal cortex in one monkey, and from the precentral motor cortex and the prefrontal cortex in another monkey. At this preliminary stage of the study, insufficient data have been collected from both associative cortical areas to permit valid statistical analyses. Data obtained from the precentral cortex alone are reported here. Recordings were made from about 109 neurons in which variations in the rate of discharge were observed to be clearly related to pointing movements of the contralateral arm. It was possible to record the activity of 56 of these cells (51%) for the full duration of the experimental procedure thereby permitting their activity to be exhaustively

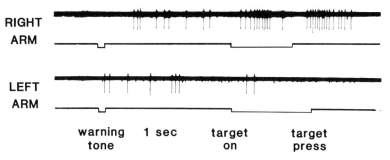

Fig. 1. Example of the "presetting" activity of a cell of the left motor cortex. This cell was activated during the pointing movement of the right arm and, then, when the hand was coming back from the target to the lever. A slight activity of this cell was triggered by the warning tone whatever the responding arm was, since during this preparatory period left and right responses were equiprobable and hence the animal did not know which target would be illuminated and hence which response would be required

analyzed. Of this sample, 21 cells (37%) had a mean firing rate of less than 5/sec prior to movement and were classified as "phasic" cells, whereas the remaining 35 cells (63%) had a firing rate greater than 5/sec and were classified as "tonic" cells. Thirty-six (65%) cells were activated in association with the pointing movements while 20 (35%) were inhibited. These differences seemed to be independent of the "phasic/tonic" classification. Among the 56 cells considered, 19 (32%) were classified as "presetting" neurons because their rate of firing during the PP varied in relation to the probability of the pointing movement to be performed and was correlated with RT.

Figure 1 shows an example of a "presetting" phasic unit recorded in the left precentral cortex during a block of trials in which the probabilities for left and right responses were equal. This cell, which was identified as controlling right biceps activation, was inactive prior to the warning tone presentation. It discharged slightly during the PP and fired firstly, when the monkey's right arm released the lever and pointed at the target, and secondly, on the cessation of the pointing movement and prior to pressing the lever to initiate a new trial. Both of these releasing movements required biceps activation. This movement-related activity did not appear during pointing movements of the left arm. However, in such cases, anticipatory activity appeared in the cell, since during the PP the probability that a right arm response would be required was only .50.

Figure 2 shows an analysis of the same "presetting" cell according to different right/left response probability biases. Rasters (trials being ordered from top to bottom according to increasing RT) and averaged frequency histograms, time-locked to the warning and response signals, are shown separately for left and right responses with corresponding mean RTs for each block of 64 trials. When the response was performed by the right arm, the average discharge frequency increased during the PP to reach a rate at the time of the response signal that was correlated with the mean RT. It will be noted that on this session, although RT was longer when the response probability was 1.0 than when it was 0.75, this discrepancy could be predicted by the discharge frequency. Moreover, it is clear from the rasters associated with each block of trials that as spike frequency decreased during the PP, RT increased. When the response was performed by the left arm, the average discharge frequency during the PP did not increase as the response probability increased and hence as the left arm RT decreased. However, the discharge frequency of the cell did show a tendency to increase as the complementary probability and hence the requirements for a right arm response increased. Relationships between the amount of "presetting" activity of this cell and RT for right and left pointing movements were calculated over the entire session and disregarding response probabilities. As suggested by data presented in Figure 2, a significant correlation ($r = .67$; $p < .01$) was found between discharge frequency during a time window extending from 750 msec before the RS to 50 msec before lever release, and RT, for the right arm only.

DISCUSSION

Thirty-two per cent of the analyzed samples of precentral cells in which activity was clearly related to pointing movements of the contralateral arm exhibited firing rates during the foreperiod that were significantly correlated, either positively or negatively, with RT. On this basis, these cells are said to be sensitive to presetting mechanisms. Because this anticipatory activity was unrelated to RT in the ipsilateral arm, it may be concluded that it was specifically associated with preparing the movement which it controlled for activity and that it did not reflect a general arousal process. The percentage of such cells observed in the present study differs from those (61% for pyramidal tract neurons and 44% for non PTNs) reported by TANJI and EVARTS (1976). However the different behavioral procedure employed in that study (the warning signal was fully informative about which of two possible antagonistic movements was required) as well as the criterion employed for classifying a cell as "presetting" (differential activity change triggered by prior instruction) makes a valid statistical comparison difficult. On the

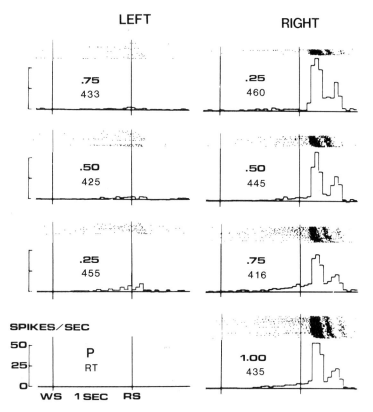

Fig. 2. Presetting activity of the same cell as in Figure 1, according to the different right/left response probability biases (from .25 to 1.00, by steps of .25) employed during a whole series of trials. For each block of 64 trials, the following data are shown separately for responses performed by the left and right arms : 1) rasters indicating cell firing with trials being ordered from top to bottom according to increasing RT, 2) the averaged histograms summarizing the data in 1), time-locked either to the warning (WS) and response (RS) signals, 3) the mean RTs

other hand, our findings do confirm those obtained by KUBOTA and HAMADA (1979) in a visual tracking task, where a negative correlation between spontaneous changes in the firing rate during the preparatory period and the time to initiate the movement was found in 31% of the neurons of the hand and arm motor areas.

This presetting activity seems to occur independently of the cell's basic discharge pattern (phasic or tonic) and whether it was activated or inhibited during movement. Although the number of cells analyzed is too low to permit a precise mapping of their cortical anatomical distribution, our observations suggest that they are preferentially located in the peripheral zones of area 4. This area has been reported in recent maps to control elbow and shoulder movements (MURPHY, KWAN, McKAY and WONG, 1978 ; WONG, KWAN, McKAY and MURPHY, 1978). Further studies are required to clarify these anatomical characteristics as well as the functional characteristics of the "presetting" cells, especially with regard to their relationship to the pyramidal tract. However, these findings suggest that motor cortex is a crucial structure in motor preparation and, as such, conform well with the emerging conception according to which motor cortex should not only be considered as specialized in the control of spinal motoneurons during motor command, but also probably is responsible for integrating more complex "cognitive" functions (WISE and EVARTS, 1981).

A problem raised in interpreting the functional significance of these presetting activities is to determine which brain structures exert modulating influences upon motor cortex so far in advance of the movement process. One can suggest that this role might be played by associative cortical structures. Evidence for such a function of associative cortex has already been provided for the posterior parietal areas, in which the activation of the so-called "reaching" cells seem to be closely related to the "goal-directed" feature of an expected action (MOUNTCASTLE, LYNCH, GEORGOPOULOS, SAKATA and ACUNA, 1975 ; LEINONEN, HYVARINEN, NYMAN and LINNANKOSKI, 1979), and for the prefrontal cortex, from which changes in unit activity anticipating motor responses have recently been reported, especially by KUBOTA, TONOIKE and MIKAMI (1980) and by WATANABE (1981) in delayed-conditioned discrimination tasks. Along the same line, anatomical studies have shown that both prefrontal and posterior parietal areas send information to the motor cortex (MATSUMURA and KUBOTA, 1979 ; MUAKKASSA and STRICK, 1979 ; STRICK and KIM, 1978 ; ZARZECKI, STRICK and ASANUMA, 1978). Using the same behavioral procedure we are now investigating the time course of single-cell activity changes in these areas.

SUMMARY

A number of single-cell recordings in monkeys trained to perform sensorimotor tasks have shown that neurons in precentral motor areas and associative areas are activated prior to movement. The purpose of this study was to systematically investigate these anticipatory neuronal discharges using a paradigm in which the level of preparation for response was controlled.

Two monkeys (Macaca fascicularis) were trained to perform a between-hand, choice-reaction time (RT) task initiated by a warning signal, in which the animal was required to point at a target. The probability of each hand performing this movement was varied in blocks of trials from 0 to 1.0 within each session. This manipulation is well-known to result in an inverse relationship between RT and response probability while movement duration remains constant, and this effect was confirmed here. A chamber was then attached to the skull, allowing microelectrode recording in the precentral cortex.

Preliminary results were based on an extensive analysis of about 56 cells which were activated during the pointing movement performed by the contralateral arm. They show that about 32% of these neurons, especially in the periphery of area 4, have firing rates which either increase or decrease during the foreperiod of 1 sec. duration, in correlation with the decrease in RT produced by an increase in response probability. That some of these changes appeared prior to ipsilateral movement - but without correlation with RT - could be further evidence for selective presetting processes triggered by the warning signal.

It is proposed that brain structures which exert modulating influences upon the functional state of motor cotex so far in advance of the movement process could be the associative cortical areas, as has already been suggested for the posterior parietal cortex and prefrontal cortex.

REFERENCES

EVARTS EV, TANJI J (1974) Gating of motor cortex reflexes by prior instruction. Brain Res 71:479-494

GANTCHEV GN (1978) Neuronal activity in the sensorimotor cortex of monkey related to the preparation for performing movement. Activ nerv sup (Praha) 20:195-202

GODSCHALK M, LEMON RN, NIJS HGT, KUYPERS HGJM (1981) Behaviour of neurons in monkey peri-arcuate and precentral cortex before and during visually guided arm and hand movements. Exp Brain Res 44:113-116

KUBOTA K, HAMADA I (1979) Preparatory activity of monkey pyramidal tract neurons related to quick movement onset during visual tracking performance. Brain Res 168:435-439

KUBOTA K, TONOIKE M, MIKAMI A (1980) Neuronal activity in the monkey dorsolateral prefrontal cortex during a discrimination task with delay. Brain Res 183:29-42

LEINONEN L, HYVARINEN J, NYMAN G, LINNANKOSKI I (1979) Functional properties of neurons in lateral part of associate area 7 in awake monkey. Exp Brain Res 34:299-320

MATSUMURA M, KUBOTA K (1979) Cortical projection to hand-arm motor area from post-arcuate area in macaque monkeys. A histological study of retrograde transport of horseradish peroxydase. Neurosci Letters 11:241-246

MOUNTCASTLE VB, LYNCH JC, GEORGOPOULOS A, SAKATA H, ACUNA C (1975) Posterior parietal association cortex of the monkey : command functions for operations within extrapersonal space. J Neurophysiol 38:871-908

MUKKASSA KF, STRICK PL (1979) Frontal lobe inputs to primate motor cortex. Evidence for four somatotopically organized premotor areas. Brain Res 177:176-182

MURPHY JT, KWAN HC, McKAY WA, YOUNG YC (1978) Spatial organization of precentral cortex in awake primates. II. Input-output coupling. J Neurophysiol 41:1132-1139

NEAFSEY EJ, HULL CD, BUCHWALD NA (1978a) Preparation for movement in the cat. I. Unit activity in the cerebral cortex. Electroenceph clin Neurophysiol 44:706-713

NEAFSEY EJ, HULL CD, BUCHWALD NA (1978b) Preparation for movement in the cat. II. Unit activity in the basal ganglia and thalamus. Electroenceph clin Neurophysiol 44:714-723

REQUIN J (1980) Toward a psychobiology of prepration for action. In: STELMACH GE, REQUIN J (eds) Tutorials in motor behavior. North Holland Publishing Co, Amsterdam, pp 373-398

SCHMIDT EM, JOST RG, DAVIS KK (1974) Cortical cell discharge patterns in anticipation of a trained movement. Brain Res 75:309-311

STRICK PL (1979) Control of peripheral input to the dentate nucleus by motor preparation. In: MASSION J, SASAKI K (eds) Cerebro-cerebellar interactions. Elsevier North Holland, Amsterdam, pp 185-201

STRICK PL, KIM CC (1978) Input to primate motor cortex from posterior parietal cortex (area 5). I. Demonstration by retrograde transport. Brain Res 157:325-330

TANJI J, EVARTS EV (1976) Anticipatory activity of motor cortex neurons in relation to direction of an intended movement. J Neurophysiol 39:1062-1068

TANJI J, TANIGUCHI K, SAKA T (1980) Supplementary motor area : neuronal response to motor instructions. J Neurophysiol 44:60-68

THACH WT (1978) Correlation of neural discharge with pattern and force of muscular activity, joint position and direction of intended next movement in motor cortex and cerebellum. J Neurophysiol 41:654-676

THEIOS J (1975) The components of response latency in simple information processing tasks. In: RABBITT P, DORNIC S (eds) Attention and Performance V. Academic Press, London, pp 418-440

WATANABE M (1981) Prefrontal unit activity during delayed conditional discriminations in monkey. Brain Res 225:51-65

WISE SP, EVARTS EV (1981) The role of the cerebral cortex in movement. Trends in Neurosc 4:297-300

WONG YC, KWAN HC, McKAY WA, MURPHY JT (1978) Spatial organization of precentral cortex in awake primates. I. Somatosensory inputs. J. Neurophysiol 41:1107-1119

ZARZECKI P, STRICK PL, ASANUMA H (1978) Input to primate motor cortex form posterior parietal cortex (area 5). II. Identification by antidromic activation. Brain Res 157:331-335

Facilitation of the H-Reflex in a Simple and Choice Reaction Time Situation

A. Eichenberger and D.G. Rüegg

Institute of Physiology, University of Fribourg, CH-1700 Fribourg, Switzerland

INTRODUCTION

The time course of the preparation and the initiation of a movement can be easily investigated in a reaction time (RT) situation in which the onset of the preparation is defined by the stimulus. If the conditioned movement is a plantar flexion of the foot the preparation of the movement can be further analysed by eliciting monosynaptic reflexes (H-reflex) in the same muscles which are participating in the movement. The H-reflex is known to increase in size before any changes in the electromyographic (EMG) activity occur (PIERROT-DESEILLIGNY et al., 1971 ; COQUERY and COULMANCE, 1971 ; MICHIE et al., 1976 ; KOTS, 1977). It is, however, not known how this facilitation is influenced by different experimental conditions and the performance of the subject. In this report, two of its properties have been studied namely (1) whether the onset of the facilitation was specific for the limb involved in the movement, and (2) whether the time course of the facilitation depended on RT.

METHOD

The experiments were performed with one female and three male healthy subjects 21 to 35 years old. The experimental set-up was consistent with the standards described by DESMEDT (1973). The required voluntary movement, a plantar flexion of the foot, was elicited by a visual stimulus. In a simple RT situation, always the same foot had to be moved in successive trials in a choice RT-situation, either the right or left foot had to be moved in random order. The stimulation strength to elicit H-reflexes was adjusted before a session so that half maximal amplitudes were obtained. An H-reflex was elicited for control purposes 7 to 10 s before each trial. A test H-reflex stimulus was applied at variable intervals following the light stimulus (go-signal). The sequence of the intervals (between 0 and 400 ms) was arranged randomly. Fourty movements in a simple RT situation (20 on the right and 20 on the left side) and 40 movements in a choice RT situation (on left or right side) were tested and recorded during a session. The sequence of the three blocks was at random. Each subject was tested in about 20 sessions.

The light stimulus, the H-reflex stimulus, the pressure executed by each foot and the EMG of each leg were recorded on-line by a HP-1000 computer system. RT was defined as the interval between onset of the visual stimulus and onset of increased EMG activity. All the test H-reflexes were normalised in relation to the mean control H-reflex amplitudes obtained from one block of data. Differences between the legs were eliminated by pooling data from trials with the movement on the right and left side.

RESULTS

Specificity of the H-reflex facilitation

In two subjects who were tested in a simple RT-situation, a facilitation of the H-reflex was only obvious in the leg which was going to move (results from one subject in Fig. 1). The facilitation reached significant levels ($p < .05$) 100 ms before the onset of the EMG activity (end of RT) and values of up to 150% at the end of RT. Similar results were obtained in the choice RT situation (not illustrated). The facilitation began about 40 ms earlier than in the simple RT situation ($p < .05$). In the other two subjects, a light facilitation occurred also on the side which was not involved in the movement. However, the specific portion of the facilitation defined as the difference between the facilitation on the involved and the non-involved side remained significant. In summary, the specific portion of the H-reflex facilitation was in all four subjects significant in a simple as well in a choice RT situation.

Dependence of the H-reflex facilitation on RT

The RT can be divided into two parts : the interval from the onset of the light sitmulus till the onset of the H-reflex facilitation (I1) and the interval from the onset of the facilitation till the onset of EMG activity (I2). In order to study how the relative lengths of I1 and I2 depend on the duration of the RT two populations of RTs have been selected from each subject. The first one included the short RTs (from 0 to mean - 20 ms) the second the long RTs (from mean + 20 ms to 500 ms). The facilitation of the H-reflex obtained in trials with short RTs has been compared with that

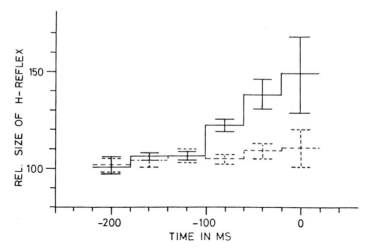

Fig. 1. Specificity of the H-reflex facilitation in a simple RT situation (mean + confidential limits, p=.05). Pooled data from the right and left side on one subject. Continous line : H-reflex on the involved side (voluntary movement), dashed line : H-reflex on the non-involved side. Abscissa : time before and after onset of EMG (end of RT), ordinate : size of the H-reflex in % of the control values

obtained in trials with long RTs. Figure 2 shows the pooled results from the right and left side of the four subjects in a choice RT situation. For short RTs, the H-reflex facilitation started 90 ms before EMG onset (Fig. 2A), for long RTs, a significant facilitation occurred already 120 ms before EMG onset (Fig. 2B). The interval I2 is thus 30 ms shorter for short RT as compared to long RTs. The medians of the first and second population of RTs were 240 ms and 340 ms, respectively. It follows from these results that part but not all of the difference between short and long RTs can be attributed to an increase of the interval I2. This has been verified by plotting the same data taking as time reference not the RT as in Figure 2 but the onset of the light stimulus. It could be estimated that about half of the difference can be attributed to an increase of I1 and about half to an increase of I2.

CONCLUSIONS AND SUMMARY

A facilitation of the H-reflex before movement initiation was in two subjects confined only to the leg which had been moved. In two other subjects, it was partly bilateral but it was significantly larger on the side on which the movement was carried out. These results are in agreement with those from

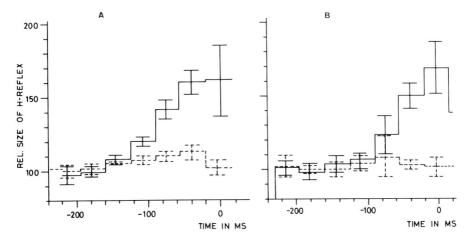

Fig. 2. H-reflex in a complex RT situation (mean + confidential limits, p=.05). Pooled data from the right and left side on 4 subjects. Facilitation in trials with RT shorter than mean - 20 ms in A and longer than mean + 20 ms in B. Continous line : H-reflex on the involved side, dashed line : H-reflex on the non-involved side. Abscissa and ordinate see Fig. 1

PIERROT-DESEILLIGNY et al. (1971) obtained in a simple RT situation. From the finding that the facilitation was also specific in a choice RT situation it can be concluded that the decision which leg had to be moved was already made at the onset of the facilitation. RT was therefore divided into two intervals the first one of which (from stimulus onset till onset of facilitation) includes the decision making process the second one (from onset of facilita- tion till EMG onset) the setting of the motor system for the movement to be executed. It was found that both intervals are dependent on RT.

ACKNOWLEDGMENT

Financial support was reveived from the Swiss National Science Foundation (grant n° 3.722-1.80).

REFERENCES

COQUERY JM, COULMANCE M (1971) Variations d'amplitude des réflexes avant un mouvement volontaire. Physiol Behav 6:65-69

DESMEDT JE (1973) A discussion of the methodology of the triceps surae T- and H-reflexes. New developments in electromyography and clinical neurophysiolo- gy. S Karger, Basel, volume 3, pp 773-780

KOTS YM (1977) The organization of voluntary movement. Neurophysiological mechanisms. Plenum Press, New York, London

MICHIE PT, CLARKE AM, SINDEN JD, GLUE LCT (1976) Reaction time and spinal excitability in a simple reaction time task. Physiol Behav 16:311-315

PIERROT-DESEILLIGNY E, LACERT P, CATHALA HP (1971) Amplitude et variabilité des réflexes monosynaptiques avant un mouvement volontaire. Physiol Behav 7:495-508

Changes in Mechanical Impedance and Gain of the Myotatic Response During Transitions Between Two Motor Tasks

F. Lacquaniti and J. F. Soechting

Istituto di Fisiologia dei Centri Nervosi, CNR, Via Mario Bianco, 9 - 20131 Milano, Italy

The mechanical impedance (stiffness and viscosity) of a limb depends on both the inherent mechanical properties of muscle and on contribution by the myotatic response. Under steady state conditions, it has been shown that both components are task dependent. Thus, the mechanical impedance of a limb is larger when a subject is instructed to resist imposed perturbations than when he does not (cf. STARK, 1968 ; DUFRESNE et al., 1978). The amplitude of the myotatic response is also larger when the subject resists applied perturbations (cf. HAMMOND, 1956 ; EVARTS and TANJI, 1974 ; MARSDEN et al., 1976 ; DUFRESNE et al., 1978).

The suggestion has been made (HOUK, 1978) that these two factors contributing to overall limb impedance are not independent variables, the increase in muscular impedance and the increase in amplitude of the myotatic response both resulting from an increased level of activation of motor units. If so, one would expect the changes in mechanical impedance, myotatic response amplitude and motor unit activity to evolve in parallel as the motor task changes. Furthermore, one should find the same temporal relationship among these variables during any task requiring a change in the level of motor unit activity.

To test for this possibility, we performed a series of experiments in which human subjects were instructed initially not to resist applied perturbations consisting of a pseudo-random sequence of torque pulses and then to resist them upon hearing a tone. The impulse responses of forearm angular position, biceps and triceps EMG were recovered by cross-correlation methods at 20 ms intervals beginning from the onset of the torque pulses (SOECHTING et al., 1981). Figure 1 shows a set of such impulse responses for one experiment. The oblique axis represents time measured from the onset of the perturbations, and each trace represents the impulse response measured at that time. The impulse responses obtained from the time the signal to begin to resist was

136

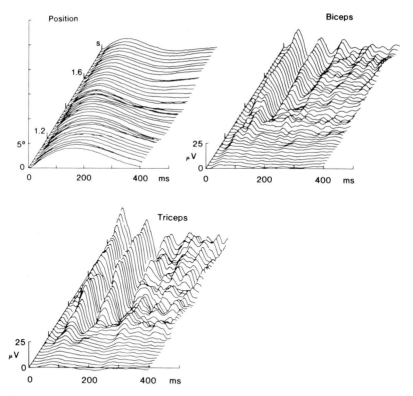

Fig. 1. Temporal evolution of the impulse responses of position, biceps and triceps EMG during the transition between the states specified by the instruction "do not resist" the applied perturbations and "resist" them. Each trace of the plots represents the response of the indicated variable to a pulse 20 ms in duration occurring 0 to 400 ms before the time indicated on the oblique axis. As plotted, biceps and triceps traces represent the response of full-wave rectified EMG activity in that muscle to a pulse tending to stretch it. The signal to begin to resist was given at 1 sec

given (at 1 s after the onset) up to 0.8 s later are shown. The horizontal time scale denotes the time before that indicated on the oblique scale at which a 20 ms pulse occurred. For example, the first trace in each plot depicts the average contribution of 20 ms pulses tending to displace the forearm occurring from 0 to 400 ms prior to 1 s (i.e. between 0.6 and 1 s after the onset of the perturbations).

It can be seen, in agreement with previous results, that the mechanical impedance of the forearm increases as the subject resists the applied perturbations ; the maximum amplitude of the impulse response of position decreases by about 50%, as does the time to peak (LACQUANITI et al., 1982). The amplitude of the myotatic response of biceps and triceps also increases after the subject begins to resist.

Figure 2 shows the representation in the frequency domain of the same data as in Figure 1. The top-left plot in the figure shows the power spectra of the impulse responses of position, that is the variation in time of the gain of the overall system. The individual traces have the general appearance of a second order system, the gain dropping asymptotically by 40dB/decade. Furthermore, the natural frequency increases from about 1.5 Hz to about 3 Hz and the system becomes more underdamped.

The other two panels show the changes with time of the gain of the myotatic feedback of biceps and triceps, defined as the gain of the transfer function with position taken as the input and EMG response as the output (DUFRESNE et al., 1978). They thus depict the contribution to forearm mechanical impedance due to feedback action, measured at the level of the alpha-motoneuron output. Both the gain and the dynamics of the feedback vary considerably with time ; the gain being about 20 dB or tenfold larger when the subject is resisting the perturbations.

Despite the fact that the subjects were instructed to begin to resist as quickly as possible, the described changes occurred very gradually. For example, the full development of the myotatic response amplitude was reached only 250 to 400 ms after it had begun to increase. It is during this transitional phase that changes in the dynamics of the myotatic feedback are most prominent, the slope of the gain curve being greater during this time (see especially triceps in Fig. 2).

The changes of various parameters were evaluated in the following way. As a measure of the myotatic response amplitude, the maximum deviation from a base line of EMG impulse responses was calculated over the first 100 ms (the base line was the mean level of the impulse response for the first 20 ms). The amplitude of overall EMG activity was instead evaluated from the average of full-wave rectified EMG activity of all the trials (thus, it included both activity correlated with the perturbations as well as activity uncorrelated with them, the latter resulting from agonist-antagonist co-contraction). The rate of change of these parameters was quantified by fitting exponentials (SOECHTING et al., 1981 ; LACQUANITI et al., 1982). The main finding was that there were considerable and consistent differences in the values of the time

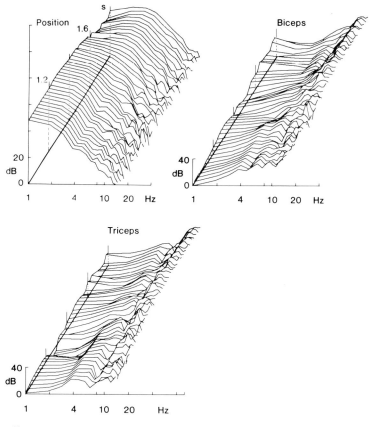

Fig. 2. Changes in the gain of the overall system and of the myotatic feedback for the same experiment as in Fig. 1.
The top-left panel represents the Fourier Transform of the position impulse responses ; the other two panels show the gain of the transfer function of position taken as the input and EMG as the output

constants for the various parameters. On average, the time constant for the increase in the myotatic response amplitude was 250 ms, while that for overall EMG activity was 110 ms (SOECHTING et al., 1981). Given the low-pass filter properties of muscle, muscle tension increases more slowly, the equivalent time constants being 320 ms and 250 ms, respectively. Time constants for the increase in limb stiffness and viscosity were found to be 240 ms and 320 ms, respectively. Thus, the changes in gain of the myotatic feedback do not parallel those in the impedance of the forelimb.

Given the different time course in the increase in gain of the myotatic feedback and the increase in alpha-motoneuron activity, one can conclude that the former can be controlled independently of the latter. This conclusion is reinforced by the fact that the temporal relationship between these two variables is highly task-dependent (SOECHTING et al., 1981). For example, in a tracking task, the changes in gain of the myotatic feedback lead those in overall EMG activity.

Our results also indicate that the mechanical impedance of a limb is not uniquely related to a given level of muscle tension when this latter parameter is permitted to vary in time, since impedance and tension do not evolve in parallel.

ACKNOWLEDGEMENT

This work was supported in part by USPHS Grant NS-15018

REFERENCES

DUFRESNE JR, SOECHTING JF, TERZUOLO CA (1978) Electromyographic response to pseudo-random torque disturbances of human forearm position. Neurosci 3:1213-1226

EVARTS EV, TANJI J (1974) Gating of motor cortex reflexes by prior instruction. Brain Res 71:479-494

HAMMOND PH (1956) The influence of prior instruction to the subject on an apparently involuntary neuromuscular response. J Physiol (London) 132:17-18P

HOUK JC (1978) Participation of reflex mechanisms and reaction time processes in the compensatory adjustments to mechanical disturbances. Progr Clin Neurophysiol 4:193-215

LACQUANITI F, LICATA F, SOECHTING JF (1982) The mechanical behavior of the human forearm in response to transient perturbations. Biol Cybern 44:35-46

MARSDEN CD, MERTON PA, MORTON HB (1976) Servo action in the human thumb. J Physiol (London) 257:1-44

SOECHTING JF, DUFRESNE JR, LACQUANITI F (1981) Time-varying properties of myotatic response in man during some simple motor tasks. J Neurophysiol 46:1226-1243

STARK L (1968) Neurological control systems. Plenum Press, New York, 428 p

A Comparison of Neuronal Discharge Recorded in the Sensori-Motor Cortex, Parietal Cortex and Dentate Nucleus of the Monkey During Arm Movements Triggered by Light, Sound or Somesthetic Stimuli

Y. Lamarre, G. Spidalieri, and C.E. Chapman

Université de Montréal, Faculté de Médecine, Centre de recherche en sciences neurologiques, Case Postale 6128, Succ. A, Montréal, Québec H3C 3J7

INTRODUCTION

It is now well established that neurons in the motor cortex change their discharge frequency before the onset of movement, suggesting that they are causally involved in initiating movements (EVARTS, 1974). In the situation where movements are initiated in response to a sensory signal, where and how is the stimulus transformed into a command to move ? Since muscle activity for equivalent movements is always the same irrespective of the sensory modality of the triggering signal, one can hypothesize that the different sensory pathways must eventually converge upon structures elaborating the motor command. To study this we have trained monkeys to perform identical movements of the arm in response to 3 different conditioning stimuli : visual, auditory and somesthetic, while recording from neurons in motor and parietal cortical areas and in the dentate nucleus of the cerebellum. In analyzing the activity of the neurons from these different brain regions we have attempted to determine if the activity was mainly related to the per- formance of the movement or mainly related to the sensory cues. It was expected that this information would provide some insight into the role of these areas in the initiation of triggered movements.

The results presented here support the hypothesis that the parietal cortex, the neocerebellum and the precentral cortex are hierarchically involved in the chain of events which transforms a conditioning sensory input into a motor command. Reports of some findings of this study have been given (LAMARRE, SPIDALIERI, BUSBY and LUND, 1980 ; LAMARRE, SPIDALIERI and LUND, 1981).

Experimental Brain Research, Suppl. 7
© Springer-Verlag Berlin · Heidelberg 1983

METHODS

The experiments were performed on four adult macaque monkeys seated in a primate chair. Recordings were obtained in the cerebral cortex of two macaca mulatta and in the cerebellar nuclei of two macaca fascicularis. The upper arm was extended horizontally from the shoulder at an angle of about 25° in front of the coronal plane and lay comfortably in a shallow trough which was hinged about the elbow joint. During training sessions the animals learned to perform flexion and extension movements of the forearm in response to each of the stimuli. Three conditioning stimuli were randomly alternated : a light (LEDs unless otherwise indicated), a tone, and a small torque applied at the elbow, in either the flexion or extension direction, via a torque motor. The displacement produced by this pulse was usually less than 1°. Fruit juice rewards were delivered when movements of sufficient amplitude (15-30°) in the required direction were initiated within 500 ms. There were no reference points for starting or stopping.

After training, the animals were anesthetized with pentobarbital and a cylindrical plastic chamber was attached to the skull under aseptic conditions to allow microelectrode recordings to be made (LAMARRE et al., 1970). Multistranded stainless steel wires insulated with Teflon were implanted into selected arm muscles and passed under the skin to a multichannel connector attached to the skull. In two animals, electro-oculograms and neck muscle activity were also recorded. Glass-coated tungsten microelectrodes were used to record neuronal activity during the performance of the tasks. The outputs of the angular displacement transducer, EMG wires, and microelectrode were amplified in a conventional manner and displayed on an oscilloscope. Selected data were recorded on multichannel magnetic tape or directly on photographic paper. On-line date acquisition was performed by a PDP-9 computer which was also programmed to control the task. Neural spike intervals, pulse replicas of the EMG activity (EVARTS, 1974), and the angular displacement (digitized at 200 Hz) were stored on Dec tapes. During recording sessions, the motor response was occasionally extinguished by withholding the reward. Since animals usually ceased to move after 2 or 3 unrewarded trials, it was possible to test the response of the same unit both with and without the conditioned movement.

At the conclusion of the last recording session, the monkeys were killed with an overdose of pentobarbital. For cortical recordings, the dura mater was removed from the depth of the recording chamber and reference points, at known stereotaxic coordinates, were marked on the surface of the cortex by penetrations of a microelectrode dipped in India ink. A photograph was made of the surface of the brain and the coordinates of the point of entry of each microelectrode track were marked upon the photograph. For dentate recordings, small electrolytic lesions were left in some of the tracks at known stereotaxic coordinates. The location of electrode tracks was verified in serial 20 μm sections of the fixed brains.

RESULTS

Unitary discharge was recorded from 715 neurons in the cerebral cortex of two macaca mulatta and from 491 cells in the dentate nucleus of two macaca fascicularis. Detailed analyses were performed for 369 units in the pre- and post-central cortex, 91 in areas 5 and 7 of the parietal cortex and 237 in the dentate nucleus of the cerebellum. A summary of some selected results is presented here for each of the five regions that we investigated.

Motor cortex

Figure 1 illustrates the discharge of a motor cortex (area 4) neuron in relation to flexion of the contralateral elbow. In addition to changes in firing frequency linked to the performance of the movement. this neuron responded directly to the three triggering stimuli. These sensory responses occurred at a fixed latency after the conditioning stimuli. They were most easily differentiated from the later "voluntary" bursts when the trials were ranked in order of increasing reaction time (RT) and aligned with respect to stimulus onset (line at 0.5s) as shown in Figure 1 (left). The irregular line running through the rasters indicates the time of onset of elbow displacement. This method of displaying the data is most convenient to separate changes in activity linked to the sensory cues from those linked to the performance of the movement. When the trials were aligned with the onset of movement (line at 0.5s) as shown in the right part of Figure 1, the sensory responses were not as evident. This display demonstrates, however, that the movement-related discharge of this neuron preceded the onset of elbow displacement as was the case for the great majority of precentral cortex neurons (mean 110 ms).

The neuron illustrated in Figure 1 is one of the few motor cortex cells which responded to all three of the sensory cues. Most neurons responded to only one or two sensory inputs - somesthetic responses were by far the most frequently observed (30%), followed by auditory (12%) and visual (4%).

DAL49

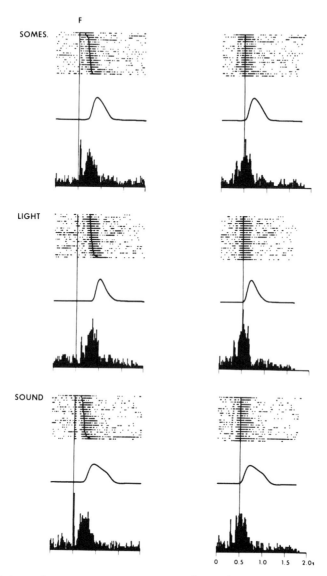

Fig. 1 Activity of a motor cortex neuron (DAL49) during flexion (F) of the contralateral elbow. Rasters and histograms (bin width 10 ms in this and all other figures) are aligned with the presentation of the cue (left) and the onset of movement (right). For further details see text

DAL35

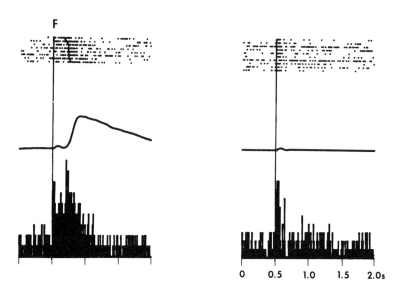

Fig. 2. Comparison of the response to the somesthetic stimulus in a motor cortex neuron (DAL35) during movement (left) and after movement was extinguished (right). Trials are aligned with the stimulus. Note that the sensory response was unchanged after extinction

In this, and in all other movement related neurons in the precentral cortex, the pattern of discharge associated with movement was independent of the modality of the conditioning stimulus. The early sensory responses, however, differed both in latency and intensity. In this example, the response to light was weak and had a long latency (100 ms, including about 35 ms required for filament heating) as compared to the responses to sound (15 ms) and to somesthetic stimulation (25 ms). The mean latencies of the sensory responses were 30 ms (somesthetic), 39 ms (visual) and 22 ms (auditory). These sensory responses appeared to be totally independent of the later bursts associated with the "voluntary" activity, except when they merged at the shortest RT. Furthermore, the latency, duration and intensity of these responses were never correlated with RT and, whenever tested, they persisted after extinction of the motor response (Fig. 2). These and other observations suggest that the motor cortex itself is little involved in the early processing of sensory information required for planning and initiating the type of triggered movements that we are studying (LAMARRE et al., 1980).

DAL110

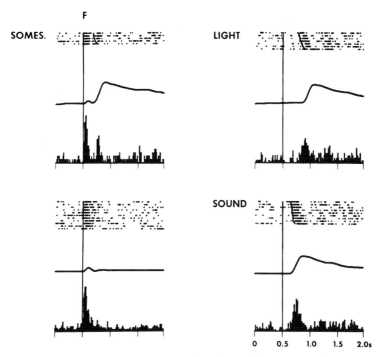

Fig. 3. Discharge of a neuron in area SI (DAL110) in the 3-input paradigm. Trials are aligned with the stimulus. There was an early response to the somesthetic cue (40 ms) followed by a burst of activity during movement. The sensory response persisted, unchanged, after extinction of the motor response (bottom left)

Sensory cortex

From previous studies (EVARTS, 1972 ; 1974 ; BIOULAC and LAMARRE, 1979) we know that in the postcentral cortex (area SI) movement related discharges occur later that in the precentral cortex. This was confirmed in the present experiments where postcentral units modfied their discharge frequency on the average 20 ms before onset of displacement as compared to the mean value of 110 ms found for units of the precentral cortex.

Sensory responses to the somesthetic stimulus were found for 35% of the neurons with a mean latency of 32 ms. As in the motor cortex, these responses were not significantly altered during extinction (Fig. 3, left). As expected, we found no response to the visual and auditory stimuli in SI. These data again are in agreement with the view that the primary sensory cortex does not play any significant role in the initiation of movement.

Area 5

Most area 5 units were recorded in the anterior bank of the intraparietal sulcus. As a whole these neurons discharged later than the motor cortex cells, the mean interval between the beginning of the modification in discharge rate and movement onset being 40 ms, i.e. about 70 ms later than the average for cells of the motor cortex. This confirms previous findings (BIOULAC and LAMARRE, 1979).

In about the same proportion (35%) as in the sensory cortex, area 5 neurons also responded directly to the somesthetic stimulus but not to the visual and auditory cues. The mean latency of these responses was 44 ms, i.e. 12 ms longer than the mean value found in SI. Contrary to what was found in the motor and primary sensory cortex however, the somesthetic responses in area 5 were very much contingent upon the performance of the movement. Extinction of the motor response almost entirely abolished the effect of the somesthetic stimulus in all neurons tested. This is illustrated in Figure 4. The significance of this finding is not yet clear but it indicates that the responsiveness of area 5 neurons can be strongly modulated by the state of the animal, and that the activity of these neurons could play a role in the early processing of somesthetic information leading to movement initiation.

Area 7

Neurons recorded in the bottom and in the posterior bank of the intraparietal sulcus all showed early responses to the sensory cues that were dependent upon the subsequent execution of the movement. In agreement with previous works (MOUNTCASTLE et al., 1975 ; LYNCH et al., 1977 ; ROBINSON and GOLDBERG, 1978) the vast majority of cells (95%) showed some respones linked to the visual stimulus with a mean latency of 105 ms (including about 35 ms required for filament heating). About 65% of these neurons responded only to light. One example is shown in Figure 5. There was a response linked to light presentation (Fig. 5, top left) but not to auditory (Fig. 5, top right) or somesthetic (not shown) stimuli. These visual responses did not appear to depend on eye movements made towards the light source (LAMARRE et al., 1980) and did not occur in the absence of the conditioned arm movement (Fig. 5, bottom right). In order to investigate the significance of such responses

DAL112

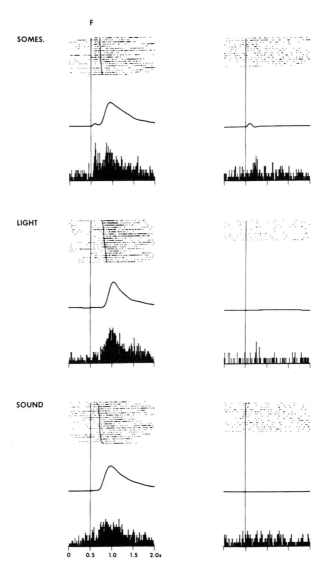

Fig. 4. Activity of a neuron in area 5 (DAL112) during movement (left) and after movement was extinguished (right). Trials are aligned on the presentation of the sensory stimulus. There was both an early response to the somesthetic stimulus (60 ms) and a second burst during movement. In contrast to SI (Fig. 3), the sensory response was almost abolished after extinction

DAL311

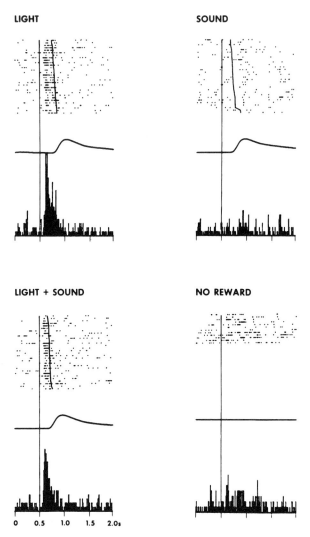

Fig. 5. Responsiveness of an area 7 neuron (DAL311) to the visual cue. Trials are aligned on the stimulus. Note that the duration of the sensory response was decreased when RTs were reduced by presenting both light and sound simultaneously (bottom left) and that it was greatly attenuated when the motor response was extinguished (bottom right)

DAL434

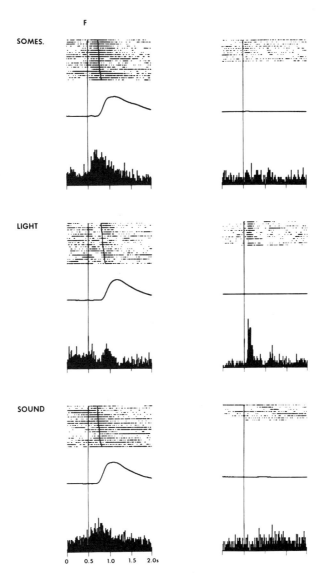

Fig. 6. Activity of an area 7 neuron (DAL434) during movement (left) and after the motor response was extinguished (right). Trials are aligned on the stimulus. See text for details

with respect to movement initiation, both light and sound were presented simultaneously (Fig. 5, bottom left). With sound alone, the mean reaction time was 80 ms shorter than with light alone (RT for light : 305 ms ; RT for sound : 225 ms). When both stimuli were presented simultaneously, the reaction time was the same as that observed with sound alone suggesting that, in this situation, the animal was in fact moving in response to sound. The sensory response had the same latency as with the light stimulus alone (Fig. 5, bottom left) but the duration of the response was significantly decreased when movements were initiated with a shorter reaction time due to the sound stimulus. In both conditions the sensory discharge ended at about the onset of movement. This observation was taken as evidence in favor of a possible role played by such neurons in the initiation of light-triggered movements.

Other neurons recorded from area 7 had more complex responses to the three sensory inputs. About 30% were modulated by both visual and somesthetic inputs and some (20%) responded to all three inputs. For all of these units the neural response to the conditioning stimuli was also dependent on the performance of the conditioned motor response. In the example shown in Figure 6 (left) somesthetic and auditory stimuli caused an early excitation (40 to 60 ms) which continued during the movement. Following presentation of the visual cue, there was a weak inhibition and subsequent excitation during the movement. Extinction (Fig. 6, right) abolished the responses to the somesthetic and auditory stimuli, while the visual stimulus now produced an early excitation with a latency of 60 to 70 ms. Whether such responses which are related to both the sensory and the motor components of the task represent a motor command or merely a complex sensory response is not known at the present time. The discharge properties of these neurons suggest, however, that they may be involved in movement initiation at an early stage of sensory processing rather than close to the final execution phase.

Dentate nucleus

The view that the dentate nucleus is involved in the initiation of rapid voluntary movements is supported by electrophysiological and lesion studies (MEYER-LOHMANN et al., 1977 ; LAMARRE and JACKS, 1978 ; BEAUBATON et al., 1978). Also, in view of the interconnections between the associative cortical areas and the neocerebellum (MASSION, 1973) we decided to investigate the behavior of dentate neurons during the same three input paradigm which was used to study cerebral cortex neurons. As a rule, task-related dentate neurons modified their discharge rate before the onset of movement (mean 122 ms). In two-thirds of the neurons analyzed, the initial change in activity was linked to one or more of the sensory cues (mean latencies of 60 to 90 ms). The latter were found mainly in the caudal one-half of the nucleus. Responses to light and/or sound were most commonly encountered. These sensory responses, which often ended at the onset of movement, were abolished, like those in parietal associative cortex, when movement was extinguished. Contrary to what was found in areas 5 and 7, however, the onset, duration and intensity of the dentate responses were often strongly correlated with reaction time as illustrated in Figure 7. The properties of the early "sensory" responses observed in the dentate nucleus suggest that the lateral cerebellar system plays a role in the initiation of some rapid triggered movements. The relative timing of the early discharges recorded in the parietal association cortex and in the dentate nucleus does not rule out, however, the possibility that the parietal cortex is at the origin of the early dentate activity (MASSION, 1973). We know, on the other hand, that the dentate cannot be responsible for the parietal cortex activity since we have found (unpublished observations) that lesions of the dentate, which delay area 4 activity, do not affect the early "sensory" discharges in area 7.

DISCUSSION

The results presented in this paper support the view that the parietal associative cortex (areas 5 and 7) and the neocerebellum are involved early in the chain of events which transforms a conditioning sensory cue into a command to move while the motor cortex appears to lie closer to the final execution phase (EVARTS and THACH, 1969 ; MASSION, 1973 ; ALLEN and TSUKAHARA, 1974). The primary sensory cortex which displays only somesthetic feedback properties (at least area 3b and 1 that were investigated in these experiments) is not likely to contribute directly to the initiation of movement as has also been suggested by the results from deafferentation experiments (BIOULAC and LAMARRE, 1979). Our finding that the sensory responses of SI neurons are not modified during extinction of the motor response is in agreement with the work of HYVARINEN et al. (1980) who showed that the responses of most SI neurons, in awake monkeys, do not vary with respect to relevant and irrelevant stimulus conditions, and are not sensitive to variations in attentive behavior.

In our experimental situation, there was no warning stimulus and we did not observe any significant modification of the sensory responses in the motor cortex when movement was extinguished. This is in contrast with the modulation of the spontaneous and evoked activity of area 4 neurons which has been observed with paradigms involving a preparatory signal (TANJI and EVARTS,

PLA63

LIGHT and SOUND

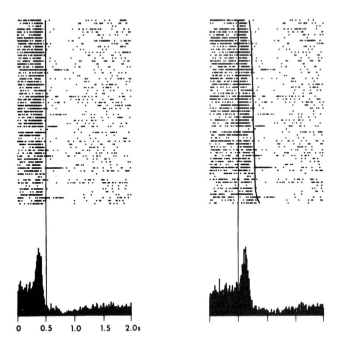

0   0.5   1.0   1.5   2.0s

SPIKES/s

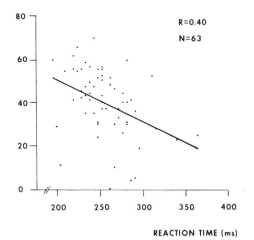

R=0.40

N=63

REACTION TIME (ms)

1976 ; EVARTS and TANJI, 1976 ; KUBOTA and HAMADA, 1979). Our data from the motor cortex are also at variance with the results of KWAN et al. (1981) and MURPHY et al. (1982) who found that the majority of task-related neurons showed visual cue responses with a mean latency of 150 ms, the earliest onset latency being 70 ms. We observed similar values (mean 120 ms, range 70-200) but, in all instances, the neural responses were temporally locked to the arm movement, i.e. progressively longer reaction times were associated with progressively longer latencies of the unitary response. These data are, however, in full agreement with those of EVARTS (1966). We found only a small proportion of units (4%) with real "photic" responses and these occurred at short latencies of 30-60 ms (mean 39 ms). These values are comparable to the latencies observed in animals anesthetized with chloralose (BUSER and ASCHER, 1960). Our data thus support the contention that the command for voluntary movements is elaborated mainly outside the motor cortex.

Neurons of area 5 responded, like neurons of area SI, only to somesthetic input. However, contrary to what was seen in SI, the sensory responses in area 5 were strongly context-dependent. When the motor response was extinguished, the sensory response to the somesthetic cue was abolished or greatly reduced. These data are in accordance with the results of other investigators (DUFFY and BURCHFIEL, 1971 ; SAKATA et al., 1973). Also MOUNTCASTLE et al. (1975) studied extensively the properties of neurons of area 5 and found that nearly 90% respond to somatic stimuli and that their responsiveness varies greatly with changes in the state of alertness of the animal.

Despite the strong state-dependence of the sensory response of the neurons of area 5, they would seem to come into play rather late to be involved significantly in the initiation of movement (BIOULAC and LAMARRE, 1979). However, recent experiments by SEAL et al. (this symposium) have shown that some neurons of area 5 can discharge as early as 280 ms before onset of movement thus strongly suggesting that they could play a role in the

◀ Fig. 7. Response of a dentate neuron (PLA63) to the visual and auditory cues. Flexion and extension trials are combined since the response was the same for both and are aligned with the onset of movement (left) and the stimulus (middle). Light and sound, but not the somesthetic cue (not shown), produced an early burst (40 ms) which ended before the onset of movement. There was a significant correlation (p < 0.01) between the intensity of the response (measured from 40 ms after the cue to 40 ms before movement onset) and the duration of the reaction time (right)

generation of movement as well as being involved in some complex sensory processing during manual exploration (MOUNTCASTLE et al., 1975).

LYNCH (1980) has recently reviewed the evidence in favor of the participation of the posterior parietal cortex neurons in the generation of movements. There is certainly no one simple function that can be attributed to the neurons of this region of the brain which display both some "sensory" and some "motor" properties (see also HYVARINEN and PORANEN, 1979 ; MOUNTCASTLE et al., pp 520-522 in LYNCH, 1980). In our experimental paradigm, the pattern of the motor response was, as far as could be determined, the same irrespective of the modality of the sensory cue. Furthermore, the animals were not overtrained to perform complex motor tasks nor were they required to detect and interpret any particular complex pattern of sensory stimuli. In particular, there was no bias toward the visual sensory input and yet nearly all responsive neurons of area 7 (95%) were influenced, in one way or another, by light. On the other hand, the old idea of polymodality attributed to this cortical area finds support from our observation that a proportion of these neurons also responded to somesthetic (30%) and auditory (25%) inputs. The fact that the responses of these neurons were contingent upon the performance of the movement suggests that they are involved in some higher level integrative function which cannot be considered as being purely motor or purely sensory in nature. It does, however, appear unlikely that the discharge of the neurons of area 7 represents a direct motor command since we did not find any correlation with the reaction time or with the parameters of movements. It might be more appropriate to think that the neurons of area 7 take part, along with several other systems, in the integration of internal and external information whereby the decision is taken between two alternatives : moving or not moving in response to the stimulus.

The interpretation of the results obtained in the dentate nucleus is somewhat easier than for those obtained in area 7. Dentate neurons showed responses (mainly to light and sound) that, as in the posterior parietal cortex, were abolished when the movement was extinguished by withholding the reward. Unlike in the parietal cortex, however, the "sensory" responses in dentate could be correlated with the reaction time and some other parameters of movement. These properties of dentate neurons suggest a more direct involvement in the initiation of movement as has been indicated by other studies (MEYER-LOHMANN et al., 1977 ; LAMARRE and JACKS, 1978 ; SASAKI et al., 1979).

In summary, the observations presented in this paper indicate that in area 4, the sensory responses evoked by the conditioning stimuli are independent of the motor responses, suggesting that the motor cortex, like the spinal motoneurons, lies at the end of the chain of events which transforms a conditioning sensory cue into a motor command. Neurons of area SI show pure sensory responses to the somesthetic stimuli and thus are not likely to contribute directly to the generation of movements. Neurons of the posterior parietal cortex (areas 5 and 7) show "sensory" responses to the conditioning stimuli that are context-dependent but not directly related to the subsequent motor output, suggesting that they may be involved only at a very early stage of the processing of sensory input which is required for planning and initiating movements. The dentate neurons show an early modulation of their discharge which is related to the sensory input as well as to the reaction time and parameters of the subsequent motor response. These properties of dentate neurons are compatible with a more direct role in the initiation of the movement.

ACKNOWLEDGEMENTS

This research was supported by a grant form the Medical Research Council of Canada. The authors wish to thank M.T. PARENT and R. BOUCHOUX for technical assistance.

REFERENCES

ALLEN GI, TSUKAHARA N (1974) Cerebrocerebellar communication systems. Physiol Rev 54:957-1006

BEAUBATON D, TROUCHE E, AMATO G., GRANGETTO A (1978) Dentate cooling in monkeys performing a visuo-motor pointing task. Neuroscience Letters 8:225-229

BIOULAC R, LAMARRE Y (1979) Activity of postcentral cortical neurons of the monkey during conditioned movements of a deafferented limb. Brain Res 172:427-437

BUSER P, ASCHER PL (1960) Mise en jeu réflexe du système pyramidal chez le chat. Arch ital Biol 98:123-164

DUFFY FH, BUCHFIEL JL (1971) Somatosensory system : organizational hierarchy from single units in monkey area 5. Science 172:272-275

EVARTS EV (1966) Pyramidal tract activity associated with a conditioned hand movement in the monkey. J Neurophysiol 29:1011-1027

EVARTS EV (1972) Contrast between activity of precentral and postcentral neurons of cerebral cortex during movement in the monkey. Brain Res 40:25-31

LAMARRE Y, JACKS B (1978) Involvement of the cerebellum in the initiation of fast ballistic movement in the monkey. EEG clin Neurophysiol 34:442-447

LAMARRE Y, JOFFROY J, FILION M, BOUCHOUX R (1970) A stereotaxic method for repeated sessions of central unit recording in the paralysed or moving animal. Rev Can Biol 29:371-376

LAMARRE V, SPIDALIERI G, BUSBY L, LUND JP (1980) Programming of initiation and execution of ballistic arm movements in the monkey. In: KORNHUBER HH, DEECKE L. (eds) Motivation, motor and sensory processes of the brain. Progr in Brain Res. Elsevier/North-Holland Biomedical Press, vol 54 pp 157-169

LAMARRE Y, SPIDALIERI G, LUND JP (1981) Patterns of muscular and motor cortical activity during a simple arm movement in the monkey. Can J Physiol Pharmacol 59:748-756

LYNCH JC (1980) The functional organization of posterior parietal association cortex. Behav Brain Sci 3:485-534

LYNCH JC, MOUNTCASTLE VB, TALBOT WH, YIN TCT (1977) Parietal lobe mechanisms for directed visual attention. J Neurophysiol 40:362-389

MASSION J (1973) Intervention des voies cérébello-corticales et cortico-cérébelleuses dans l'organisation et la régulation du mouvement. J Physiol, Paris, 67:117-170

MEYER-LOHMANN J, HORE J, BROOKS VB (1977) Cerebellar participation in generation of prompt arm movements. J Neurophysiol 40:1038-1050

MOUNTCASTLE VB, LYNCH JC, GEORGOPOULOS A, SASAKA H, ACUNA C (1975) Posterior parietal association cortex of the monkey : command functions for operations within extrapersonal space. J Neurophysiol 38:870-908

MURPHY JT, KWAN HC, MACKAY WA, WONG YC (1982) Activity of primate precentral neurons during voluntary movements triggered by visual signals. Brain Res 236:429-449

ROBINSON DL, GOLDBERG ME (1978) Sensory and behavioral properties of neurons in posterior parietal cortex of the awake, trained monkey. Fed Proc 37:2258-2261

SAKATA H, TAKAOKA Y, KOVARASAKI A, SHIBUTANI H (1973) Somatosensory properties of neurons in the superior parietal cortex (area 5) of the rhesus monkey. Brain Res 64:85-102

SASAKI K, GEMBA H, HASHIMOTO S, MIZUMO N (1979) Influences of cerebellar hemispherectomy on slow potentials in the motor cortex preceding self-paced hand movements in the monkey. Neuroscience Letters 15:23-28

SEAL J, GROSS C, BIOULAC B (This symposium) Different neuronal populations within area 5 of the monkey

TANJI J, EVARTS EV (1976) Anticipatory activity of motor cortex neurons in relation to direction of an intended movement. J Neurophysiol 39: 1062-1068

Different Neuronal Populations Within Area 5 of the Monkey

J. Seal, C. Gross, and B. Bioulac

Groupe Motricité, Laboratoire de Neurophysiologie, Université de Bordeaux II, 146, rue Léo Saignat, 33076 BORDEAUX Cedex

INTRODUCTION

The posterior parietal association cortex (areas 5 and 7) has been classically considered to be a higher order association area. Following posterior
parietal lobe lesions in man and animals, there occurs a wide range of
behavioural deficits which concern selective attention, perception and
sensation (DENNY-BROWN and CHAMBERS, 1958 ; ETTLINGER and KALSBECK, 1962).
The responses of parietal neurons to somaesthetic and other sensory stimuli
in awake monkeys have confirmed that this cortical area is the site of higher
order processing of sensory information (HYVARINEN and PORANEN, 1974 ;
MOUNTCASTLE et al., 1975 ; SAKATA et al., 1973). However, parietal lesions
also lead to deficits in the initiation of voluntary movement and manipulation. Furthermore, anatomical studies have shown that the parietal association cortex does not only receive inputs from sensory structures. Area 5 is
richly interconnected with other ipsi- and contra-lateral cortical areas as
well as a considerable number of sub-cortical structures (JONES et al.,
1978). In addition to a sensory input, there are direct and indirect
projections to motor structures such as the precentral motor cortex and the
basal ganglia (JONES et al., 1977 ; STRICK and KIM, 1978 ; ZARZECKI et al.,
1978). Recently, recordings of unit activity in areas 5 and 7 in monkeys
performing a conditioned movement have demonstrated several functional categories of neurons (MOUNTCASTLE et al., 1975). Apart from neurons with somaesthe-
tic-like properties similar to or more complex than the primary somaesthetic
cortex, a novel population of neurons was described. These neurons were
active only in relation to and preceding the behavioural act of arm projection and hand manipulation. MOUNTCASTLE et al. (1975) concluded that the
functional organization of the posterior parietal association cortex may
include mechanisms for the generation of movement as well as for the
processing of sensory information.

METHODS

In order to examine, in detail, the sensory and motor functions of area 5, we have recorded unit activity of neurons located in this cortical area during the performance of a simple motor task with the contralateral forelimb. Recordings were made in monkeys (Macaca mulatta) before and after unilateral dorsal rhizotomy C_1 to T_7 which effectively suppressed all sensory input from the trained limb. The task consisted of a flexion or extension movement of the forearm about the elbow in response to the respective auditory signal. It should be noted that the animal was unable to see the trained limb during experimental runs. With this experimental model, neuronal activity could be precisely aligned to the onset of forearm displacement and the onset of the auditory signal. For each neuron recorded, the responses to ipsi- and con-tra-lateral somaesthetic, visual and auditory stimuli were systematically tested. The experiments were monitored via a PDP8/E computer.

RESULTS

Recordings were obtained for 243 neurons in area 5 which had consistent changes of activity related to the onset of the arm movement. Of these cells, 63% (n = 153) presented modifications of activity after the onset of movement and a somaesthetic input, often complex, was identified for each of these neurons. After deafferentation, such cells were no longer encountered. A second population (32%, n = 78) of movement-related neurons presented modifications of activity which, in general, preceded the movement and occurred up to 280 msec before movement. These cells were unresponsive to all forms of sensory input and were still encountered after deafferentation (Fig. 1).

The discharge characteristics of this second population of neurons included a high precocity of change in activity with modification of activity only when the movement was performed as a conditioned response to the signal and irrespective of the direction of movement. The activity of over half of this population of neurons showed a different pattern of discharge when the unit activity was aligned to the onset of the auditory signal although the signal alone was ineffective. Such cells were considered to have a bimodal pattern of discharge (Fig. 2).The neuronal changes related to the signal consisted of both excitation and inhibition. A third but much smaller population (5%, = 12) of area 5 cells which was not observed after deafferentation had a pattern of discharge related to both the signal and the movement although the movement-related activity occurred after the onset of movement (Fig. 3).

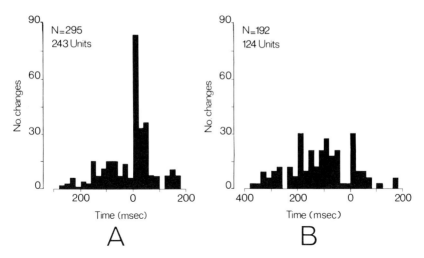

Fig. 1. Histograms showing the time of change in neuronal activity in relation to the onset of contralateral arm displacement.

A. Distribution of neuronal changes for movement-related units located exclusively in area 5, normal animals,

B. Distribution of neuronal changes for movement-related units located in area 5 after deafferentation of the contralateral arm.

The abscissa is the time of change in neuronal activity (at intervals of 20 ms) before or after the onset of arm displacement (time 0). The ordinate is the number of neuronal changes, one value for the movement of extension and another for flexion. It was not always possible to record the modification of neuronal activity of the same neuron for both movements

DISCUSSION

These results suggest that there are at least three different functional populations of neurons in area 5. The majority of cells subserve a complex somaesthetic function during movement and their absence after deafferentation has shown that these cells are influenced by peripheral feedback (BIOULAC and LAMARRE, 1979). A further population of cells appears to play a role in the generation of movement but at a stage higher than that of the primary motor cortex. The hypothesis of "sensory enhancement", as described by ROBINSON et al. (1978) for cells in area 7, cannot be used to explain the characteristics of such area 5 cells for the following reasons. These cells were unresponsive to all forms of sensory input and the modification in activity occurred only in the context of a sound-triggered arm movement ; the auditory stimulus without a subsequent movement or spontaneous arm movements was without effect

160

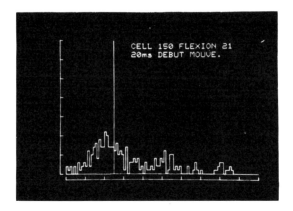

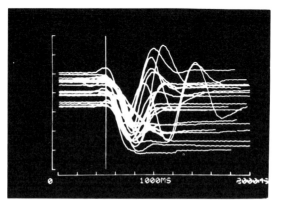

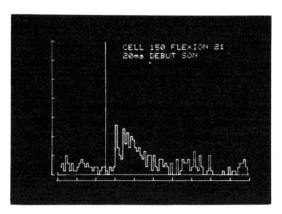

Fig. 2. Pattern of discharge for a neuron in area 5 during a sound-triggered displacement of the contralateral forearm. It can be seen that the neuron has a bimodal pattern of discharge. Top : histogram (bin width 20 msec) of neuronal activity in relation to the onset of movement. Middle : mechanograms of the individual flexion movements. Ordinate marked at intervals of 20°. Bottom : histogram (bin width 20 msec) of neuronal activity in relation to the onset of the auditory signal

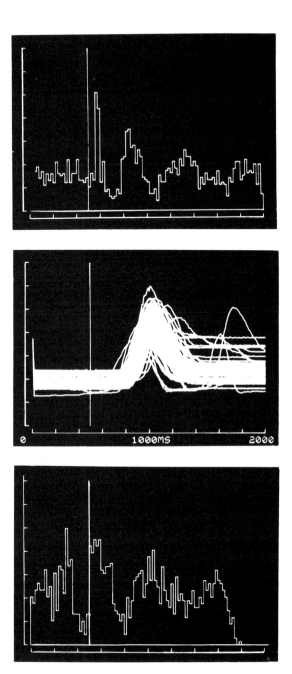

Fig. 3. Pattern of discharge for a neuron located in area 5 which showed two
different patterns of discharge ; one in which the neuronal change occurred
after the onset of movement (bottom) and a second related to the onset of the
signal (top). Top and bottom : histograms (bin width 20 msec) of neuronal
activity. Middle : mechanograms showing the individual movements aligned to
the onset of the auditory signal. Ordinate marked at intervals of 20°

162

on the activity of these cells. These cells are neither sensory nor motor as has been highlighted by several authors (LYNCH, 1980). The observation that the activity of some of these cells, the bimodal cells, is related to the onset of the signal but dependent on the forthcoming movement further emphasizes the position of these as an intermediate stage between the sensory and motor processes. Neurons with similar characteristics have been observed in the precentral cortex (KWAN et al., 1981) and the thalamus (ROLLS et al., 1981). The third population of area 5 neurons may correspond to cells involved in the generation of movement, yet which are informed on the execution of the motor act via peripheral feedback.

In conclusion, the characteristics of these three populations of cells may reflect the central processing, represented as a functional transformation, which occurs in area 5 between recognition of a signal and execution of a motor act.

REFERENCES

BIOULAC B, LAMARRE Y (1979) Activity of postcentral cortical neurons of the monkey during conditioned movements of a deafferented limb. Brain Res 172:427-437

DENNY-BROWN D, CHAMBERS RA (1958) The parietal lobe and behavior. Res Publ Assoc Nerv Ment Dis 36:35-117

ETTLINGER G, KALSBECK JE (1962) Changes in tactile discrimination and in visual reaching after successive and simultaneous bilateral posterior parietal ablations in the monkey. J Neurol Neurosurg Psychiatry 25:256-268

HYVARINEN J, PORANEN A (1974) Function of the parietal associative area 7 as revealed from cellular discharges in alert monkey. Brain 97:673-692

JONES EG, COULTER JD, BURTON H, PORTER R (1977) Cells of origin and terminal distribution of corticostriatal fibres arising in the sensory-motor cortex of monkeys. J Comp Neurol 173:58-80

JONES EG, COULTER JD, HENDRY SHC (1978) Intracortical connectivity of architectonic fields in the somatic sensory, motor and parietal cortex of monkeys. J Comp Neurol 181:291-348

KWAN HC, MacKAY WA, MURPHY JT, WONG YC (1981) Distribution of responses to visual cues for movement in precentral cortex of awake primates. Neurosci Letters 24:123-128

LYNCH JC (1980) The functional organization of posterior parietal association cortex. Behav Brain Sci 3:485-534

MOUNTCASTLE VB, LYNCH JC, GEORGOPOULOS A, SAKATA H, ACUNA C (1975) Posterior parietal association cortex of the monkey : command functions for operations within extrapersonal space. J Neurophysiol 38:871-908

ROBINSON DL, GOLDBERG ME, STANTON GB (1978) Parietal association cortex in the primate : sensory mechanisms and behavioural modulations. J Neurophysiol 41:910-932

ROLLS ET, CAAN AW, PERRETT DI, WILSON FAW (1981) Neuronal activity related to long-term memory. Acta neurol scand Suppl 89:121-127

SAKATA H, TAKAOKA Y, KAWARASAKI A, SHIBUTANI H (1973) Somatosensory properties of neurons in the superior parietal cortex (area 5) of the rhesus monkey. Brain Res 64:85-102

STRICK PL, KIM CC (1978) Input to primate motor cortex from posterior parietal cortex (area 5). I. Demonstration by retrograde transport. Brain Res 157:325-330

ZARZECKI P, STRICK PL, ASANUMA H (1978) Input to primate motor cortex from posterior parietal cortex (area 5). II. Identification by antidromic activation. Brain Res 157:331-335

Effects of Lesion of Posterior Parietal Area 7 on Visually Guided Movements in Monkeys

S. Faugier-Grimaud and C. Frenois

Laboratoire de Neuropsychologie Expérimentale, INSERM, U94, 16, avenue du Doyen Lépine, 69500 Bron, France

INTRODUCTION

Within the last few years several clinical and experimental data have suggested that the posterior parietal cortex in primate plays a role in the mediation of visually guided behaviour (HEILMAN, 1979 ; LYNCH, 1980). In a previous study (FAUGIER-GRIMAUD et al., 1978) we found that a unilateral lesion of parietal cortex restricted to area 7 in monkeys produced temporary deficits in the hand contralateral to the lesion. These deficits were manifested by : a refusal to use spontaneously the hand, a misreaching and a modification of the shaping of the hand when approaching the target. The present work studies the effects of the same type of lesion upon 2 parameters of a visually-guided movement : accuracy and reaction time (RT).

METHODS

Six naive macaque monkeys were trained to position a vertical rod in front of target lights spaced 20° apart on a concave screen. The rod supports a 22 mm length line of 9 phototransistors (1,5 mm diameter each). The cells are activated and induce a reward pulse when they happen to be in line with one of the infrared lights placed on the vertical axis of each target light. A computer was used to monitor the experiment, to record and average stimulus position and movement amplitude and reaction time. After the animals had reached 80% correct responses they received a 2-stage bilateral lesion restricted to parietal cortical area 7. The interval between the two lesions varied from 0 to 426 days depending on the animals. Retesting the monkeys on the visually guided task began within 1-2 days post-operatively. At the end of the experiment the animals were overdosed with Nembutal and given intracardiac perfusion of a 10% formalin solution. The brains were removed and lesions were reconstructed.

Experimental Brain Research, Suppl. 7
© Springer-Verlag Berlin · Heidelberg 1983

RESULTS

The lesions of area 7 were never found to be total and especially they never included the whole depth of the posterior part of the intraparietal sulcus.

A posterior parietal cortex lesion was found to affect visually guided movement parameters in all the monkeys. However, the effects of the first and second lesion were not similar for the 2 parameters studied, accuracy and RT.

1) Effects of the first lesion :

A unilateral lesion of parietal area 7 produced two main changes in visually-guided behaviour :

- A marked decrease in percentage of correct responses occurred for the hand contralateral to the lesion (Fig. 1). This deficit corresponded to the inability for the monkey to position accurately the rod in front of the target light. The animal made systematic errors up to several degrees towards the side of the lesion. This deficit was consistent but temporary and resolved within about three weeks.

- Simultaneously movement RT increased for the hand contralateral to the lesion (Fig. 2). In normal animals mean RT varied between 280 ms and 600 ms. After a lesion of area 7 this mean value was significantly increased between 400 ms and 1 sec. according to the animal.

These changes in movement RT were temporary but lasted longer than the accuracy deficit since it took about eight weeks for movement RT to return to preoperative values.

2) Effects of the second lesion :

The second lesion of the intact parietal cortex in the hemisphere contralateral to the first lesion did not affect movement parameters in the same way as the first lesion would do. Although the effects on the movement accuracy were found to be similar (and symmetrical) to those found after the first lesion, the changes in movement RT were found to be different according to the time interval between the 2 lesions.

The second lesion significantly increased movement RT of the contralateral hand if the time interval between the two lesions was short (less than 40

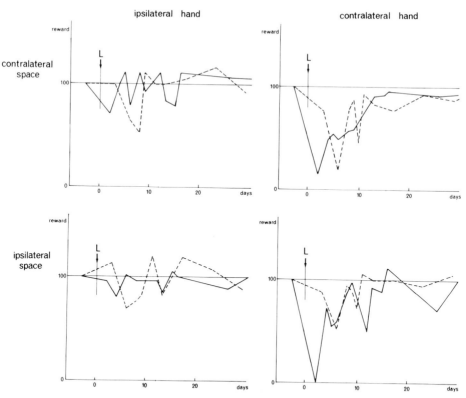

Fig. 1. Performance of two different monkeys (solid and dashed lines) on a visually-guided task with both hands, before and after parietal lesion (L), in both visual spaces. The mean percentage of reward for 3 days before lesions corresponds to a reward level of 100%. After lesion each value represents :

$$\frac{100 \times \text{post operative \% reward}}{\text{pre operative \% reward}}$$

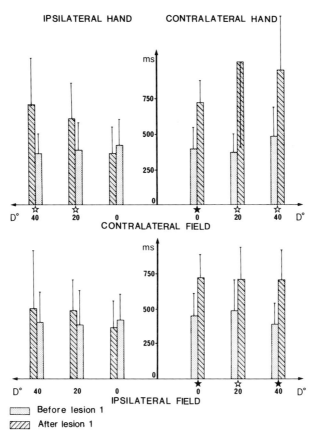

Fig. 2. Movement reaction time (ms, ordinates) before and after the first parietal lesion as a function of target location (degrees, abscissae) for one monkey. Each column represents the mean RT value for 2 days before lesion (30 trials) and one day after lesion (15 trials). The post operative day has been chosen to be that with maximum changes. Vertical lines correspond to standard deviation. The student t-test was used to test statistical differences. ☆ $p < 0.01$; ★ $p < 0.001$

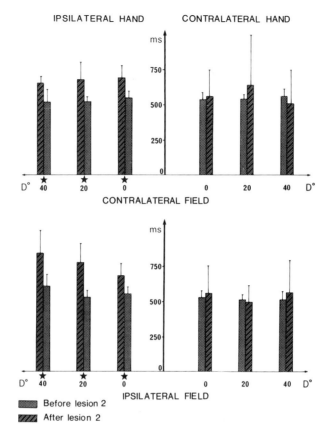

IPSILATERAL HAND   CONTRALATERAL HAND

CONTRALATERAL FIELD

IPSILATERAL FIELD

▨ Before lesion 2
▧ After lesion 2

Fig. 3. Effects of the second parietal lesion on movement reaction time (ms, ordinates) as a function of target location (degrees abscissae) in one monkey. Same legend as Fig. 2

days). On the contrary, when the second lesion occurred more than two months after the first one, the RT increased for movements made with the hand ipsilateral to the second lesion (Fig. 3).

In all cases the effects were temporary and RT finally recovered the same mean value as found before the second lesion.

DISCUSSION AND CONCLUSION

Posterior parietal lesion restricted to area 7 clearly modifies visual-ly-guided movement parameters by increasing movement RT and decreasing accuracy.

Accuracy deficits are always found in the arm contralateral to the more recent lesion for both lesions. RT changes are also generally observed in the arm contralateral to the more recent lesion. However if the time interval between the two lesions is longer than 2 months RT changes are only seen for the arm ipsilateral to the second lesion. For both parameters these changes are very consistent, but temporary. It is to be noted that latency takes longer to return to preoperative values than accuracy.

Thus a two stage bilateral lesion of the posterior parietal cortex affects movement RT and movement accuracy in different ways. These results suggest that area 7 plays a role in visually guided behaviour by acting at two separate levels : on the movement itself, and on the phase preceding the movement. Such a duality is supported by electrophysiological data found in the literature. First area 7 has been suggested to command arm and eye movements (MOUNTCASTLE et al., 1975) and to guide motor acts towards targets of interest (HYVARINEN and PORANEN, 1974 ; LEINONEN et al., 1979). Second, the same area could participate in visual attention mechanisms as proposed by LYNCH et al. (1977) ; ROBINSON et al. (1981) ; BUSHNELL et al. (1981).

The accuracy deficit observed in our monkeys after area 7 lesion could result from a loss of those neurons involved in the motor act itself. The RT changes seen after the same lesion which were ·found to be independent of accuracy changes might thus reflect the visual attention defect.

REFERENCES

BUSHNELL MC, GOLDBERG ME, ROBINSON DL (1981) Behavioural enhancement of visual responses in monkey cerebral cortex. I. Modulation in posterior parietal cortex related to selective visual attention. J Neurophysiol 46:755-772

FAUGIER-GRIMAUD S, FRENOIS C, STEIN DG (1978) Effects of posterior parietal lesions on visually guided behavior in monkeys. Neuropsychologia 16:151-168

HEILMAN KM (1979) Neglect and related disorders. In: HEILMAN KM, VALENSTEIN E (eds) Clinical Neuropsychology. Oxford University Press, New-York, pp 268-307

HYVARINEN J, PORANEN A (1974) Function of the parietal associative area 7 as revealed from cellular discharges in alert monkeys. Brain 97:673-692

LEINONEN L, HYVARINEN J, NYMAN G, LINNANKOSKI I (1979) Functional properties of neurons in lateral part of associative area 7 in awake monkeys. Exp Brain Res 34:299-320

LYNCH JC (1980) The functional organization of posterior parietal association cortex. Behav Brain Sci 3:485-534

LYNCH JC, MOUNTCASTLE VB, TALBOT WH, YIN TCT (1977) Parietal lobe mechanisms for directed visual attention. J Neurophysiol 40:362-389

MOUNTCASTLE VB, LYNCH JC, GEORGOPOULOS A, SAKATA H, ACUNA C (1975) Posterior parietal association cortex of the monkey : command functions for operations within extrapersonal space. J Neurophysiol 38:871-908

ROBINSON DL, BUSHNELL MC, GOLDBERG ME (1981) The role of posterior parietal cortex in selective visual attention. In: FUCHS A, BECKER W (eds) Progress in oculomotor research. Elsevier, New-York, pp 203-310

The Encoding of Motor Acts by the Substantia Nigra

W. Schultz, P. Aebischer, and A. Ruffieux

Institut de Physiologie, Université de Fribourg, CH-1700 Fribourg, Switzerland

INTRODUCTION

The interest in the substantia nigra (SN) concerns mostly the nigrostriatal dopamine (DA) system : neurons of the pars compacta of the SN project to the striatum and liberate the neurotransmitter DA. The functioning of this system is impaired in Parkinsonism and affected by the action of neuroleptic drugs employed for treatment of psychoses. Less spectacular, but not to be underestimated, is the role of the non-DA neurons of the pars reticulata of the SN. These cells provide a major output of the basal ganglia by virtue of their projections to thalamus, superior colliculus and some nuclei in the reticular formation (GRAYBIEL and RAGSDALE, 1979). For assessing the respective roles of the two parts of the SN, we will present data on the activity of their neurons in monkeys performing in a motor task in response to sensory signals. Before this, we will briefly review results on the impairment of nigral mechanisms in human diseases and after experimental lesions because these data provide indications about the role of the SN in behavior.

IMPAIRED FUNCTION OF NIGRAL DOPAMINE NEURONS

Destruction of the DA containing cells of the SN, pars compacta leads to profound deficits in motor behavior. This is documented by the impairments seen in human Parkinsonism. Of the three main symptoms of this disease - hypokinesia, tremor and rigidity - hypokinesia is the one which is most closely related to nigral destruction (BERNHEIMER et al., 1973). Hypokinesia also occurs after experimental lesions of the monkey SN, whereas tremor and rigidity develop only after additional destruction of other motor nuclei (PECHADRE et al., 1976). Thus, hypokinesia appears to most closely represent the negative image of the normal function of nigral DA neurons.

Experimental Brain Research, Suppl. 7
© Springer-Verlag Berlin · Heidelberg 1983

Studies on the pathophysiology of hypokinesia in Parkinsonian patients provide details of this motor deficit and help to further characterize the role of the SN in movements. In a reaction time (RT) paradigm, the interval between the stimulus and the onset of movement concerns the period of initiation of the response, whereas the subsequent movement towards a target (movement time, MT) represents the execution phase. Earlier studies reported mainly an increase of RT in Parkinsonian patients. More recent studies, however, found considerable inconsistencies and variability in RT impairment (DRAPER and JOHNS, 1964 ; EVARTS et al., 1981). In many Parkinsonian patients, simple RT is reported to be essentially normal (KING, 1959 ; WIESENDANGER et al., 1969 ; TERAVAINEN and CALNE, 1981). The MT phase, however, is much more consistently prolonged, indicating defective mechanisms during the execution of movements (KING, 1959 ; DRAPER and JOHNS, 1964 ; WIESENDANGER et al., 1969 ; FLOWERS, 1978 ; HALLETT and KHOSHBIN, 1980 ; EVARTS et al., 1981 ; TERAVAINEN and CALNE, 1981). It is also the defect in MT that is more reproducibly ameliorated after L-DOPA therapy, rather than the RT (VELASCO and VELASCO, 1973). The prolongation of MT is due to a reduction of the necessary phasic muscular activation, independent of the degree of rigidity (HALLETT and KHOSHBIN, 1980 ; EVARTS et al., 1981). The deficit becomes particularly apparent in rapid movements of large amplitude, which require considerable muscular activation (DRAPER and JOHNS, 1964 ; FLOWERS, 1978 ; HALLETT and KHOSHBIN, 1980). This is well described as a lack of "energizing the appropriate muscles required to make the movement" (HALLETT and KHOSHBIN, 1980). Thus, the increased RT in many Parkinsonian patients also may partly be due to a prolonged interval between the onset of EMG activity and the ensuing movement, due to the deficient phasic muscular activation (EVARTS et al., 1981). (It should be noted that RT is measured in relation to the onset of movement and not in relation to the - earlier - onset of EMG activity). In summary, Parkinsonian hypokinesia is, to a large extent, due to the consistently impaired execution phase of movements, whereas deficiencies of the preparatory processes during the initiation phase are less certain in simple RT situations.

The brain reacts to the decrease of nigrostriatal DA transmission by employing several mechanisms (Fig. 1) which serve to maintain a certain degree of dopaminergic function in the striatum (for review see SCHULTZ, 1982). Minor striatal DA depletions of about 25% are already compensated for by an increased metabolic activity of DA neurons, probably leading to an increased amount of released DA per individual neuron (AGID et al., 1973). A further reduction of nigrostriatal terminals leads to a reduced reuptake of DA in the striatum, thereby counteracting the DA depletion ("presynaptic supersensitivi-

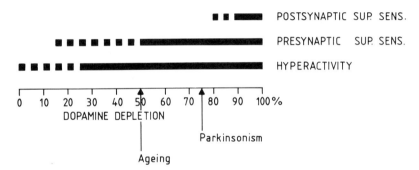

Fig. 1. Mechanisms of adaptation to striatal dopamine depletion. The solid lines indicate the operational range of each of the three main processes in relation to the degree of striatal dopamine depletion. Interrupted lines ahead denote estimated or controversial lower limits of onset. For references see text

ty" : GOLDSTEIN et al., 1969 ; KRUEGER et al., 1976). A true postsynaptic receptor supersensitivity is measured with more than 80 to 90% DA reductions (UNGERSTEDT, 1971 ; CREESE et al., 1977 ; SCHULTZ and UNGERSTEDT, 1978). These adaptative processes are responsible for the fact that hypokinesia in man and monkey only becomes apparent after at least three quarters of the nigrostriatal DA system have been destroyed (BERNHEIMER et al., 1973). The deficits after a further DA depletion in a certain range can be counteracted by the therapeutic administration of DA agonists. This has a beneficial effect mostly on hypokinesia, whereas tremor and rigidity are less readily reversed (BERNHEIMER et al., 1973 ; PECHADRE et al., 1976). Experimental transplants of DA neurons into SN-lesioned animals also considerably ameliorate the sensorimotor deficits (PERLOW et al., 1979 ; BJORKLUND et al., 1981). These data indicate that striatal DA receptor stimulation is the variable that is to be controlled and maintained for adaptation and recuperation after nigrostriatal damage. It seems that DA receptor stimulation has to reach a critical limit for movements to occur.

NEURONAL ACTIVITY IN THE SUBSTANTIA NIGRA

In order to gain a direct insight into the normal functions of the SN we recorded the impulse activity of its neurons in monkeys during sensorimotor behavior. Macaca fascicularis monkeys, seated in a primate chair, kept their hand on a telegraph key. Depending upon the illumination of one of two colored lights the monkey had either to remain on the telegraph key or to release it in order to collect a piece of food from a box placed ahead or laterally (GO-NOGO paradigm). The light signal itself was preceded by a tone (500 msec fixed interval) to indicate onset of the trial. After monkeys were proficient in the task, the extracellular activity of single neurons was recorded in the substantia nigra in daily sessions by using standard techniques (EVARTS, 1968). Recordings close to cell somata were discriminated from fiber recordings using conventional criteria (HELLWEG et al., 1977), including the latter's discharges of very short duration which, in addition, were often initially positive. Neuronal discharges, EMG activity from surface or chronically implanted electrodes, sensory signals and markers of the movement sequence, including photobeam interruptions by the monkey's hand, were recorded by a laboratory computer. The locations of neurons were reconstructed afterwards from histological sections using multiple small lesions placed during or after recording sessions at the positions of selected neurons or at a known distance from them. To avoid tissue damage in the SN, no more than two small marking lesions were placed into the confines of the nucleus of one hemisphere. Neighboring parallel tracks without lesions were only reconstructed when they were within a distance of less than 1.5 mm.

Most neurons recorded within the anatomical boundaries of the SN were assigned to one of two groups. Slowly discharging neurons (0 to 8 impulses per second) with impulses of comparatively longer duration (1.0 to 2.0 msec at 300 Hz -3dB filtering) were mostly found in the pars compacta, while more rapidly discharging neurons (30 to 110 impulses per second) with shorter discharges (0.6 to 1.0 msec) were recorded predominantly in the pars reticula. Only pars compacta neurons, but not reticulata neurons, in the monkey SN, were found to be depressed in their activity by the systemic administration of the DA agonist apomorphine, (to be published). In analogy to the situation in the rat, the compacta neurons of this study most probably represent the dopaminergic neurons of the SN, whereas the reticulata type corresponds to the non-DA nigral neuron mainly projecting outside of the basal ganglia (GUYENET and AGHAJANIAN, 1978 ; RUFFIEUX and SCHULTZ, 1980). Neurons not belonging to these two groups (n=38) discharged impulses of short duration at a low frequency and were distributed rather evenly over the entire SN. Some of them may also represent reticulata neurons (GUYENET and AGHAJANIAN, 1978 ; RUFFIEUX and SCHULTZ, 1980). These neurons will presently not be further evaluated because of their uncertain identity.

The discharge of more than half of nigral compacta neurons in 7 hemispheres was modulated while the monkey performed in the paradigm : 30 out of 68 tested neurons were activated and 10 depressed during reaching movements of

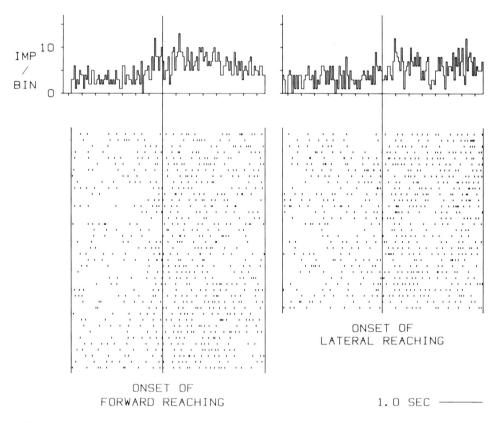

Fig. 2. Activity of a typical pars compacta neuron in the monkey substantia nigra during performance in a sensory-motor paradigm. The activity is increased during contralateral arm movement, in some trials preceding the onset of reaching. The monkey's arm is reaching towards a food containing box placed ahead of him (left) or at a 45° angle laterally (right). In virtually every single trial, the impulse counts are higher during the movement phase as compared to the resting state, independent of the direction of the movement. Total increases are 90% and 75% in the left and right histograms, respectively

the contralateral arm (Fig. 2). There were no activity changes related to any of the behaviorally relevant sensory stimuli before each movement. Onset of the modulations was about 250 ms before to 250 ms after key release. The changes in activity remained during the whole reaching phase and continued or subsided partially or completely after the food had been brought to the mouth. In this way the modulation occurred rather slowly, and maximal discharge rates never surpassed 20 impulses/sec. In the NOGO situation, modulations did not occur until the monkey made a late reaching movement for reward. There were no detectable changes of activity with minor arm or hand movements nor with the usual minor postural adjustments. The latter finding is in accord with the lack of modulation when the monkey made small, well controlled arm movements in an earlier study (DELONG and GEORGOPOULOS, 1979).

Pars reticulata neurons, in contrast, displayed a great variety in their relations to the different events in the paradigm. Of 106 cells tested, the discharge of 69 was modulated (Fig. 3A,B) ; most of these (n=60) showed sharp phasic activations or depressions in relation to contralateral movements. Somewhat fewer cells were modulated in response to the sensory events (n=38), and several of these were also modulated in relation to the movements (n=28). Very few cells were seen that changed their activity only during distal hand movements or chewing. The discharges of most movement related cells in the pars reticulata were also modified by ipsilateral arm movements, often but not always in a symmetric fashion. Eye movement related cells, as reported before by others (HIKOSAKA and WURTZ, 1981), were seen in addition but not further investigated.

SUMMARY AND CONCLUSIONS

Pars compacta cells in the primate SN of presumably dopaminergic nature are modulated, mostly activated, in their discharge rate in relation to large reaching movements. The activations were rather moderate and occurred predominantly during the execution rather than before movement onset. In this way they appear to represent a positive image of the decreased muscular activation of Parkinsonian patients during the execution phase of movements (see above).

Increased nigrostriatal impulse activity leads to an increased release of DA in the striatum (CHIUEH and MOORE, 1973). Through this mechanism, striatal DA liberation, and consequently DA receptor stimulation, will be augmented during the movement related increase in impulse activity of compacta cells. After substantial nigrostriatal damage, the extracellular concentration of DA in the striatum and the DA receptor stimulation is decreased tonically as well as phasically during movements. As a consequence, the activity of neurons in the striatum is conceivably also altered in this situation. The changes are likely to be transmitted via pallidum and thalamus to premotor and motor cortices. Motor cortex cells in monkeys indeed show a change in the movement-related activity after nigral lesions (GROSS et al., this volume). The alteration consists in a diminished but prolonged activation of cells

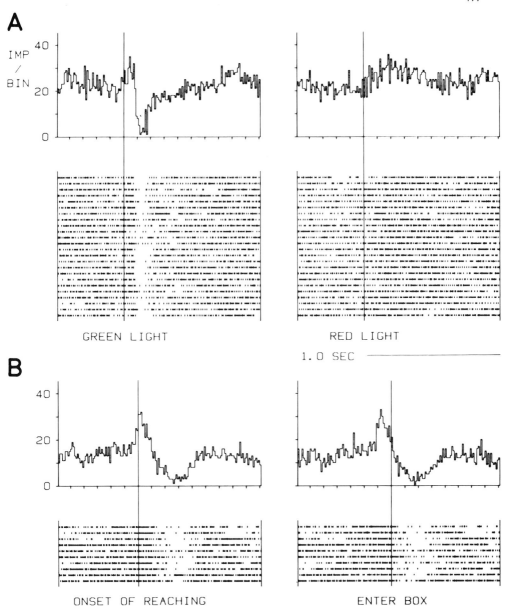

Fig. 3. The activity of two neurons in the pars reticulata. In A, activity is depressed after appearance of the green light signalling the "GO"-situation, with a latency of less than 100 msec. There is virtually no response or a slight activation after the red light signalling the "NOGO"-situation. The cell is thus differentially modulated in relation to the significance of the light stimuli. The cell in B is phasically activated during the arm's reaching towards the box but depressed during hand manipulation after having entered it

during the execution of bradykinetic movements. The altered activation of the motor cortex may explain the reduced EMG build-up in Parkinsonian patients during movements (EVARTS et al., 1981). From the combined data on impaired and normal nigral functioning we may therefore postulate that the necessary amounts of DA receptor stimulation in the striatum are higher during muscular activity than during other behavioral phases. This condition is met with larger movements by phasically increasing the impulse activity of nigrostriatal DA neurons. Minor muscular activation with more limited movements may be carried out in the presence of already available DA released with spontaneously occurring impulses and through local presynaptic interactions (CHERAMY et al., 1977 ; GIORGUIEFF et al., 1977 ; NIEOULLON et al., this volume). This may explain why DELONG and GEORGOPOULOS (1979) and we in the present study have failed to detect changes in compacta cell activity when the animal performed only small movements.

In conclusion, nigrostriatal DA neurons, with their profuse ramifications in the striatum (ANDEN et al., 1966), do not seem to be engaged in a precise cell-to-cell information transmission as are probably neurons in the specific sensory systems and in parts of the motor system. By their impulses flow and by presynaptic mechanisms in the striatum, they rather appear to phasically control the striatal DA concentration, and consequently the amount of DA receptor stimulation, according to the needs imposed by the behavioral situation. Neurons in the striatum under the influence of DA and other synaptically related elements of the motor system may then perform the more discrete algorithms necessary for controlled movements.

Cells in the pars reticulata of the SN show much more obvious changes in relation to the various events in the paradigm. From these data, and through their location at the output of the basal ganglia, they appear to be much more closely linked to the details of the behavioral situation than compacta neurons. Since we know less about this part of the SN, more details need to be evaluated in order to gain a more profound understanding of their role in movement-related processes.

ACKNOWLEDGEMENTS

We acknowledge the technical support of B. AEBISCHER, A. GAILLARD, P. HUBSCHER, E. REGLI and P. SCHOUWEY. The study is supported by the Swiss National Science Foundation, grant n° 3.226-0.77, 3.752-0.80.

REFERENCES

AGID Y, JAVOY F, GLOWINSKI J (1979) Hyperactivity of remaining dopaminergic neurons after partial destruction of the nigro-striatal dopaminergic system in the cat. Nature New Biology 245:150-151

ANDEN NE, FUXE K, HAMBERGER B, HOKFELT T (1966) A quantitative study on the nigro-neostriatal dopamine neuron system in the rat. Acta Physiol Scand 67:306-312

BERNHEIMER H, BIRKMAYER W, HORNYKIEWICZ O, JELLINGER K, SEITELBERGER F (1973) Brain dopamine and the syndromes of Parkinson and Huntington : clinical, morphological and neurochemical correlations. J Neurol Sci 20:415-455

BJORKLUND A, STENEVIU, DUNNETT SB, IVERSEN SD (1981) Functional reactivation of the deafferented neostriatum by nigral transplants. Nature 289:497-499

CHERAMY A, NIEOULLON A., GLOWINSKI J (1977) Stimulating effects of gamma-hydroxybutyrate on dopamine release from the caudate nucleus and the substantia nigra of the cat. J Pharmacol exp Ther 203:283-293

CHIUEH CC, MOORE KE (1973) Release of endogenously synthesized catechols from the caudate nucleus by stimulation of the nigro-striatal pathway and by the administration of d-amphetamine. Brain Res 50:221-225

CREESE I, BURT DR, SNYDER SH (1977) Dopamine receptor binding enhancement accompanies lesion-induced behavioral supersensitivity. Science 197:596-598

DELONG M, GEORGOPOULOS A (1979) Motor functions of the basal ganglia as revealed by studies of single cell activity in the behaving primates. Adv Neurol 24:131-140

DRAPER JT, JOHNS RJ (1964) The disordered movement in parkinsonism and the effect of drug treatment. Bull Johns Hopkins Hosp 115:465-480

EVARTS EV (1968) A technique for recording activity of subcortical neurons in moving animals. Electroenceph Clin Neurophysiol 24:83-86

EVARTS EV, TERAVAINEN H, CALNE DB (1981) Reaction time in Parkinson's disease. Brain 104:167-186

FLOWERS KA (1978) Some frequency response characteristics of Parkinsonism on pursuit tracking. Brain 101:19-34

GIORGUIEFF MF, KEMEL ML, GLOWINSKI J (1977) Presynaptic effect of 1-glutamic acid on the release of dopamine in rat striatal slices. Neurosc Letters 6:73-77

GOLDSTEIN M, ANAGNOSTE B, BATTISTA AF, OWEN WS, NAKATANI S (1969) Studies of amines in the striatum in monkeys with nigral lesions. J Neurochem 16:645-653

GRAYBIEL AM, RAGSDALE CW (1979) Fiber connections of the basal ganglia. In: CUENOD M, KREUTZBERG GW, BLOOM FE (eds) Development and chemical specificity of neurons. Elsevier, Amsterdam, pp 239-283

GUYENET PG, AGHAJANIAN GK (1978) Antidromic identification of dopaminergic and other output neurons of the rat substantia nigra. Brain Res 150:69-84

HALLETT M, KHOSHBIN S (1980) A physiological mechanism of bradykinesia. Brain 103:301-314

HELLWEG FC, SCHULTZ W, CREUTZFELDT O (1977) Extracellular and intracellular recordings from cat's cortical whisker projection area : thalamocortical response transformation. J Neurophysiol 40:463-479

HIKOSAKA O, WURTZ RH (1981) The role of the substantia nigra in the initiation of saccadic eye movements. In: FUCHS AF, BECKER B (eds) Progress in oculo-motor research. Elsevier, Amsterdam, pp 145-152

KING HE (1959) Defective psychomotor movement in Parkinson's disease : exploratory observations. Percept Motor Skills 9:326

KRUEGER BK, FORN J, WALTERS JR, ROTH RH, GREENGARD P (1976) Stimulation by dopamine of adenosine cyclic 3,5 monophosphate formation in rat caudate nucleus : effect of lesions of the nigro-neostriatal pathway. Molec Pharmacol 12:639-648

PECHADRE JC, LAROCHELLE L, POIRIER LJ (1976) Parkinsonian akinesia, rigidity and tremor in the monkey. J Neurol Sci 28:147-157

PERLOW MJ, FREED WJ, HOFFER BJ, SEIGER A, OLSON L, WYATT RJ (1979) Brain grafts reduce motor abnormalities produced by destruction of nigrostriatal dopamine system. Science 204:643-647

RUFFIEUX A, SCHULTZ W (1980) Dopaminergic activation of reticulata neurons in the substantia nigra. Nature 285:240-241

SCHULTZ W (1982) Depletion of dopamine in the striatum as an experimental model of parkinsonism : direct effects and adaptive mechanisms. Progr Neurobiology 18:121-166

SCHULTZ W, UNGERSTEDT U (1978) Striatal cell supersensitivity to apomorphine in dopamine-lesioned rats correlated to behaviour. Neuropharmacol 17:349-353

STARR MS (1978) GABA potentiates potassium-stimulated ^{3}H-dopamine release from slices of rat substantia nigra and corpus striatum. Europ J Pharmacol 48:325-328

TERAVAINEN H, CALNE DB (1981) Assessment of hypokinesia in parkinsonism. J Neural Trans 51:149-159

UNGERSTEDT U (1971) Postsynaptic supersensitivity after 6-hydroxydopamine induced degeneration of the nigrostriatal dopamine system. Acta Physiol Scand Suppl 367:69-93

VELASCO F, VELASCO M (1973) A quantitative evaluation of the effects of L-DOPA on Parkinson's disease. Neuropharmacol 12:89-99

WIESENDANGER M, SCHNEIDER P, VILLOZ JP (1969) Electromyographic analysis of a rapid volitional movement. Am J Physic Med 48:17-24

Neuronal Activity in Area 4 and Movement Parameters Recorded in Trained Monkeys After Unilateral Lesion of the Substantia Nigra

Ch. Gross, J. Feger*, J. Seal, Ph. Haramburu, and B. Bioulac

Groupe Motricité, Laboratoire de Neurophysiologie, Université de Bordeaux II, 146, rue Léo Saignat, 33076 Bordeaux Cedex, France
*U.E.R. de Psychologie, Université R. Descartes, 28, rue Serpente, 75006 Paris, France

INTRODUCTION

The French clinician BRISSAUD (1895) was the first to propose that Parkinson's disease was related to a lesion of the locus niger of SOEMMERING. This hypothesis was based on the well-known observations by BLOCQ and MARINESCO (1893). These authors described the case of a patient presenting a hemisyndrome of Parkinson with destruction of the substantia nigra by a tuberculoma. Later, it was clearly demonstrated that the neuropathological trait of Parkinson's disease was a degenerative process of the substantia nigra (ESCOUROLLE et al., 1971).

From this pioneering work, the substantia nigra became a member of the extrapyramidal system which is highly implicated in motor processes. In fact, nowadays, the substantia nigra has to be included in the nigro-neostriatal or nigro-striato-pallidal complex. In this complex, the dopaminergic nigro-neostriatal pathway occupies a privileged position (see reviews by DRAY, 1979 and FEGER, 1981).

The functional role of the dopaminergic nigro-neostriatal pathway has mainly been studied using neurochemical and neuropharmacological approaches. Furthermore, the majority of these experiments have been carried out in vitro or in vivo but with small animals such as the rat or the cat (see reviews by NIEOULLON, 1978 and DRAY, 1979). Incidentally, with the abundance of data on the dopaminergic nigral neurons, one should not forget the non-dopaminergic nigral efferents, mainly the nigro-thalamic, nigro-tectal and nigro-reticular pathways.

Few experiments have been performed on awake subhuman primates in an attempt to establish the relationship between neuronal activity of the substantia nigra and the execution of a motor task. A change in discharge rate during movement was observed for certain of the neurons recorded (DE LONG and GEORGOPOULOS, 1978). Results obtained from this type of experiment could be interpreted in relation to different aspects of motor behaviour, especially motivation or execution. Indeed, changes in nigral activity have been related to the latter aspect (SCHULTZ et al., 1981) and not directly to the motivational state of the animal (ROLLS et al., 1979). The question remains open as regards possible mechanisms of activation due to the involvement of proprioceptive input to the substantia nigra during the execution of movement (FEGER et al., 1978).

We propose another method to detect the role of the nigro-neostriatal system in aimed movement i.e. the analysis of neuronal activity in area 4 of a monkey trained to perform a well-defined forearm displacement before and after unilateral destruction of the substantia nigra.

Since the extensive works by EVARTS (1966 ; 1968 ; 1981), the main functional characteristics of these neurons during the performance of a motor act are well established. Moreover, the neurons of area 4 represent a site of convergence for messages from the basal ganglia and the neocerebellum via the thalamic relays (KORNHUBER, 1971).

Therefore, suppression of the influences coming from the substantia nigra may allow a better appreciation of the functional role played by this structure in the build-up of the patterns of discharge of area 4 neurons in relation to movement.

METHODS

The methods used have been described in detail elsewhere (LAMARRE et al., 1970 ; BIOULAC and LAMARRE, 1979 ; FEGER et al., 1975).

The main characteristics can be summarized as follows (Fig. 1) :

1°) Movement

The monkeys were trained to perform a rapid elbow movement of extension (X) or flexion (F) in response to an auditory signal, 1000 Hz, and 400 Hz respectively. An arm displacement in excess of 30° was rewarded with fruit juice. Occasionally, a displacement less than 30° was accepted in the lesioned monkeys because these animals showed an apparent difficulty in performing the arm movement. Since a nigral involvement in motivation has

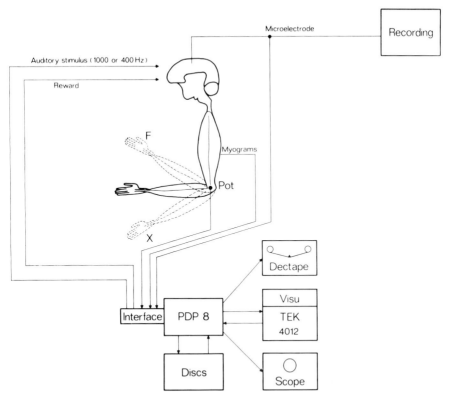

Fig. 1. Diagram showing the experimental design. The unit activity in area 4 was continuously recorded. The interface of the computer ensured monitoring of the experiment and the digitalization of recorded data

been discussed, special attention was made to avoid differences in motivation : the experimental sessions were at the same time each day and the same number of movements were performed.

2°) Recording and data processing of cortical unit activity

Cortical units were recorded in the animals following the technique of LAMARRE et al. (1970). Data were processed "on line" with a DIGITAL PDP8/E computer, and unit activity from 500 msec before to 1500 msec after the beginning of the auditory signal were displayed and stored.

3°) Nigral lesion and histological control

A single large electrolytic lesion was performed unilaterally at the level of the substantia nigra. The localization of the tip of a monopolar electrode

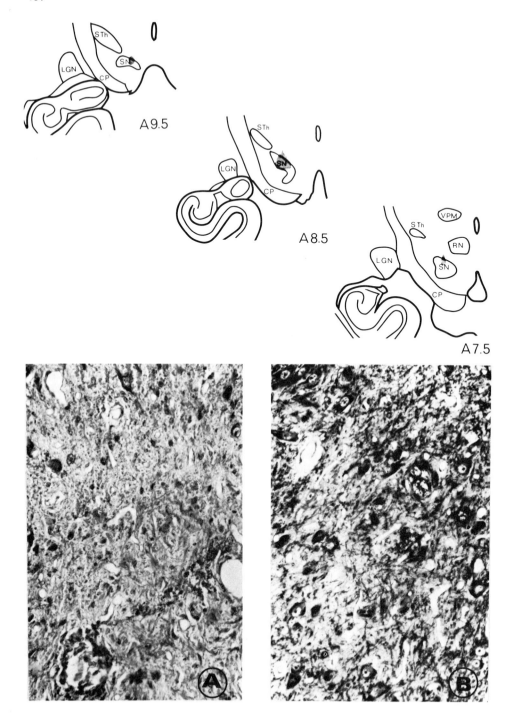

was determined on the basis of ventriculographic data (FRANCOIS, 1979). The technique of lesioning with multiple penetrations of the coagulating electrode was not employed because we wished to minimize damage to the premotor cortex which lies above the substantia nigra. At the end of the experiments, the brain of each animal was processed for histological observation and on the basis of this, we estimated that between a third and one half of the substantia nigra was destroyed. An illustration showing the extent of a nigral lesion is given in Figure 2. Close examination of the lesion site revealed an important neuronal depopulation of the substantia nigra. The lesions were essentially of the zona compacta although, in the monkey, this structure is diffuse and intermingled with the zona reticulata (FEGER, 1981).

RESULTS

Two groups of results have been studied, firstly those related to the changes in neuronal activity in area 4, secondly those related to the modification of movement parameters. Statistical analysis of the results was performed using the student t-test.

1°) NEURONAL ACTIVITY IN AREA 4

In normal animals, 110 neurons located in area 4 and which had an activity clearly related to movement were studied. The pattern of discharge of these neurons presented the clear increase of activity prior to the onset of movement (Fig. 3) described by EVARTS (1966 ; 1968 ; 1981). The mean value of this early change (T_B in Fig. 5) was 151 $\pm$ 43 msec before the beginning of displacement. Generally, the level of activity returned to resting levels with the onset of forearm displacement. The duration of the modification in neuronal activity ($T_B + T_C$) was 234 $\pm$ 75 msec.

◄ Fig. 2.
Top : The localization of an electrolytic lesion of the substantia nigra is represented on the corresponding frontal sections drawn from the atlas of SNIDER and LEE (1961). The shaded region represents the site of the lesion which extended over 2 mm.
LGN : lateral geniculate nucleus, STh : subthalamic nucleus, SN : substantia nigra, CP : cerebral peduncule, RN : red nucleus, VPM : ventro-posterio-medial nucleus.
Bottom : Photomicrographs of the substantia nigra showing the effects of nigral lesion. The electrolytic lesion resulted in an important neuronal depopulation (A). Control, intact substantia nigra (B). Magnification, 180 times

186

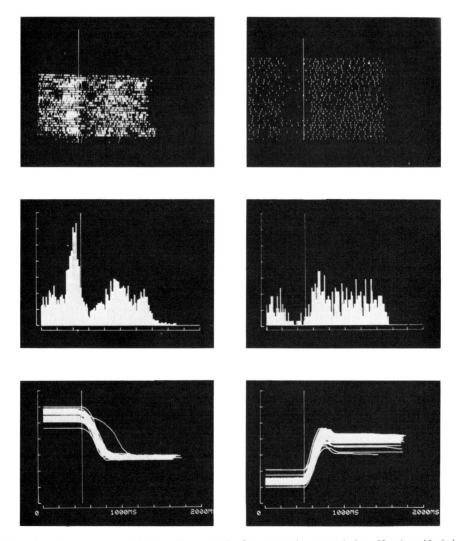

Fig. 3. Changes in activity of a cortical neuron in area 4 for flexion (left) and extension (right) in normal monkey.
Top : The spike discharges related to successive movements are represented in the form of a raster display. The vertical bar indicates the beginning of movement.
Middle : Same data cumulated into histograms each bin corresponds to 10 msec. In these two representations, the reciprocal organization of cellular activity appears clearly.
Bottom : The superimposed traces corresponding to successive mechanograms

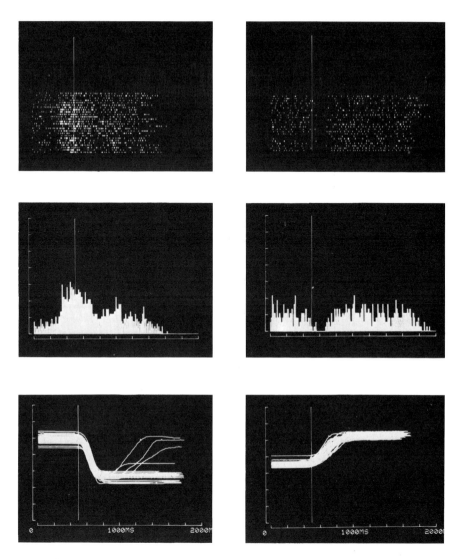

Fig. 4. Cortical unit activity and mechanograms recorded in a monkey after nigral lesion. Same representation as in figure 3. Note the increase in the duration yet the reduction in frequency of discharge for the burst of activity related to the flexion movement. The reciprocal organization is altered.
The comparison of this figure with figure 3 reveals the effect of nigral lesion on the duration of neuronal activity and movement time

In lesioned animals, 130 neurons of area 4 were studied under the same experimental conditions.

The following results were observed (Fig. 4).

a) The cellular reaction time (T_A in Fig. 5) was unchanged after nigral lesion. This time was not significantly different for flexion or extension movements ($p > 0.1$) and the mean value was 275 ± 91 msec in normal animals and 276 ± 59 msec in lesioned animals.

b) The latency between the onset of neuronal change and the beginning of forearm displacement was significantly increased in lesioned animals (mean : normal animals, T_B : 151 ± 43 msec : lesioned animals, T_B : 202 ± 44 msec, $p < 0.05$).

c) Moreover, the neuronal change which normally returned to resting values with the onset of movement was prolonged well beyond the onset of displacement (Fig. 4) and thus the duration of this activity was statistically increased ($p < 0.05$) (T_C in Fig. 5) ; mean : normal animals, T_C : 83 ± 67 msec : lesioned animals, T_C : 319 ± 95 msec. Thus the mean overall duration of the movement-related activity ($T_B + T_C$) was increased by 123% compared to normal animals. It is important to note that in lesioned animals, the maximum discharge frequency within this prolonged activity was lower (35 ± 15 spikes/second) than in normal animals (52 ± 25 spikes/second). This difference was significant, $p < 0.01$. However, the total number of action potentials during the movement-related activity was approximately the same for normal and lesioned animals.

2°) PARAMETERS OF MOVEMENT

We have considered only two parameters of the arm movement performed by normal and lesioned animals : behavioural reaction time and movement time (Fig. 5). The behavioural reaction time after nigral lesion was significantly increased for both extension and flexion movements ($p < 0.05$).

There was also an increase in the movement time after nigral lesion. However, in contrast to the behavioural reaction time, the effect varied according to the movement performed. There was a moderate increase in the case of flexion ; mean movement time, normal animals : 335 ± 39 msec, lesioned animals : 364 ± 79 msec (no significant difference $p > 0.1$) whereas in the case of extension this value changed from 330 ± 43 msec in normal animals, to 585 ± 62 msec in lesioned animals (significantly different $p < 0.05$).

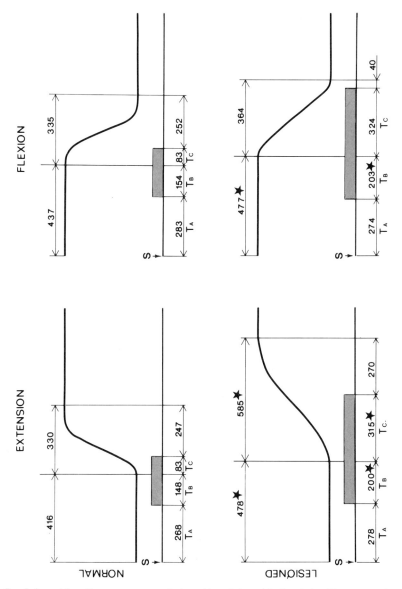

Fig. 5. Schematic diagram summarizing the data obtained in the present work : for each part of the figure : Top : representation of the forearm displacement (mechanogram) with the mean value of the behavioural reaction time (left) and the mean value of the movement time (right). Bottom : representation of the neuronal change related to movement (shaded area). The vertical bar indicates the onset of forearm displacement. auditory cue : S ; mean value of cellular reaction time : (T_A) ; changes of neuronal activity preceding (T_B) and following (T_C) the onset of movement. An asterisk indicates that there is a statistical difference (student t-test, p < 0.05) between the value obtained in normal and lesioned animals

The change in movement time for a given amplitude of arm displacement resulted in a reduction of the mean velocity of movement (decrease in mean movement velocity ; flexion 13%, extension 56%).

DISCUSSION

The present work leads to two main observations : (1) after lesion of the substantia nigra, the neurons of area 4 presented a clear disturbance in their patterns of discharge during the performance of a simple forearm movement. (2) In lesioned animals, although the cellular reaction time (T_A) was unchanged in comparison with normal animals, there was an increase in the behavioural reaction time ($T_A + T_B$).

- 1) The neurons recorded in area 4 of normal monkeys exhibited a change in activity prior to the onset of a motor task (EVARTS, 1966 ; 1968 ; 1981 ; LAMARRE et al., 1978). After destruction of the substantia nigra, the neurons of the ipsilateral motor cortex still presented a change of activity preceding the subsequent movement. However, the duration of this modification of activity greatly exceeded that observed in normal animals (mean : normal animals : 234 ± 75 msec : lesioned animals : 521 ± 124 msec). In consequence, the change in activity lasted well beyond the onset of movement which was not the case in normal animals. This implies that the substantia nigra, and the nigro-neostriatal system in general, may function as a "time-marker" to control the duration of the movement-related neuronal discharge in area 4. This role of a "time-marker" appears to operate by terminating the neuronal discharge because the time of onset of movement-related neuronal activity is not influenced by nigral lesion.

Several studies on central coding of motor output have suggested a functional relationship between the duration of neuronal discharge in a given motor structure and the duration of the specific movement generated by that structu-re (GOLDBERG and WURTZ, 1972 ; HIKOSAKA and WURTZ, 1981 ; EVARTS, 1972 ; 1981). Thus, it can be proposed that the prolonged discharge we recorded for certain area 4 neurons may result in the long lasting movements observed in lesioned animals. This phenomenon would correspond, at the clinical level, to bradykinesia, a symptom of Parkinson's disease.

Furthermore, this central message appears to contain the same "quantity" of information. Indeed, if the duration of the burst of activity exhibited by neurons of area 4 was drastically prolonged in lesioned animals, the internal frequency of discharge of this burst was decreased. In gross terms, this observation indicates that the number of action potentials produced by the neuron, in anticipation of movement, is unchanged. The modification induced by nigral lesion bears upon the temporal organization of the burst. One may assume that, in terms of coding, although the same quantity of central information may be "produced", its expression over time is greatly modified (maximum frequency of discharge for movement-related activity, normal animals, 52 ± 25 spikes/second ; lesioned animals, 35 ± 15 spikes/second). The "temporal dilution" of the central message may account for its fading efficacy and the subsequent slowing down of movement i.e. bradykinesia.

- 2) The second main feature to discuss arises from the comparison between unit changes and the onset of movement. The cellular reaction time was unchanged whereas the behavioural reaction time or the delay in movement was increased for both extension and flexion movements. The observed increase of behavioural reaction time is in agreement with the results of VIALLET et al. (1981) in monkeys and EVARTS and TERAVAINEN (1981) in humans suffering from Parkinson's disease. Since the timing of the onset of neuronal activity within area 4 is unchanged, it can be hypothesized that the nigral lesion does not affect the central processes which occur between perception of the auditory cue and the onset of discharge of movement-related neurons in this motor area. Moreover, we can speculate that the substantia nigra is not involved in the so-called "initiation of movement phase" or "motivational function" which is in agreement with data reported by ROLLS et al. (1979). It seems more likely that nigral lesion induces a perturbation in the build up of motor cortical area output i.e. a disturbance of the "execution phase" of the motor process.

ACKNOWLEDGMENT

This project was supported by the C.N.R.S. (ERA 493 and ATP 3620) and the Unité I.N.S.E.R.M. U 176.

REFERENCES

BIOULAC B, LAMARRE Y (1979) Activity of postcentral cortical neurons of the monkey during conditioned movement of a deafferented limb. Brain Res 172:427-437

BLOCQ P, MARINESCO G (1893) Sur un cas de tremblement parkinsonien hémiplégique, symptomatique d'une tumeur du pédoncule cérébral. CR Soc Biol (Paris) 5:105-111

BRISSAUD E (1895) Leçons sur les maladies nerveuses (Salpêtrière, 1893- 1894) MEIGE H (ed). Masson, Paris

DRAY A (1979) The striatum and substantia nigra, a commentary on their relationships. Neuroscience 4:1407-1439

ESCOUROLLE R, DE RECONDO J, GRAY F (1971) Etude anatomo-pathologique des syndromes parkinsoniens. In: Monoamines, noyaux gris centraux et syndrome de Parkinson. Symp Bel Air IV (Genève). Masson, Paris 1, pp 173-229

EVARTS EV (1966) Pyramidal tract activity associated with a conditioned hand movement in the monkey. J Neurophysiol 29:1011-1027

EVARTS EV (1968) Relation of pyramidal tract activity to force exerted during voluntary movement. J Neurophysiol 31:14-27

EVARTS EV (1981) Role of motor cortex in voluntary movements in primates. In: GEIGER SR (ed) Handbook Physiol The nervous system II. Am Physiol Soc, Bethesda, pp 1083-1120

EVARTS EV, TERAVAINEN H, CALNE DB (1981) Reaction time in Parkinson's disease. Brain 104:167-186

FEGER J, OHYE C, GALLOUIN F, ALBE-FESSARD D (1975) Stereotaxic techniques for stimulation and recordings in nonanesthetized monkeys : application to the determination of connection between caudate nucleus and substantia nigra. In: MELDRUM BS, MARSDEN CD (eds) Primate models of neurological disorders. Raven Press, New York (Adv Neurol vol 10 pp 35-45)

FEGER J, JACQUEMIN J, OHYE C (1978) Peripheral excitatory input to substantia nigra. Exp Neurol 59:351-360

FEGER J (1981) Les ganglions de la base : aspects anatomiques et électrophysiologiques. J Physiol (Paris) 77:7-44

FRANCOIS C (1979) Anatomie topographique, subdivision cytoarchitectonique type neuronaux de la substantia nigra et localisation des neurones nigrostriés chez le primate. Thèse de Doctorat en Sciences, Paris

GOLDBERG ME, WURTZ RH (1972) Activity of superior colliculus in behaving monkey. II Effect of attention on neuronal responses. J Neurophysiol 35:560-574

HIKOSAKA O, WURTZ RH (1981) The role of substantia nigra in the initiation of saccadic eye movements. In: FUCHS P, BECKER J (eds) Progress in oculomotor research. Elsevier, Amsterdam, pp 145-152

KORNHUBER HH (1971) Motor functions of the cerebellum and basal ganglia : the cerebello-cortical saccadic (ballistic) clock, the cerebello-nuclear hold regulator, and the basal ganglia ramp (voluntary speed smooth movement) generators. Kybernetik 8:157-162

LAMARRE Y, JOFFROY J, FILION M, BOUCHOUX R (1970) A stereotaxic method for repeated sessions of central unit recording in the paralysed or moving animal. Revue Can Biol 29:371-376

LAMARRE Y, BIOULAC B, JACKS B (1978) Activity of precentral neurones in conscious monkeys : effects of deafferentation and cerebellar ablation. J Physiol (Paris) 74:253-264

DE LONG MR, GEORGOPOULOS AT (1978) The subthalamic nucleus and the substantia nigra of the monkey. Neuronal activity in relation to movement. Soc Neurosci abst 4:42

NIEOULLON A (1978) Etude de la régulation de l'activité de la voie dopaminergique nigro-striée. Thèse de Doctorat d'Etat en Sciences, Marseille

ROLLS ET, THORPE SJ, MADDISON S, ROPPER-HALL A, PUERTO A, PERRET D (1979) Activity of neurones in the neostriatum and related structures in the alert animal. In: DIVAC I, OBERG RGE (eds) The neostriatum. Pergamon Press, Oxford, pp 163-182

SCHULTZ W, RUFFIEUX A, AEBISCHER P (1981) Substantia nigra pars reticulata neurones in monkeys are related to arm or mouth movement. Neurosci Letters Suppl 7:S317

SNIDER RS, LEE JC (1961) A stereotaxic atlas of the monkey brain (Macaca mulatta). The University of Chicago Press, Chicago

VIALLET F, TROUCHE E, BEAUBATON D, NIEOULLON A, LEGALLET E (1981) Bradykinesia following unilateral lesions restricted to the substantia nigra in the baboon. Neurosc Letters 24:97-102

Activity of Neurones in the "Motor" Thalamus and Globus Pallidus During the Control of Isometric Finger Force in the Monkey

J.H.J.Allum, R.E.C.Anner-Baratti, and M.-C.Hepp-Reymond

Brain Research Institute, University of Zürich, CH-8029 ZURICH

INTRODUCTION

The neural coding of force by pyramidal tract, cortico-motoneuronal, and non-identified neurones lying in the hand region of the precentral cortex has been established by several investigators (EVARTS, 1968 ; SMITH et al., 1975 ; HEPP-REYMOND et al., 1978 ; CHENEY and FETZ, 1980). Force coding has not been investigated for the two subcortical structures, ventral-lateral thalamus and globus pallidus, which, via their extrinsic connections, occupy a pivotal position in the control of motor performance.

Several studies in the awake monkeys indicate that cells in the ventrolateral nuclei of the thalamus (VL_o, VL_c and VPL_o according to OLZEWISKI's (1952) terminology) alter their firing rate in relation to learned hand movements (EVARTS, 1971 ; STRICK, 1976b ; HORNE and PORTER, 1980 ; MACPHERSON et al., 1980). These thalamic areas, collectively termed "motor" thalamus (MACPHERSON et al., 1980), are reciprocally connected in a topographical manner to area 4 (STRICK, 1976a ; KUNZLE, 1976 ; KIEVIT and KUYPERS, 1977 ; AKERT and HARTMANN-VON MONAKOV, 1981) and receive connections from the cerebellar nuclei (CHAN-PALAY, 1977 ; ASANUMA et al., 1980 ; KALIL, 1981). Physiological studies have described a short-latency sensory input to the VPL_o region (LEMON and VAN DER BURG, 1979 ; HORNE and TRACEY, 1979). However, the exact modality, origin, and pathways involved are still unclear (TRACEY et al., 1980 ; ASANUMA, 1981 ; WIESENDANGER and MILES, 1982).

Globus pallidus neurones occupy a pivotal position in motor circuits as they are links in the unique output channel from the striatum (DELONG, this suppl.). Neurones in the external and internal segments of globus pallidus (GP_e and GP_i) also show modifications of their discharge rates during learned hand movements (DELONG, 1971 ; 1972 ; DELONG and GEORGOPOULOS, 1979 ; ALDRIDGE et al., 1980 ; IANSEK and PORTER 1980). Pallidothalamic afferents

Experimental Brain Research, Suppl. 7
© Springer-Verlag Berlin · Heidelberg 1983

are not however, connected to the "motor" thalamus, but to the more rostral parts of VL_o and to VA (KUO and CARPENTER, 1973 ; KIM et al., 1976). These parts of the thalamus send fibres to area 6 and not to the precentral hand area (KIEVIT and KUYPERS, 1977). Therefore GP neurones can only influence precentral cortex indirectly via the link from VL_o/VA to area 6, and then via bilateral connections from area 6 to area 4 (PANDYA and VIGNOLO, 1971 ; KUNZLE, 1978 ; MUAKKASSA and STRICK, 1979 ; MATSUMURA and KUBOTA, 1979).

On the basis of this anatomical evidence, it appears that the VL/VPL_o and GP complexes subserve different pathways for the control of hand movements and might participate differently in the control of force. In view of this, we decided to investigate the discharge characteristics of neurones in these structures during a precision grip task requiring isometric finger muscle contractions.

METHODS

The two monkeys (Macaca fascicularis) used in this study were trained to control isometric force on a force transducer held between the thumb and index finger. Each monkey was required to maintain force within a low level window (between 0.1 and 0.3N) for 1.5 s, on a light signal to increase force to within a higher level window (between 0.4 and 1.0N), and maintain this finger force for, up to, 1 s before receiving a drink reward. Visual feedback on an oscilloscope mounted 40 cm in front of the animal informed the monkey that force was within the upper or lower force window. Two horizontal bars on the oscilloscope screen were used to indicate the upper and lower bounds of the force window, and force exerted on the force transducer was displayed as the vertical excursion of a bright dot. Auditory feedback was also provided. When force lay within the lower force window a low frequency tone was heard. A higher pitched tone signalled that force was within the upper force window.

The activity of neurones within the "motor" thalamus and globus pallidus were recorded with varnished tungsten micro-electrodes extending 1-10 mm from a stainless-steel guide tube. The use of guide tubes avoided problems of localisation occurring when an electrode is deflected by the dura (MACPHERSON et al., 1981). Action potentials, force and logical signals indicating task progress were stored on FM magnetic tape for off-line data analysis (SMITH et al., 1975 ; HEEP-REYMOND et al., 1978).

Before experiments on a monkey were terminated, 6-12 electrolytic lesions (20 μA, 20-30 s) were made at different locations in the thalamus and GP. After perfusion, the brain was cut in 40 m thick frozen sections, which were stained with cresyl violet, and then used to reconstruct electrode tracts.

RESULTS

The firing pattern of 54 VL/VPL$_0$ and 53 GP neurones recorded in two monkeys showed consistent relations to the task over 10 or more trials. In order to emphasize the differences that exist between the response properties of neurones in "motor" thalamus, GP, and motor cortex finger areas, the discharge patterns were first classified into two basic types ; those atypical for cortical cells, and those typically observed in the hand region of area 4. This latter population was further subdivided into tonic, phasic-tonic, and phasic neurones on the basis of established patterns observed in area 4 (SMITH et al., 1975 ; HEPP-REYMOND et al., 1978 ; CHENEY and FETZ, 1980). Table 1 indicates that a majority of VL/VPL$_0$ and GP neurones (63% and 58% respectively) could be classified as neurones with "typical cortical" discharge patterns. In Table 1 no distinction has been made between phasic-tonic neurones whose discharge rates increase with force and those that decrease with force. Decreasing and increasing phasic neurones also comprise a single group in Table 1. Figure 1 illustrates an example of an increasing phasic-tonic cell recorded from VPL$_0$, and of a decreasing tonic cell recorded from GP$_e$.

Release cells, whose discharge rates increase phasically just before and/or after the animal releases grip on the force transducer at the end of the second holding period, comprise a small percentage of VL/VPL$_0$ and GP neurones (13 and 6% respectively). This type of discharge pattern has not been previously described for the motor cortex, though we have frequently observed it in the hand region of area 4. In one of the two monkeys used for this study 15% of area 4 discharge patterns were of the release type.

Many VL/VPL$_0$ and GP neurones (37% and 42% respectively) displayed "atypical" firing patterns during the task (Table 1). These consisted of sequences of phasic and tonic firing rate modulations which were not simply related to the force traces. Two examples of "atypical" patterns are illustrated in Figure 2. The variety and complexity of these discharge patterns made a further subdivision of the "atypical" population rather difficult and, for us, of limited usefulness since our current interest lies in an easily identifiable neural coding of force.

Table 1. TYPES OF ACTIVITY PATTERNS IN "MOTOR" THALAMUS AND GLOBUS PALLIDUS

	"ATYPICAL"	"TYPICAL"				
		Tonic Increasing	Tonic Decreasing	Phasic-tonic	Phasic	Release
"Motor" thalamus (N = 54)	37 %	20 %	11 %	11 %	8 %	13 %
Globus pallidus (N = 53)	42 %	17 %	13 %	11 %	12 %	6 %

DISCUSSION

The present study indicate that neurones in VL/VPL$_O$ ("motor" thalamus) and GP modulate their discharge rates in relation to learned hand movements, and thus confirms previous studies (STRICK, 1976b ; MACPHERSON et al., 1981 ; HORNE and PORTER, 1981 ; DELONG, 1971 ; 1972 ; ALDRIDGE et al., 1980 ; IANSEK and PORTER, 1980). Our results suggest, in addition, that a group of VL/VPL$_O$ and GP neurones alter their firing rates specifically in relation to isometric force exerted between thumb and index finger. In fact, this group, which comprised the majority of the recorded neurones, exhibited modulation of their discharge rates in a manner similar to those patterns observed in the finger region of area 4. Moreover, the largest group among "typical" cells in the structures VL/VPL$_O$ and GP, and among all area 4 neurones have tonic increasing and tonic decreasing modulation with force (Table 1 and HEPP-REYMOND et al., 1978). One difference between these subcortical and cortical structures appears to be the larger percentage of tonic and phasic-tonic increasing precentral neurones which are active during the lower and upper force holding periods. Clearly, a more quantitative analysis of force coding is required in order to assess differences precisely.

The presence of cells with complex, "atypical cortical" discharge patterns indicates that the VL/VPL$_O$ and GP are coding aspects of the task which are not simply related to force generated during the precision grip. Our histological reconstruction provided no evidence that cells with "typical" and "atypical" discharge patterns lie in distinct regions of these two structures. For example, the cells shown on the left of Figures 1 and 2 were recorded within 300 μm of each other.

Our study also suggests that, within the restricted sample of neurones, little difference exists between activity patterns, in relation to force, in the "motor" thalamus and GP. An answer to the question whether this indicates that the two structures are functionally closely connected, and by which pathways, must await future investigation. Current anatomical evidence provides no basis for a link.

An attractive interpretation for the existence of "typical" and "atypical" neurones in the motor thalamus is suggested by the fact that thalamocortical afferents to area 4 in the cat are of two types ; endings localised within a small area, and those with widely divergent axonal branching (RISPAL-PADEL et al., 1973 ; ASANUMA et al., 1974). If a similar duality in the connectivity exists in the monkey, then one could speculate that "typical" thalamic

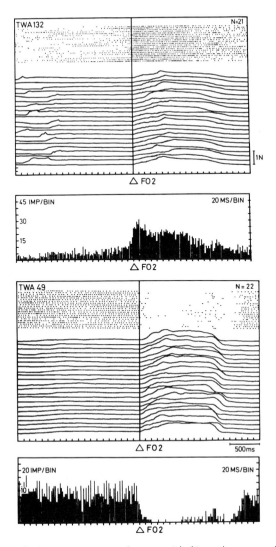

Fig. 1. Examples of two neurones whose activity changes with force in a manner typical for cells in the hand area of the motor cortex. On the top (TWA 132) : neurone located in VPL_o and showing a phasic tonic increasing relation to the force trace. On the bottom (TWA 49) : neurone located in GP_e and having a tonic decreasing relation to force. The dot rasters shown in the upper set of traces indicate the occurrence of action potentials and correspond in order from top to bottom to the force curves illustrated in the middle part of the figures. Both the dot raster and the force curves are aligned with onset of force increase from one level to the next (FO2). The lower part of the figure shows periresponse time histograms aligned also with FO2. Total display period 4 s

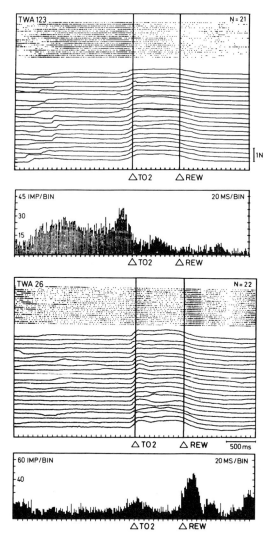

Fig. 2. Examples of two neurones whose activity changes with the task in a manner atypical for cells in the hand area of motor cortex. On the top (TWA 123) : neurone located in VPL_o and having first a phasic increase and then a tonic decrease in activity as force increased. On the bottom (TWA 26) : neurone located in GP_i showing a phasic increase as force increases and a further increase as the animal released its grip on the force transducer. The dot rasters, force curves and histograms have been aligned with the entry point into the upper force window (TO2). REW indicates the time of the reward. Total display period 5 s

neurones influence a specific group of corticomotoneuronal cells controlling one muscle via the localised thalamo-cortical system, and that neurones with "atypical" activity patterns might signal synergistic characteristics of a movement to many groups of corticofugal cells via the diffuse pathway.

ACKNOWLEDGEMENTS

The authors gratefully acknowledge the assitance provided by the technical staff of the Brain Research Institute, and in particular by R. KAEGI, M. PADUA and C. WUEST.

This research was supported by Swiss National Science Foundation grants 3.505.79 and 3.585.79, the Eric Slack-Gyr Foundation, and the Sandoz Foundation.

REFERENCES

AKERT K, HARTMANN-VON MONAKOV K (1981) Relationships of precentral, premotor and prefrontal cortex to the mediodorsal and intralaminar nuclei of the monkey thalamus. Acta Neurobiol exp 40:7-25

ALDRIDGE JW, ANDERSON RJ, MURPHY JT (1980) Sensory-motor processing in the caudate nucleus and globus pallidus : a single-unit study in behaving primates. Can J Physiol Pharmacol 58:1192-1201

ASANUMA C, THACH WT, JONES EG (1980) Patterns of termination of the cerebello-thalamic pathway in the monkey. Soc Neurosci Abstr 6:512

ASANUMA H, FERNANDEZ J, SCHEIBEL ME, SCHEIBEL AR (1974) Characteristics of projections from the nucleus ventralis lateralis to the motor cortex in cats : an anatomical and physiological study. Exp Brain Res 20:315-330

ASANUMA H (1981) Functional role of sensory inputs to the motor cortex. Prog Neurobiol 16:241-262

CHAN-PALAY V (1977) Cerebellar dentate nucleus : organisation, cytology and transmitters. Springer, Berlin Heidelberg New-York

CHENEY PD, FETZ EE (1980) Functional classes of primate corticomotoneuronal cells and their relation to active force. J Neurophysiol 44:773-791

DELONG MR (1971) Activity of pallidal neurons during movement. J Neurophysiol 34:414-427

DELONG MR (1972) Activity of basal ganglia neurones during movement. Brain Res 40:127-135

DELONG MR, GEORGOPOULOS AP (1979) Motor function of the basal ganglia as revealed by studies of single cell activity in behaving primate. Adv Neurol 24:131-140

EVARTS EV (1968) Relation of pyramidal tract activity to force exerted during voluntary movement. J Neurophysiol 31:14-27

EVARTS EV (1971) Activity of thalamic and cortical neurons in relation to learned movement in the monkey. Intern J Neurol 8:321-326

HEPP-REYMOND MC, WYSS UR, ANNER R (1978) Neuronal coding of static force in the primate motor cortex. J Physiol (Paris) 74:287-291

HORNE MK, TRACEY DJ (1979) The afferents and projections of the ventroposterolateral thalamus in the monkey. Exp Brain Res 36:129-141

HORNE MK, PORTER R (1980) The discharges during movement of cells in the ventrolateral thalamus of the conscious monkey. J Physiol (London) 304:349-372

IANSEK R, PORTER R (1980) The monkey globus pallidus : neuronal discharge properties in relation to movement. J Physiol (London) 301:439-455

KALIL K (1981) Projections of the cerebellar and dorsal column nuclei upon the thalamus of the rhesus monkey. J comp Neurol 195:25-50

KIEVIT J, KUYPERS HGJM (1977) Organization of the thalamocortical connexions to the frontal lobe in the rhesus monkey. Exp Brain Res 29:299-322

KIM R, NAKANO K, JAYARAMAN A, CARPENTER MB (1976) Projections of the globus pallidus and adjacent structures : an autoradiographic study in the monkey. J comp Neurol 169:263-290

KUNZLE H (1976) Thalamic projections from the precentral motor cortex in Macaca fascicularis. Brain Res 105:253-267

KUNZLE H (1978) An autoradiographic analysis of the efferent connections from premotor and adjacent prefrontal regions (areas 6 and 9) in Macaca fascicularis. Brain Beh Evol 15:185-234

KUO JS, CARPENTER MB (1973) Organization of pallido-thalamic projections in the rhesus monkey. J comp Neurol 151:201-236

LEMON RH, VAN DER BURG J (1979) Short latency peripheral inputs to thalamic neurons projecting to the motor cortex in the monkey. Exp Brain Res 36:445-462

MACPHERSON JM, RASMUSSON DD, MURPHY JT (1980) Activities of neurones in "motor" thalamus during control of limb movement in the primate. J Neurophysiol 44:11-28

MATSUMURA M, KUBOTA K (1979) Cortical projection to hand-arm motor area from post-arcuate area in macaque monkeys : a histological study of retrograde transport of horse-radish peroxidase. Neurosci Lett 11:241-246

MUAKKASSA KF, STRICK PL (1979) Frontal lobe inputs to primate motor cortex : evidence for somatotopically organized "premotor" areas. Brain Res 177:176-182

OLSZEWSKI J (1952) The thalamus of the Macaca mulatta. Karger, Basel

PANDYA DN, VIGNOLO LA (1971) Intra- and interhemispheric projections of the precentral, premotor and arcuate areas in the rhesus monkey. Brain Res 26:217-233

RISPAL-PADEL L, MASSION J, GRANGETTO A (1973) Relations between the ventrolateral thalamic nucleus and motor cortex and their possible role in the central organization of motor control. Brain Res 60:1-20

SMITH AM, HEPP-REYMOND MC, WYSS UR (1975) Relation of activity in precentral cortical neurons to force and rate of force change during isometric contraction of finger muscles. Exp Brain Res 23:315-332

STRICK PL (1976a) Anatomical analysis of ventrolateral thalamic input to primate motor cortex. J Neurophysiol 39:1020-1031

STRICK PL (1976b) Activity of ventrolateral thalamic neurons during arm movement. J Neurophysiol 39:1032-1044

TRACEY DJ, ASANUMA C, JONES EG, PORTER R (1980) Thalamic relay to motor cortex : afferent pathways from the brain stem, cerebellum and spinal cord in monkeys. J Neurophysiol 44:532-554

WIESENDANGER M, MILES TS (1982) The ascending pathway of low-threshold muscle afferents to the cerebral cortex and its possible role in motor control. Physiol Rev, in press

Are Coding Schemes Actually Used? The Cooling Test Demonstration

M. Amalric, H. Condé, J. F. Dormont, and A. Schmied

Laboratoire de Neurobiologie du Développement, Université Paris Sud, 91405 Orsay France

Many investigations into the neural coding of motor performance have attempted to establish a correlation between central neural activity and some parameters of motor performance. However these correlations do not indicate the causal sequence of movement initiation, and even if the activation of peripheral receptors can be excluded, one cannot eliminate corollary discharge as an important factor in determining frequency changes in the awake animal (see PERKEL and BULLOCK 1968). Blockade by cooling provides a reversible means of testing whether a particular neural activity is causally related to the motor performance. The present paper seeks to compare the results of local cooling with those of chronic unit recordings in animals trained to execute prompt movements. Are codes deduced from unitary recordings actually used as motor command ? In the ventrolateral thalamic nucleus (VL) and the red nucleus (RN) the cooling test supports a command role for the proposed code in the movement initiation whereas in the caudate nucleus (Cd) the cooling test fails to demonstrate any direct command function.

METHODS

The methods used have been described in detail previously (BENITA et al., 1979 ; SCHMIED et al., 1979). Briefly, cats were trained to execute a ballistic forelimb flexion releasing a lever as quickly as possible after a brief 10 ms auditory conditioned stimulus (CS). The reaction time (RT) was measured between the CS onset and the lever release detected by a micro-switch. Force changes on the lever were measured by strain-gauges. RTs were in the 200-400 ms range, with changes of force after the CS occurring with a latency of at least 100 ms.

After about 3 months of daily training, the animals underwent surgical preparation for either unitary recording or regional cooling. In both situations the animals were unrestrained. Local cooling was performed using

BENITA's device (BENITA, 1971). Cooling blockade with this technique permits rapid cooling onset and offset and therefore avoids recovery phenomena such as those observed after lesions. Within a certain temperature range, the synaptic transmission can be selectively blocked without impairing conduction in passing fibers (BENITA and CONDE, 1972), a point particularly useful in structures such as the red nucleus. It has been shown previously that temperature gradient is about of +1°C per 1/10th mm from the tip. The size of the cooling isotherms can be controlled by changing the tip temperature enabling changes in the motor performance to be quantitatively related to the amount of nervous tissue volume affected.

RESULTS

Unit recording studies

Unitary recordings have shown that about 40% of the neurons recorded in the VL (total : 166 neurons) or in the RN (191 neurons) showed changes of activity after the CS with a 15-60 ms latency. This was compatible with a command role in the initiation of the conditioned movement, since the earliest change of force preceding the movement occurred more than 100 ms after the CS. For the neurons which were recorded on a sufficient number of trials to be able to be studied quantitatively, it appeared that the variations in the latencies of activity changes were rather small and could only partially account for the range of RTs. Nevertheless, for certain neurons, correlations were shown between the unit discharge frequency in the 40-100 ms period after the CS and the length of the reaction time. Higher discharge frequency was inversely correlated with reaction time (Fig. 1). Moreover, for most of these neurons no change of activity occurred after the CS when the animal occasionally failed to move.

In the caudate nucleus, a total of 50 neurons were recorded and so only preliminary results can be presented. Early 20-60 ms latency changes of activity were also observed, and similar correlations between unit activity and RTs were also demonstrated (Fig. 1, right).

Since the above results suggest that the VL, RN and Cd participate in the initiation of the movement because of an approximately linear relationship between central neural activity and RT, it might be predicted that the blockade by cooling of the VL, RN or Cd efferent activity would result in a lengthening of the RTs.

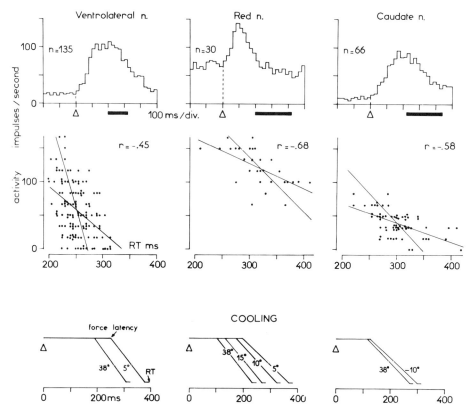

Fig. 1. top row. Averages of the activity of a single neuron recorded in the thalamic ventrolateral nucleus, in the Red Nucleus and in the Caudate nucleus respectively. The Red nucleus and the Caudate neuron were recorded in the same cat. Histograms with 20 ms bin sizes. The activity is averaged with respect to the CS occurrence (triangle). The black bars indicate the range of the reaction times, and n the number of trials. These units show a similar short (20-40 ms) latency increase of activity after the CS, occurring well before the mechanical detection of reaction time. Notice high level of activity during the foreperiod in the Red nucleus unit.

center row. Correlation between unit activity and reaction time. Each scatter diagram corresponds to individual trials from the unit which is represented above by its average activity. The activity plotted represents the average activity during the 40-100 ms period after the CS. r : Pearson's correlation coefficient. The regression lines are figured. Notice the similar correlations for these thalamic, rubral and caudate units.

bottom row. Effects of cooling blockade on motor performance for other subjects. The lines schematically represent averages of the force exerted on the lever by the animal. Each trace starts at the CS occurrence (triangle) and ends at the mechanical detection of the reaction time (RT). Arbitrary units in ordinate. Tip temperature in °C. When the thalamic (left) or rubral (center) activities are blocked by cooling, both force latency and RT are increased, in a somewhat parallel way. For the Red nucleus, where more important effects are obtained, it can be seen that these increases are quantitatively related to the tip temperature and therefore to the number of Red nucleus neurons blocked. For Caudate cooling (right) force latency is not significantly changed, although a small but significant increase in RTs is observed

Regional cooling studies

Contralateral VL cooling caused a parallel increase of force change latency (denoted force latency) and of RT. For extensive VL cooling this lengthening is about 20% of the control values (Fig. 1, bottom left).

Contralateral RN cooling also caused a parallel increase of force latency and of RT. These increases could be smoothly graduated with the cooling extension (Fig. 1, bottom center).

By contrast an extensive Cd cooling blockade failed to produce a significant modification of the force latency although a small but significant lengthening of the RTs was observed (Fig. 1, bottom right). Delayed impairments of performance have been considered elsewhere (CONDE et al., 1981).

DISCUSSION

A discussion of single unit discharge must precede consideration of the effects of regional cooling because cooling modifies both the CS evoked responses as well as the changes in spontaneous activity.

For the VL, single cell discharge during the foreperiod is of low frequency (mean : 1 to 24 impulses/s for unit activity correlated with RTs), uncorrelated with RTs, and it can be assumed that cooling affects primarily CS-triggered phasic activity. The 20% increase of force latency and of RTs during cooling shows that this phasic activity participates in the initiation of the movement, since higher discharge rates are associated with shorter reaction times and, the reduction in CS evoked activity produced by cooling is always associated with longer RTs. The cooling therefore shows that the VL participates in the movement initiation. The fact that the animals still perform CS triggered movements, although at longer latencies indicates that other systems are operating in parallel to produce these responses.

The rubro-spinal system, as analysed from unitary recordings, is obviously a candidate for participating, concomitant with the VL, in producing prompt movements (GHEZ and KUBOTA, 1977). The RN unit activity during the foreperiod is rather high (range : 1 to 90 impulses/s for unit activity correlated with RTs) and it cannot be assumed, as for the VL, that cooling affects primarily CS-triggered activity. However it has been noticed that the force amplitude and time-course during the foreperiod remained unchanged during cooling, which suggests that cooling does not affect postural mechanisms but probably the preparation of the spinal neurons during the foreperiod (TANJI and EVARTS, 1976) and the movement initiation itself. The graded effects of cooling temperatures indicates that the reaction time lengthening is related to the number of RN neurons affected and that cooling does not have an all-or-none effect.

Parallel involvement of the thalamo-cortico-spinal and of rubro-spinal system is supported by their common input from the cerebellar interposate nucleus, and by their possible excitatory convergence on propriospinal neurons monosynaptically connected to the forelimb motoneurons (ILLERT et al., 1976). With Cd cooling, the effects were limited to a small lengthening of the RTs without any change in force latency, which indicated that the movement initiation is not serially processed through the Cd, but rather that the Cd output modulates the initiation program. Therefore the "intensity" code which was suggested on the basis of unitary recordings is not validated by the cooling test. However an extensive exploration of the Cd is required before the results of our cooling (3 cats) and recording (1 cat) experiments involving only the central part of this nucleus (A 15 L 5) can be generalized to all parts of the Cd.

In conclusion, the combined discussion of reversible cooling effects and of single unit discharge in the same structures in animals trained to perform the same task is a worthwhile method in attempting to establish causal relations between central unit activity and performance.

ACKNOWLEDGEMENTS

The invaluable secretarial and technical assistance of S. SOURIOU and D. FARIN is gratefully acknowledged. This reseach was supported by the CNRS (LA 89) and the DGRST (DN P111).

REFERENCES

BENITA M (1971) Appareil adapté aux refroidissements localisés des structures nerveuses. Electroenceph Clin Neurophysiol 32:90-94

BENITA M, CONDE H (1972) Effects of local cooling upon conduction and synaptic transmission. Brain Res 36:133-151

BENITA M, CONDE H, DORMONT JF, SCHMIED A (1979) Effects of cooling the thalamic ventrolateral nucleus of cats on a reaction time task. Exp Brain Res 34:433-452

CONDE H, BENITA M, DORMONT JF, SCHMIED A, CADORET A (1981) Control of reaction time performance involves the striatum. J Physiol (Paris) 77:97-105

GHEZ C, KUBOTA K (1977) Activity of red nucleus neurons associated with a skilled forelimb movement in the cat. Brain Res 131:383-388

ILLERT M, LUNDBERG A, TANAKA R (1976) Integration in descending motor pathways controlling the forelimb in the cat. 2. Convergence on neurones mediating disynaptic cortico-motoneuronal excitation. Exp Brain Res 26:521-540

PERKEL DH, BULLOCK TH (1968) Neural coding. Neurosciences Res Prog Bull, 6:226-343

SCHMIED A, BENITA M, CONDE H, DORMONT JF (1979) Activity of ventrolateral thalamic neurons in relation to a simple reaction time task in the cat. Exp Brain Res 36:285-300

TANJI J, EVARTS EV (1976) Anticipatory activity of motor cortex neurons in relation to direction of an intended movement. J Neurophysiol 39: 1062-1068

Structural Coding:
Prewired Addressing

Neocerebellar Synergies

L. Rispal-Padel, F. Cicirata, and J.-C. Pons

Departement de Neurophysiologie générale, INP, CNRS, B.P. 71, 31, chemin Joseph Aiguier, 13277 Marseille Cedex 9, France

INTRODUCTION

Two questions are often asked concerning the neocerebellar control of movement. First, what types of movements are controlled by the dentate nucleus ? Second, is the cerebello-thalamo-cortical pathway involved in the control of movements induced by the dentate stimulation ?

The first question has arisen from the well known observation of motor incoordination in cerebellar patients. Contradictory hypotheses are given to explain this deficit : according to BABINSKI (1899) it is a fundamental deficit and he named it "the cerebellar asynergy". In other words asynergy would be the consequence of a programming error concerning the distribution of the activity in muscles fixing joints during coordinated movements (RONDOT et al., 1979).

In contrast, HOLMES (1939) considered the asynergy as a secondary deficit due to the hypotonia affecting each elementary movement making up the complex movement.

In order to determine what type of control the neocerebellum exerts on the musculature, punctate stimulation of the dentate nucleus was peformed. If the neocerebellum is involved in motor synergies, one might expect that the stimulation of the dentate nucleus would provoke synergistic effects.

The second question concerned the dentate efferent pathway transmitting cerebellar information to the musculature. Two distinct pathways could be involved : the dentato-reticulo-spinal (BANTLI and BLOEDEL, 1975) and the dentato-thalamo-cortical paths. The latter is well known for its central role in the cerebello-cerebral loop (ALLEN and TSUKAHARA, 1974 ; EVARTS and THACH, 1969) but its action at the spinal level is still uncertain. Limb movements

Experimental Brain Research, Suppl. 7
© Springer-Verlag Berlin · Heidelberg 1983

induced by dentate stimulation have been reported (SCHULTZ et al., 1979) after motor cortical lesion implying that dentate outputs are in part transmitted to the spinal cord by the reticulo-spinal tract. However, these data can not completely exclude the participation of the dentato-thalamo-cortical circuit. The question arises as to what extent the dentato-thalamo-cortical path could also transmit motor effects induced by dentate stimulation to spinal centres. It may be asked more particularly if the internal organization of the cerebellum confers upon it a role in the elaboration of motor synergies.

METHODS

To answer the two questions posed above, punctate stimulation of the neocerebellar region was performed in seven awake baboons with chronically implanted electrodes. Motor effects evoked by the stimulations were either examined by two separate observers or filmed and studied later. Moreover changes in the activity of the motor cortex, the pyramidal tract and the muscular activity (eight muscles) were systematically monitored. The cerebellum was stimulated with monopolar nickel-chrome electrodes, a train of stimuli was applied (eight shocks of 0.5 msec and 100 µA at 300 Hz). When a movement was induced, the threshold was determined and the spatial distribution of the responses was established with this just liminar stimulation. But in order to measure the response latencies the stimulus was fixed at two times threshold. A map was drawn for the cortical responses accompanying each movement. The marks made by an iron deposit (present as an impurity in the nickel-chrome alloy) which were made at the end of each trajectory across the dentate nucleus, were subsequently located in serial histological sections, thus permitting exact localization of stimulation points. Only the data gathered when the stimulation was applied inside the neuronal region of the dentate nucleus have been analyzed in the present work.

RESULTS

A - Types of movements observed

Two types of movements were observed in more or less equal numbers : simple movements (44) involving the head or a single joint of the limb, and complex movements (47) involving several body regions (RISPAL-PADEL and coll., 1982).

The simple movements visually observed were characterized by a brief and unidirectional displacement of a single segment of the body (Fig. 1B). On

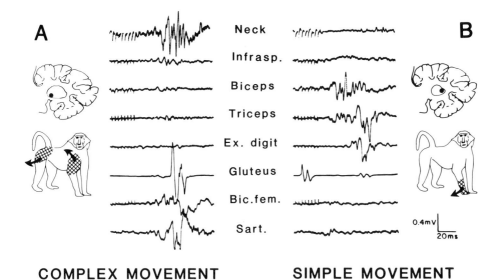

A   Neck   **B**

Infrasp.

Biceps

Triceps

Ex. digit

Gluteus

Bic.fem.

Sart.

0.4mv

20ms

COMPLEX MOVEMENT   SIMPLE MOVEMENT

Fig. 1. Myographic responses in complex and simple movements
A - Above left : the dentate point stimulated is shown on a schematic
sagittal section at L 6.5.
    Below : On the diagram of the animal, the movement elicited by the
stimulus is indicated by an arrow, and the moving limb segment is shaded.
    In the middle are shown simultaneous myographic recordings from a neck
extensor and from infraspinatus, biceps, triceps, extensor digitorum, gluteus, biceps femoris, sartorius. The complex movement involved shoulder and
hip. This "rostro-caudal synergy" corresponded to almost simultaneous activation of neck, shoulder and hindlimb muscles.
B - The simple movement (dorsiflexion of wrist) was accompanied by an
activation of the extensor digitorum but in addition by a co-contraction of
biceps and triceps

electromyographic analysis a burst of about 50 msec appeared in the muscles
of the moving segment (here extensor digitorum). Moreover a co-contraction
was also observed in the muscles of the neighbouring segment (triceps and
biceps).

The complex movements like the simple ones were exclusively ipsilateral and
were also perfectly stable and stereotyped.

They were grouped around two or three neighbouring joints but frequently they
involved distinct and separate regions of the body (Fig. 1A). Electromyography confirmed the visual observation : the punctate rostromedial dentate
stimulation produced activation in a large number of muscles localized in
"non contiguous" muscular groups (neck, shoulder and hip).

Such motor effects sometimes had the features of several simple movements. Nevertheless they were indissociable into their elementary components and they were induced with all or none properties with a just liminar stimulation.

The muscular responses were almost simultaneous in all muscles. The slight latency difference observed between the infra-spinatus and the gluteus responses can be explained by the different distances between the cerebellar sites and the recorded muscles.

B - Topographical arrangement of the motor effects

From a functional point of view, strictly related to motor localization, it appears that the dentate nucleus can not be considered as a homogeneous structure. The sites of origin of simple and complex movements are not mixed in the nucleus (Fig. 2). Complex movements were obtained by stimulation applied in the more rostral and medial regions of the dentate nucleus, whereas simple movements were induced from the posterior and lateral parts of this nucleus.

Thus, according to the kind of movement controlled, two functionally distinct regions are distinguished within the neocerebellar nucleus.

C - Cerebello-thalamo-cortical participation in movements induced by dentate stimulation

To establish if the dentato-thalamo-cortical path contributes to the elaboration of simple and complex movements, several arguments were considered. They were :

1. The concomitance between the muscular and cortical responses. 2. The chronological aspects of the dentate efferent effects and 3. The spatial aspects of the dentate efferent effects.

1. The concomitance between muscular and cortical responses

One muscular excitation always coincided with an almost simultaneous cortical evoked potential (Fig. 3C upper traces). On the other hand when the muscular response was absent a cortical activation never appeared (lower traces).

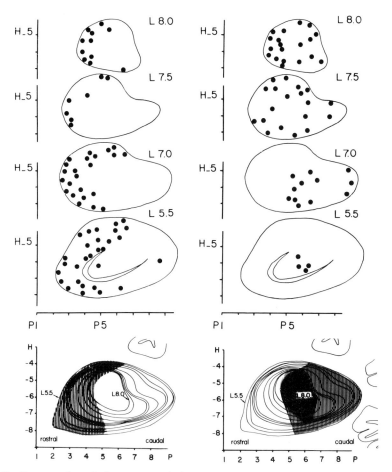

Fig. 2. Topography of dentate-evoked movements
Complex movements are represented in the left column, simple movements in the right one.
Four parasagittal sections through the dentate nucleus between L 5.5 and L 8.0 : the dots indicate the sites from which movements were elicited. The antero-posterior co-ordinates are shown below each section, the vertical co-ordinates are on the left.
On the lower part of the figure are two contoured reconstructions, at 250 μm intervals of the dentate nucleus between L 5.5 and L 8.0 ; on the left map, the region giving rise to complex movements is shaded ; it occupies the whole anteromedial part of the nucleus. On the right, the shaded area is the zone controlling simple movement. Inside this zone the darkest part is the motor area for the hand

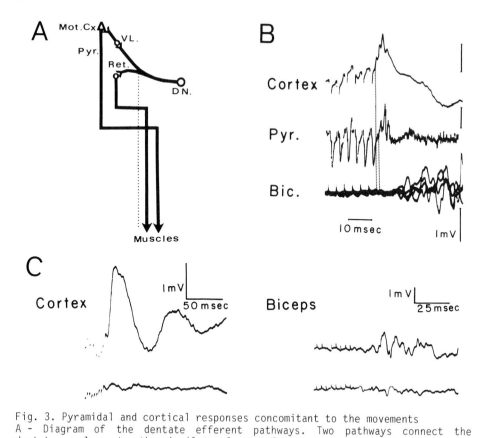

Fig. 3. Pyramidal and cortical responses concomitant to the movements
A - Diagram of the dentate efferent pathways. Two pathways connect the
dentate nucleus to the ipsilateral musculature : one is relayed in the
reticular formation, the other transmits the dentate effects to the spinal
centers via the thalamus and the motor cortex. DN = dentate nucleus ; Ret =
reticular nucleus ; VL = ventro-lateral nucleus ; Mot.Cx = motor cortex.
B - Responses observed during a dentate stimulation (6 shocks of 0.5 msec and
30 μA at 300 Hz). Simultaneous cortical (Cortex), pyramidal (Pyr.) and biceps
(Bic.) activations are observed. The dotted lines marked the latency differences between the three evoked responses.
C - The two upper traces sh the coincidence between the presence of the
cortical and muscular responses. The two lower traces indicate that when the
muscular response is absent, the evoked cortical potential does not appear

2. The chronological aspects of the dentate efferent effects

The chronological aspects are represented in Figure 3B. The movement presence
illustrated by the biceps recording was accompanied by cortical and pyramidal
activation. The latencies observed were respectively 3 msec for the cortical
evoked potential, 4.2 msec for the pyramidal response and 11 msec for the
muscular activation. Allowing for synaptic delays, the timing of the responses observed at the three different recording sites along the path indicated

a constant velocity and latency differences compatible with a dentato-thalamo-cortical transmission of the neocerebellar output.

3. The spatial aspects of the dentate efferent effects

The spatial aspect of the dentate projection has been examined with the
following experimental procedure : we have tested the activity of twelve
distinct motor cortical sites simultaneously with eight electromyographic
recordings or to the observation of the movement. Afterwards, the sites from
which evoked potentials were obtained were in turn stimulated and the sum of
the movements induced in this way was then compared to the movement elicited
by dentate stimulation.

The spatial distribution of the dentato-cortical projections which accompany
simple and complex movements is illustrated in Figure 4. Precise relations
exist between dentate sites and the motor cortex : the map of the cortical
evoked potentials varied according to the stimulus localization in the
cerebellar nucleus. In addition the cortical projection of a given site
seemed to be related to the movement induced from this site (Fig. 4A). A
large number of evoked cortical potentials were observed simultaneous to a
rostro-caudal synergy (shoulder-hip movement). They were localized in two
functional motor cortical areas in which stimulation induced five distinct
movements. These latter were the tail (point 1), the hip (point 2), the thigh
(point 4), the shoulder (point 8) and the hand (point 11).

It thus appears that from a single cerebellar focus, a coordinated hip-shoul-
der movement is induced at the same time as responses are evoked on the
cortical zones from which the same elementary movements could be induced.

Concerning the sites producing simple movements, their projections were
limited to a small number of cortical points. In Figure 4B only two responses
were observed in a focalized cortical region, producing after stimulation,
shoulder (point 8) and hand movements (point 11). In the right part of the
Figure (4A, B), the two summarized schemas show that a movement produced by a
given site in the dentate nucleus is similar to the sum of movements induced
by stimulation of each cortical point receiving excitatory projections from
the same dentate focus.

Thus, these arguments concerning the timing and the organization of the
dentate-cortical projections support the idea that the motor effects induced
by the dentate stimulation can be transmitted to the musculature by the
cerebello-thalamo-cortico-spinal circuit.

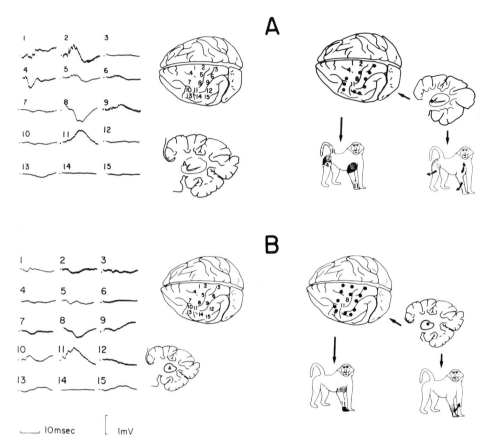

Fig. 4. Organization of the dentato-cortical projections

A - Example concerning complex movement : Map of the cortical potentials evoked from a dentate site at the origin of a rostro-caudal synergy. Five responses were observed in two distinct cortical motor areas : the first area included the sites 1,2,4 ; the second area contained the sites 8 and 11. Afterwards successive stimulation of each of the five sites respectively induced tail (1), hip (2), thigh (4), shoulder (8) and hand (11) movements. The sum of these movements involved the same parts of the musculature which were activated by the stimulation of the dentate site.

B Example for a simple movement : Stimulation of another site of the dentate induced simple movement of the hand, the repartition of evoked potentials is mainly limited to a cortical zone where the forelimb is represented (sites 8 and 11)

DISCUSSION

The neocerebellum seems to be able to play a role in the execution of motor synergies. Indeed the complex movements induced by dentate stimulation can be defined as motor synergy : they are stable, perfectly stereotyped, indissociable into their elementary components and they are not of reflex nature. These characteristics suggest that complex movements could be implemented by a single central command. In this way, the cerebellar asynergy could be considered as a fundamental deficit (BABINSKI, 1899) or as a programming error for a coordinated movement. The consequence could be a faulty spatial and temporal distribution of muscular activity (RONDOT et al., 1979).

Some data obtained on chronic preparations can give information concerning the role of the dentate nucleus in the elaboration of motor synergies : the unitary discharges which are linked to a simple movement are rarely coded with the patterns of the ongoing muscular activity, they are related to other parameters of the intended movements such as presetting (STRICK, 1979 ; THACH, 1978). It is also shown that the dentate could be concerned in different movements or in a more complex task (ROBERTSON and GRIMM, 1975).

Among the efferent pathways from the dentate nucleus, an organization exists at several levels which could be recognized as the morphological substrate of motor synergies. Thus the present work demonstrates that the dentato-thalamo-cortical system participates in the performance of these movements. Furthermore, the present work shows, on one hand, that also the dentato-thalamo-cortical system like the reticulo-spinal circuit (BANTLI and BLOEDEL, 1976 ; SCHULTZ et al., 1979) participates in the performance of the movement induced by cerebellar stimulation. On the other hand, it shows that the motor synergy is accompanied by a simultaneous activation of diverging projections onto multiple zones of the motor cortex. The circuitry on which these synergies depend has been analyzed at the cellular level in the cat. It is characterized by an organization which exhibits divergence and convergence throughout the cerebello-thalamo-cortical pathway (RISPAL-PADEL and GRANGETTO, 1977 ; RISPAL-PADEL et al., 1973).

This same property accomplished through branching axons, has been shown in several other pathways such as the corticospinal, reticulospinal and propriospinal ones, which have been reported to play a role in the distribution of cerebellar influences in distinct spinal centers (LUNDBERG, 1975 ; PETERSON et al., 1975 ; SHINODA et al., 1976).

Referring to the sites at the origin of simple and complex movements, two regions have been delineated in the dentate nucleus. Notwithstanding the fact that stimulation evidences mainly the efferent pathway organization, it appears that the anteromedial region at the origin of motor synergies has a different function with respect to the posterolateral one which produces simple movements. In fact the two regions differentiated in this experiment

222

have the same boundaries as those separating the magno and the parvocellular portions of the human dentate nucleus (DEMOLE, 1927). The antero-medial part would correspond to the magnocellular one and the postero-lateral to the parvocellular one. In his review of the anatomical, phylogenetical and ontogenetical studies, DEMOLE (1927) presented the hypothesis that the antero-medial (magnocellular) part is older than the postero-lateral (parvocellular) portion. Only the latter, where the hand motor area is included, would be purely neocerebellar.

SUMMARY

In order to clarify the role of the neocerebellum in the elaboration of motor synergies the spatial organization of the cerebellar effects in relation to the musculature has been studied. Simultaneous recordings of eight muscles (located in forelimb, neck and hindlimb) were obtained in chronically implanted baboons (Papio-papio) during punctate cerebellar stimulation.

Two kinds of motor effects were observed : 1) Unidirectional movements of a single joint. 2) Complex movements which involved simultaneously several segments of the body. These complex movements have the characteristics of motor synergies and they appear to result from a single central command.

Some data reveal that the cerebello-thalamo-cortical pathway participates in this command. A. During realization of a motor synergy, cortical and pyramidal responses can be observed simultaneously with the muscular activation. The response latencies show that the effects are partly transmitted through the dentato-thalamo-cortical pathway. B. The complex movement which is produced by stimulation of a site in the dentate nucleus is similar to the sum of movements induced by stimulation of each cortical point which receives excitatory projections from the same dentate focus.

Two regions could be distinguished within the dentate nucleus in relation to the motor localization : a) a rostromedial region, from which synergistic effects were elicited. b) a posterolateral portion from which simple movements were induced.

ACKNOWLEDGEMENT

We acknowledge Dr. A. TROIANI for her help in English translation.
This work was supported by grant from D.G.R.S.T. n° 79 7 1079

REFERENCES

ALLEN GI, TSUKAHARA N (1974) Cerebro-cerebellar communication systems. Physiol Rev 54:957-1006

BABINSKI J (1899) De l'asynergie cérébelleuse. Rev Neurol 7:806-816

BANTLI H, BLOEDEL JR (1976) Characteristics of the output from the dentate nucleus to spinal neurons via pathways which do not involve the primary sensorimotor cortex. Exp Brain Res 25:199-220

DEMOLE V (1927) Structures et connections des noyaux dentelés du cervelet. Schweitz Arch Neurol Neurochir Psychiat 271:293-315

EVARTS EV, THACH WT (1969) Motor mechanisms of the CNS : cerebro-cerebellar interrelations. Ann Rev Physiol 31:451-498

HOLMES G (1939) The cerebellum of the man. Brain 62:1-29

LUNDBERG A (1975) Control of spinal mechanisms from the brain. In: TOWER DB (ed) The nervous system. Vol. I. The basic neurosciences. Raven Press, New York, pp 253-265

PETERSON BW, MAUNZ RA, PITTS NG, MACKEL RG (1975) Patterns of projection and branching of reticulospinal neurons. Exp Brain Res 23:333-351

RISPAL-PADEL L, CICIRATA F, PONS C (1982) Cerebellar nuclear topography of simple and synergistic movements in the alert baboon (Papio papio). Exp Brain Res 47:365-380

RISPAL-PADEL L, MASSION J, GRANGETTO A (1973) Relations between ventrolateral thalamic nucleus and motor cortex and their possible role in the central organization of motor control. Brain Res. 60:1-20

RISPAL-PADEL L, GRANGETTO A (1977) The cerebello-thalamo-cortical pathway. Topographical investigation at the unitary level in the cat. Exp Brain res 28:101-123

ROBERTSON LT, GRIMM RJ (1975) Responses of primate dentate neurons to different trajectories of the limb. Exp Brain Res 23:447-463

RONDOT P, BATHIEN N, TOMA S (1979) Physiopathology of cerebellar movement. In: MASSION J, SASAKI K (eds) Cerebro-cerebellar interactions. Elsevier/North--Holland Biomedical Press, pp 203-230

SCHULTZ W, MONTGOMERY EB, MARINI R (1979) Proximal limb movements in response to microstimulation of primate dentate and interpositus nucleus mediated by brain stem structures. Brain 102:127-146

SHINODA Y, ARNOLD AP, ASANUMA H (1976) Spinal branching of cortico-spinal axons in the cat. Exp Brain Res 26:215-234

STRICK PL (1979) Control of peripheral input to the dentate nucleus by motor preparation. In: MASSION J, SASAKI K (eds) Cerebro-cerebellar interactions. Elsevier/North-Holland Biomedical Press, pp 185-201

THACH WT (1978) Correlation of neural discharge with pattern and force of muscular activity, joint position and direction of intended next movement in motor cortex and cerebellum. J Neurophysiol 41:654-676

Function of Intermediate Cerebellum in Motor Control

F. Licata, V. Perciavalle, S. Sapienza, and A. Urbano

University of Rome, Città Universitaria, 00185 Roma, Italy
Institute of Human Physiology, University of Catania, Viale Andra Doria 6, 95125 Catania, Italy

INTRODUCTION

Previous studies have shown that the motor cortex and the pars intermedia of the cerebellum (intermediate cerebellum) are linked together via brain stem and thalamic relay stations (EVARTS and THACH, 1969 ; ANGAUT, 1973 ; ALLEN and TSUKAHARA, 1974 ; MAC KAY and MURPHY, 1979). Evidence also has been provided that the intermediate cerebellum receives input from muscles, tendons, joints and skin via direct and indirect spinocerebellar pathways (OSCARSSON, 1973). On the basis of these connections it has been suggested that the intermediate cerebellum is involved in on-going corrections of evolving movement. The execution of these corrections may be initiated by the motor cortex. Such cerebellar control of the evolving movement could be mediated by a direct action on spinal centers, via the rubrospinal pathway (ECCLES et al., 1974 ; MASSION, 1973 ; ALLEN and TSUKAHARA, 1974). According to this functional schema, the intermediate cerebellum would display an "authoritative" influence on the movements initiated by the motor cortex (ECCLES, 1977).

Such an error correction is incompatible with a possible involvement of the intermediate cerebellum in a motor command pathway.

An organization of the interpositus nucleus (IN) in foci exciting single muscles of the ipsilateral limbs has been demonstrated by ASANUMA and HUNSPERGER (1975) with microstimulation experiments in awake cats. Furthermore, similar effects have been seen by GHEZ (1975) upon microstimulation of the red nucleus in the same preparations. Pyramidal tract collaterals, however, are not capable of producing movement via the cerebellum (CIONI et al., 1978). Therefore, a circuit including the intermediate cerebellum and the rubrospinal tract, that would not be fired by the motor cortex, could be responsible for precise muscle commands, in the cat.

Experimental Brain Research, Suppl. 7
© Springer-Verlag Berlin · Heidelberg 1983

Experimental results will be reported in the following sections which are consistent with such an hypothesis.

Motor effect through the Intermediate Cerebellum

In the awake cat microstimulation of cerebellar afferents running in the brachium pontis (PERCIAVALLE et al., 1977) and in the restiform body (PERCIAVALLE et al., 1978c) produces contraction of single muscles of limbs which are similar to those previously observed upon IN stimulation (ASANUMA and HUNSPERGER, 1975 ; PERCIAVALLE et al., 1978b). The effects are abolished upon brachium conjunctivum or rubrospinal tract transection, but are unaffected by prerubral decerebration and pyramidotomy (PERCIAVALLE et al., 1978a ; 1978b). Direct activation of IN is responsible for motor responses to precerebellar stimulation. In fact, responses disappear following IN lesions but not following cerebellar cortex ablation (PERCIAVALLE et al., 1978a ; 1978b ; 1979). Dorsal rhizotomy does not modify IN-induced motor responses, indicating that it is interposito-rubrospinal projections to alpha-motoneurons which are capable of triggering movement (GIUFFRIDA et al., in press).

Single muscle reciprocal organization of the Intermediate Cerebellum

Brachium pontis or restiform body activation, which elicits contraction of a given limb muscle, monosynaptically excites only IN cells located in the nuclear focus controlling that muscle (agonist cells) and inhibits IN cells located within the focus for an antagonist muscle (antagonist cells) ; the inhibition is via the cerebellar cortex. Excitatory and inhibitory influences from the two peduncles converge on singe IN cells (GIUFFRIDA et al., 1981). Furthermore, IN cells situated within an area for a given muscle are inhibited through the overlying cortex by impulses coming from force detectors in that muscle and excited by responses originating in the antagonist muscle (LICATA et al., 1978). The projections of IN to the red nucleus also are organized for single muscles and in a reciprocal manner. The agonist rubrospinal cells are monosynaptically activated from IN and the antagonist cells are di- or paucisynaptically inhibited from the same region (GIUFFRIDA et al., 1980). Similarly, IN influences the representation of single muscles in the motor cortex and in a reciprocal manner. In fact, IN stimulation, which elicits contraction of a given muscle via the rubrospinal tract, inhibits pyramidal tract neurons localized in the focus of the area 4-gamma controlling that muscle, via the ventral lateral nucleus of the thalamus ; conversely, the same stimulation produces excitation, pure or followed by inhibition, of pyramidal tract neurons belonging to the focus for its

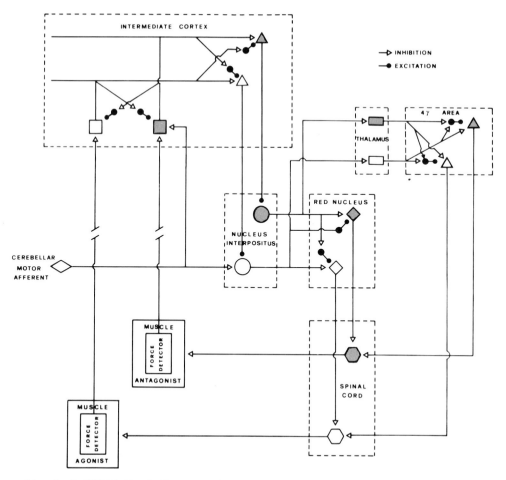

Fig. 1. FUNCTION OF INTERMEDIATE CEREBELLUM IN MOTOR CONTROL
Diagram showing input-output organization for a single muscle of the intermediate cerebellum. Full description in the text

antagonist (LI VOLSI et al., in press). On the other hand, pyramidal volleys
elicited upon medullary pyramidal tract stimulation are capable of modifying
the discharge of only 11-1? per cent of IN cells, via the pontine nuclei
(GIUFFRIDA et al., to be published).

All the described circuit operations can be best appreciated by the diagram
of Figure 1.

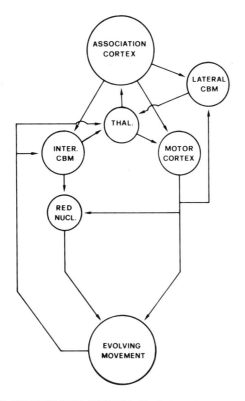

Fig. 2. FUNCTION OF INTERMEDIATE CEREBELLUM IN MOTOR CONTROL
Scheme showing cerebro-cerebellar circuits concerned with the control of voluntary movements. Abbreviations : Inter. CBM, intermediate cerebellum ; lateral CBM, lateral cerebellum ; Thal., thalamus. Full description in the text

Physiological considerations

According to the experiments described herein, the interposito-rubrospinal pathway in the cat would display all the characteristics of a circuit responsible for precise, reciprocally organized motor commands. These commands are continuously updated by muscular input from the periphery. The low percentage (11-12%) of IN cells influenced by pyramidal axon collaterals makes it unlikely that the corticospinal system could be capable of recruiting this circuit. Thus IN would not be involved in the correction of an on-going movement triggered by the motor cortex, via the interposito-thalamo-cortical pathway. The specific role of the intermediate cerebellum could be that of an interface fitting the output toward muscles, via the rubrospinal tract, to the state of muscles themselves. Concomitantly, interposito-rubral axon collaterals direct to the thalamus would depress the discharge of corticospinal neurons. The interposito-rubrospinal circuit, hence, would operate independently of the corticospinal system, likely under the influence of cortical association areas (cf. scheme of Fig. 2). If hypothetically one admits that the corticospinal and the interposito-rubrospinal pathways are fired by the same association areas, the two pathways could cooperate in the management of movement. The preferential participation of the one or the other pathway could be imposed by the peripheral conditions in every motor situation. Any involvement of the motor periphery, that reduces the contribution of the interposito-rubrospinal pathway to muscular activation, would potentiate the corticospinal discharges. In other words, the motor order would be switched from the corticospinal to the interposito-rubrospinal pathway whenever the periphery is free of perturbations. Conversely, the control of movement would be exerted by the corticospinal pathway.

SUMMARY

Evidence is provided that the intermediate cerebellum is enclosed in a motor command circuit organized for single muscles and in a reciprocal manner. It is likely that cortical association areas give origin to the impulses capable of firing this circuit. Collateral influence from intermediate cerebellum to motor cortex would play the role of switching out the corticospinal pathway.

REFERENCES

ALLEN GI, TSUKAHARA N (1974) Cerebrocerebellar communication systems. Physiol Rev 54:957-1006

ANGAUT P (1973) Bases anatomo-fonctionnelles des interrelations cérébello-cérébrale. J Physiol (Paris) 67:53A-116A

ASANUMA H, HUNSPERGER W (1975) Functional significance of projection from cerebellar nuclei to the motor cortex in the cat. Brain Res 98:73-92

CIONI M, PERCIAVALLE V, SANTANGELO F, SAPEINZA S, URBANO A (1978) Motor responses to microstimulation of the medullary pyramidal tract in the cat. Exp Neurol 61:664-679

ECCLES JC (1977) The control of movement. In: CLIFFORD R (ed) Physiological aspects of clinical neurology. Blackwell Scientific Publ, London

ECCLES JC, ITO M, SZENTAGOTHAI J (1967) The cerebellum as a neuronal machine. Springer Verlag, Berlin Heidelberg New York

EVARTS VE, THACH TW (1969) Motor mechanisms of the CNS : cerebro-cerebellar interrelations. Ann Rev Physiol 31:451-498

GHEZ C (1975) Input-output relations of the red nucleus in the cat. Brain Res 98:93-108

GIUFFRIDA R, LICATA F, LI VOLSI G, PERCIAVALLE V (in press) Motor responses evoked by microstimulation of cerebellar interpositus nucleus in cats submitted to dorsal rhizotomy. Neurosci Letters

GIUFFRIDA R, LICATA F, LI VOLSI G, PERCIAVALLE V, URBANO A (to be published) Pyramidal input to intracerebellar nuclei of the cat. Neuroscience

GIUFFRIDA R, LI VOLSI G, PANTO MR, PERCIAVALLE V, SAPIENZA S, URBANO A (1980) Single muscle organization of interposito-rubral projections. Exp Brain Res 39:261-267

GIUFFRIDA R, LI VOLSI G, PERCIAVALLE V, SANTANGELO F, URBANO A (1981) Influences of precerebellar systems triggering movement on single cells of the interpositus nucleus of the cat. Neuroscience 6:1615-1631

LICATA F, PERCIAVALLE V, SANTANGELO F, SAPIENZA S, URBANO A (1978) Input-output relationships of interpositus nucleus for single muscles. Neurosci letters (Suppl) 1:S149

LI VOLSI G, PACITTI C, PERCIAVALLE V, SAPIENZA S, URBANO A (in press) Interpositus nucleus influences on pyramidal tract neurons in the cat. Neuroscience

MAC KAY WA, MURPHY JT (1979) Cerebellar modulation of reflex gain. Prog Neurobiol 13:361-417

MASSION J (1973) Intervention des voies cérébello-corticales et cortico-cérébelleuses dans l'organisation et la régulation du mouvement. J Physiol (Paris) 67:117A-170A

OSCARSSON O (1973) Functional organization fo spinocerebellar paths. In: IGGO A (ed) Handbook of sensory physiology. vol II. Somatosensory system. Springer, Berlin Heidelberg New York, pp 339-380

PERCIAVALLE V, SANTANGELO F, SAPIENZA S, SAVOCA F, URBANO A (1977) Motor effects produced by microstimulation of brachium pontis in the cat. Brain Res 126:557-562

PERCIAVALLE V, SANTANGELO F, SAPEINZA S, SAVOCA F, URBANO A (1978a) A ponto-interposito-rubrospinal pathway for single muscle contractions in limbs of the cat. Brain Res 155:124-129

PERCIAVALLE V, SANTANGELO F, SAPIENZA S, SERAPIDE MF, URBANO A (1978b) Dentate nucleus incapability to trigger movement in the cat. Neurosci Letters (Suppl) 1:S152

PERCIAVALLE V, SANTANGELO F, SAPIENZA S, SERAPIDE MF, URBANO A (1978c) Motor responses evoked by microstimulation of restiform body in the cat. Exp Brain Res 33:241-255

PERCIAVALLE V, SANTANGELO F, SAPIENZA S, SERAPIDE MF, URBANO A (1979) Direct afferents to interpositus nucleus responsible for triggering movement. Brain Res 177:367-372

Cortical Addresses of Distal Muscles: A Study in the Conscious Monkey Using the Spike-Triggered Averaging Technique

R.N. Lemon and R.B. Muir

Department of Anatomy II, Medical Faculty Erasmus University Rotterdam P.O. Box 1738, 3000 DR Rotterdam, The Netherlands

INTRODUCTION

LEYTON and SHERRINGTON (1917) demonstrated in primates that surface stimulation of wide areas of the precentral gyrus gave rise to movements of the hand and fingers. Evidence accumulated since then has emphasized the strong link between the motor cortex and the hand. Anatomical and physiological studies have shown that some corticospinal neurones make direct excitatory connections with spinal motoneurones, and that these cortico-motoneuronal connections are strongest with the most distal muscles (for references, see PHILLIPS and PORTER, 1977). Clinical and behavioural evidence has further suggested that these direct connections are essential for the performance of the relatively independent finger movements which underlie the advanced motor repertoire of the primate hand (PENFIELD, 1954 ; LAWRENCE and KUYPERS, 1968).

We have recently been using cross-correlation techniques, developed by FETZ and his colleagues (FETZ and CHENEY, 1980), to identify, in the conscious monkey, corticospinal neurones with direct connections to the motoneurones of the small hand muscles. The behaviour of these corticomotoneuronal cells has then been studied during the performance of hand and finger movements. The clear advantage of this approach is that it gives precise information about the output target of individual corticospinal neurones and thus makes possible a direct study of the output functions of the motor cortex.

METHODS

A monkey (m. nemestrina) was trained to perform a precision grip in which two spring-loaded levers were squeezed between the thumb and index finger of the left hand. The levers, springs and potentiometers to register lever displacements were all enclosed within a box. Two slots cut in the top of this box allowed access to the levers ; the monkey flexed his ulnar fingers while

A

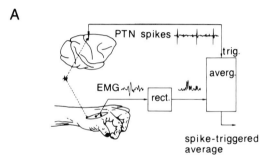

spike-triggered
average

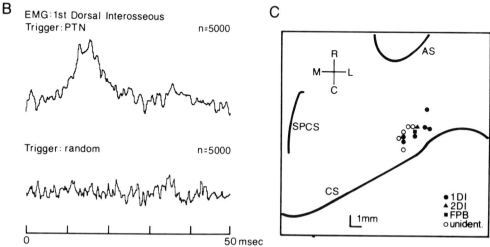

B EMG:1st Dorsal Interosseous
Trigger:PTN   n=5000

Trigger: random   n=5000

0   50 msec

C

Fig. 1.

A. Spike-triggered averaging method : the EMG is fed via a rectifier (rect.) to an averaging computer (averg.) triggered by the discharges of a PTN.

B. Above, the average of 5000 sweeps of rectified EMG from the first dorsal interosseous muscle, each sweep triggered at time zero by a PTN discharge. Below, an average of the same EMG data but triggered by pulses unrelated to the PTN spikes. The PSF in the upper average is clearly greater than the fluctuations in the randomly triggered average.

C. Microelectrode penetrations located on a surface view of the right hemisphere (CS = central sulcus, SPCS = superior precentral sulcus, AS = arcuate sulcus). Filled symbols indicate the muscle with which a PTN in that penetration yielded a PSF. Unfilled circles indicate penetrations in which PTNs yielded no detectable PSF in the muscles sampled

keeping his index finger and thumb extended to reach through the slots to the levers. The monkey had to displace each lever into a narrow target zone (1 mm) ; this required a force of 0.5 - 0.7 N. Each time the monkey kept both levers in the target zones continuously for 1.5 seconds, he received a food reward. When training was complete, the monkey underwent surgery during which a cylinder was placed over the right motor cortex and fine tungsten stimulating electrodes were implanted in the medullary pyramid for antidromic identification of pyramidal tract neurones (PTNs). Following recovery from anaesthesia extracellular recordings were made daily from PTNs in the hand region of the motor cortex. We also recorded gross EMGs from small hand muscles - 1st and 2nd dorsal interossei (1,2DI) ; flexor pollicis brevis (FPB) ; abductor pollicis brevis (AbPB) - and from long forearm muscles acting on the thumb or index finger - extensor digitorum (ED) ; flexor digitorum superficialis (FDS) ; flexor pollicis longus (FPL) and abductor pollicis longus (AbPL) - using surface electrodes or percutaneous wires.

Figure 1A shows the method used for constructing spike-triggered averages of EMG records. Rectified EMG was fed into an averaging computer triggered by the individual spikes from a single PTN. 5000-30,000 spike events were analysed off-line for each average. An example of post-spike facilitation (PSF) seen in the spike-triggered average of IDI is shown in Figure 1B. Confidence that the PSF represents a genuine spike-triggered event was gained by showing that each recorded epoch of PTN spikes and EMG yielded a reproducible PSF (i.e. similar form, amplitude and latency in each epoch). When the average was triggered by a "random" signal, temporally unrelated to the PTN discharge, averages of the same EMG data did not show any fluctuations comparable to the PSF (Fig. 1B).

RESULTS

PSF in small hand muscles. For spike-triggered averaging with EMGs, PTNs were selected which were a) recorded in cortical loci which yielded finger movements with low threshold ($< 20 \mu A$) intracortical microstimulation (ICMS) ; b) "fast" PTNs with antidromic latencies of 0.7 - 2.0 msec and thresholds ranging from 225 - 500 μA (pulse width 0.1 msec) ; c) strongly modulated during performance of the task and d) responsive to natural stimulation of the hand and fingers. We have analysed 23 PTNs satisfying these criteria ; 74 PTN-muscle combinations were studied (45 with forearm muscles and 29 with small hand muscles). Nine combinations showed a clear PSF, 8 of which were with small hand muscles (6 in IDI, 1 in 2DI and I in FPB). In each case, the PSF was clearly present in the average after

Table 1. Details of 8 PTNs yielding post-spike facilitation (PSF) in 3 intrinsic hand muscles. Aff. input : afferent input from digits I-V responding either to joint motion (J) or cutaneous stimulation (C). PSF latency measured from discharge of PTN to foot of PSF response. Rise-time from foot to peak of PSF response. ICMS effects obtained with 13 shocks, 300 Hz 5-20 µA strength. Add=adduction ; Abd=abduction ; Flx=flexion.

PTNs producing PSF in small hand muscles

		Number	1	2	3	4	5	6	7	8
PTN		Depth (mm)	1.5	1.6	1.5	4.1	1.0	1.0	1.5	7.0
		ADL (msec)	0.8	1.2	1.2	0.8	1.5	-	0.9	0.7
		Aff. input I(J)	II,III(J)	IDI	II(C)	I(C)	II(J)	II(C)	II-V(C)	-
PSF		Muscle	IDI	IDI	IDI	IDI	FPB	2DI	1DI	1DI
		Latency (msec)	12.7	9.5	10.8	7.2	7.7	6.6	10.0	14.5
		Rise-time (msec)	1.8	6.6	4.4	3.4	3.8	2.7	0.8	1.1
		% Modulation	13	29	4	6	11	18	7	10
ICM at		Digit	I	II,III	II	I	I	I	II-V	-
PTN locus		Movement	Add	Abd	Abd	Flx	Flx	Flx	Flx	-

3000-5000 PTN spike events had been sampled. Full details of PTNs and resulting PSF are given in Table 1. The PSF latency varied from 6.6 to 14.5 msec, which is consistent with the established characteristics of cortico-motoneuronal connections (LANDGREN et al., 1962 ; MUIR and PORTER, 1976) and comparable with values of 3.5 - 18.0 msec (mean 6.7 msec) reported by FETZ and CHENEY (1980) for PSFs detected in forearm muscles.

The height of the non-facilitated (background) EMG activity was measured in each average, and the incremental height of the PSF expressed as a percentage of this value. Table 1 shows that the PSF contributed by a single PTN could be as large as 29% (the mean value was 13%) of the background. This large excitatory effect is consistent with the findings of CLOUGH et al. (1968) who showed that large EPSPs could be evoked in motoneurones innervating the small hand muscles by stimulation of the motor cortex.

In all cases (except PTN 8, Table 1) when recording from a single PTN was completed, we confirmed the effect of ICMS at the recording site. We also passed single ICMS pulses, 8μA in strength and triggered the averager from the stimulus pulse (cf FETZ and CHENEY, 1978). In some cases a PSF resembling that elicited by the spontaneous spikes could be detected.

Cortical location of PTNs yielding a PSF in a small hand muscle. The 8 PTNs yielding these PSFs were recorded in the microelectrode penetrations marked with filled symbols in Figure 1C. All of these "successful" penetrations passed into the rostral bank of the central sulcus, and two of the PTNs were recorded deep in the bank (see Table 1). It is noticeable that PTNs with excitatory influences on FPB, 1 and 2DI (Table 1, units 5, 2 and 6 respectively) were recorded in closely adjacent tracks at similar depths below the pial surface. It is also interesting that 2 PTNs with a PSF in 1DI were found in penetrations made 3 mm apart. These findings are in keeping with those of ANDERSEN et al. (1975) and JANKOWSKA et al. (1975) who showed that single motoneurones supplying small hand or foot muscles could be excited monosynaptically by stimulation of large cortical territories. The open circles in Figure 1C relate to penetrations in which task-related, fast PTNs were found at loci yielding thumb or index finger movements with low threshold ICMS, but for which no PSF could be detected in the averaged EMG of the small hand muscles that we sampled. Similar "negative" results were found for a further 5 PTNs satisfying our selection criteria (see above) which were recorded in the same penetrations, and within 1 mm of PTNs which did yield a PSF (i.e. these "negative" PTNs were recorded in the penetrations in Figure 1C marked with filled symbols).

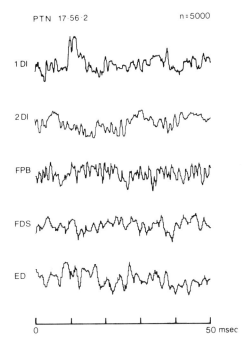

PTN 17·56·2   n=5000

1 DI

2 DI

FPB

FDS

ED

0   50 msec

Fig. 2. Spike-triggered averages of rectified EMG recorded concurrently from 5 different muscles. Each average contains 5000 sweeps triggered by the same PTN spike train. Only first dorsal interosseus yielded a clear PSF. There was no evidence of cross-talk between the EMG records

Distribution of post-spike facilitation. For 5 of the 8 PTNs which yielded a PSF we made simultaneous recordings from at least 5 different muscles (at least 3 small hand muscles). None of these 5 PTNs produced a PSF in more than one muscle. An example is shown in Figure 2 of a PTN (PTN 7 in Table 1) with a PSF in IDI, but with no comparable facilitation in the EMG averaged from 2DI, FPB, FDS or ED. These preliminary observations, suggesting a restricted pattern of projections from PTNs to the small hand muscles must now await further confirmation from a larger sample of PTNs combined with recordings from more muscles than has so far been possible.

PTN synchronisation. FETZ and CHENEY (1980) discussed in detail the possibility that short-term synchronisation of neurones within the cortex could contribute to the PSF averaged with respect to the discharges of a single PTN. The synaptic intricacy of the cortex could allow for such interactions ; two possible sources which have been clearly demonstrated are the recurrent collaterals through which a PTN influences neighbouring cells and the organisation of afferent inputs to the motor cortex which commonly results, for instance, in neighbouring cortical neurones responding to similar forms of natural stimulation (LEMON, 1981).

It remains to be resolved, first, whether such synaptic connectivity actually leads to significant levels of short-term synchronisation of motor cortex PTNs, and secondly, whether such synchronisation has a significant influence on the post-spike facilitation detected by the spike-triggered averaging method. FETZ and CHENEY (1980) have reported the results of cross-correlograms of the activity of 12 pairs of motor cortex PTNs ; only one pair showed an excitatory peak in the correlogram. In contrast, ALLUM et al. (1982) have reported correlations between 11 of 14 pairs of neurones recorded in the hand area of the motor cortex, and active during an isometric precision grip. These neurones were not identified as PTNs. Some of the cross-correlograms showed an excitatory peak at time zero, suggesting a common input to the two neurones.

On 4 occasions we have recorded the activity of two antidromically identified PTNs concurrently on the same electrode, with sufficient difference in spike amplitude to permit separation of the discharges of the two units. For 3 of these pairs, 1 PTN of each pair produced·a PSF in a hand muscle while the other, although also clearly modulated in relation to the task, did not produce a PSF. When tested for their responses to natural stimulation of the monkey's hand and fingers, one PTN of a pair could also show a quite different response from the other, suggesting a lack of common afferent input (LEMON, 1981). When subjected to cross-correlation analysis, none of the 4 pairs has shown an excitatory peak even after analysis of several thousand discharges of the PTNs. It must be stressed, however, that identification and separation of the two different spikes when they occur at, or almost at, the same instant is difficult if not impossible in the face of neural and electrical "noise" and instability in the amplitude and shape of the indivi-dual extracellular action potentials. For this reason we cannot be confident of the reliability of our cross-correlograms within a half-millisecond or so of the time zero. A similar uncertainty must apply to the results of ALLUM et al. (1982).

As to the influence of any such synchronisation, FETZ and CHENEY (1980) have calculated that the effect is likely to be weak, and would only be revealed in the EMG by averaging 20,000 - 60,000 events. If the criteria of KIRKWOOD and SEARS (1982) for determining significance from cross-correlograms are used, the excitatory peaks shown in the cross-correlograms of ALLUM et al.

(1982) suggest that between 0.2 and 6% of the discharges of one cortical neurone can be attributed with confidence to synchronisation with those of another neurone. These relatively small effects could still be significant if large numbers of cortical neurones were synchronised together. Clearly, more detailed studies are necessary to establish the significance of any synchronisation between PTNs, and this really requires unitary recordings with two separate microelectrodes.

Natural activity of PTNs. All of the PTNs producing a PSF in a small hand muscle were strikingly active during exploratory movement of the fingers, and during the fine correcting movements carried out by the monkey to bring the levers into their target zones. None of them showed any modulation of their activity during movements of the ipsilateral hand and fingers. 7 of the 8 PTNs responded reproducibly to natural stimulation of the hand while the monkey was relaxed and passive. All had small afferent input zones ; 3 were excited by movements of the index finger or thumb and 4 responded to brushing the glabrous skin of these digits (see Table 1).

Most (5 of 7) PTNs showed greater activity in relation to a fractionated precision grip between index finger and thumb than for a power grip when all digits flexed in concert, even though the muscle showing the PSF was always the more active during the power grip task. The other 2 PTNs also showed disproportionately more activity, in relation to the level of activity in their target muscles for the precision grip than for the power grip (MUIR and LEMON, in preparation ; LEMON et al., 1982).

This seems to suggest that PTNs projecting directly to the motoneurones of the intrinsic hand muscles are preferentially involved in the elaboration of relatively independent movements of the fingers. The restricted distribution of the PSF from any one corticospinal neurons combined with the specific afferent input to such neurones may well contribute to this important function.

ACKNOWLEDGEMENTS

We thank J. VAN DER BURG, E. DALM, P. VAN ALPHEN, E. KLINK and G. VAN GELDER for technical and secretarial assistance. This reseach was supported by grant 13-46-91 of the FUNGO/ZWO (Dutch Organisation for Fundamental Research in Medicine).

REFERENCES

ALLUM JHJ, HEPP-REYMOND MC, GYSIN R (1982) Cross-correlation analysis of interneuronal connectivity in the motor cortex of the monkey. Brain Res 231:325-334

ANDERSEN P, HAGAN PJ, PHILLIPS CG, POWELL TPS (1975) Mapping by microstimulation of overlapping projections from area 4 to motor units of the baboon's hand. Proc R Soc (Lond) B 188:31-60

CLOUGH JFM, KERNELL D, PHILLIPS CG (1968) The distribution of monosynaptic excitation from the pyramidal tract and from primary spindle afferents to motoneurones of the baboon's hand and forearm. J Physiol (Lond) 198:145-166

FETZ EE, CHENEY PD (1978) Muscle fields of primate corticomotoneuronal cells. J Physiol (Paris) 74:239-245

FETZ EE, CHENEY PD (1980) Post-spike facilitation of forelimb muscle activity by primate corticomotoneuronal cells. J Neurophysiol 44:751-772

JANKOWSKA E, PADEL Y, TANAKA R (1975) Projections of pyramidal tract cells to alpha-motoneurones innervating hind-limb muscles in the monkey. J Physiol (Lond) 249:637-667

KIRKWOOD PA, SEARS TA (1982) The effects of single afferent impulses on the probability of firing of external intercostal motoneurones in the cat. J Physiol (Lond) 322:315-336

LANDGREN S, PHILLIPS CG, PORTER R (1962) Minimal synaptic actions of pyramidal impulses on some alpha motoneurones of the baboon's hand and forearm. J Physiol (Lond) 161:91-111

LAWRENCE DG, KUYPERS HGJM (1968) The functional organization of the motor system in the monkey. I. The effects of bilateral pyramidal lesions. Brain 91:1-14

LEMON RN (1981) Variety of functional organisation within the monkey motor cortex. J Physiol (Lond) 311:521-540

LEMON RN, MUIR RB, GODSCHALK M, KUYPERS HGJM (1982) New data on the control of hand and finger movements in the conscious monkey. In: SPECKMAN EJ, ELGER CE (eds) Epilepsy and motor system. Urban and Schwarzenberg, Munchen, in press

LEYTON ASF, SHERRINGTON CS (1917) Observations on the excitable cortex of the chimpanzee, orang-utan and gorilla. Q Jl exp Physiol 11:135-222

MUIR RB, PORTER R (1976) The characteristics of corticomotoneuronal e.p.s.p.'s in cervical motoneurones of the anaesthetized monkey. Proc Aust physiol pharmacol Soc 7:23P

PENFIELD W (1954) Mechanisms of voluntary movement. Brain 77:1-17

PHILLIPS CG, PORTER R (1977) Corticospinal neurones. Academic Press, London

Comparison of Movement-Related Activity and Receptive Field Properties of Neurons in Primate Motor Cortex

Y. Lamour, H. Solis, and V. A. Jennings

Lab. of Neurophysiology, NIMH, Bethesda, MD 20205, USA

Monkey precentral cortex (MI) can be divided into two distinct regions based on its afferent input : a caudal part which receives predominantly cutaneous inputs and a rostral part which receives predominantly non-cutaneous inputs (STRICK and PRESTON, 1978 ; TANJI and WISE, 1981). We describe in the present report the spatial segregation and functional properties of neurons driven by non-cutaneous and cutaneous inputs in the forelimb representation of MI cortex in a behaving animal.

A monkey was trained to hold a handle and to perform isotonic movements or isometric contractions in the pronating or supinating direction in response to a visual cue. Passive movements (ramps and steps) in either the pronating or supinating direction were applied by a torque motor to the handle during periods of steady holding in both the isotonic and isometric tasks.

Single unit activity was stored on magnetic tape and analyzed offline using a PDP-11 computer. The peripheral receptive fields (RFs) of the units were examined using a variety of cutaneous and non-cutaneous stimuli. Units were accordingly classified as driven by cutaneous or non-cutaneous inputs. Several lesions were made during the last electrode penetrations to aid in the reconstruction of electrode tracks.

Of 613 neurons studied in MI of both hemispheres, 285 were found to be related to the task. RFs were examined for 154 of these neurones ; 53 received cutaneous inputs and 101 non-cutaneous inputs.

Cutaneous units were primarily (49 of 53) confined to the depths of the bank of the central sulcus corresponding to the caudal part of MI (MI/c units) while non-cutaneous units were concentrated in a more rostral MI region (MI/r). Both types tended to occur in clusters of units with similar receptive fields.

Experimental Brain Research, Suppl. 7
© Springer-Verlag Berlin · Heidelberg 1983

Cutaneous units in MI/c were characterized by a lack of sensitivity to the direction of passive movements imposed by the torque motor. These units often displayed a high discharge frequency during passive movements in both supinating and pronating direction. In contrast, non-cutaneous units in MI/r were often selectively sensitive to the direction of passive movements.

A similar lack of directional selectivity was observed for cutaneous units during active isotonic movements and isometric contractions. Cutaneous units were excited (or inhibited in a few cases) in both supinating and pronating directions whereas non-cutaneous units often displayed opposite changes in activity depending on the direction of movement or contraction. Non-cutaneous units also showed different levels of tonic activity depending on the direction of steady torque or the position of the wrist while cutaneous units exhibited mostly phasic activity during active tasks.

The latency of the change in activity following the visual cue triggering active movement was different in the two groups of units. The mean latency was 165 msec for non-cutaneous units and 226 msec for cutaneous units. A majority of non-cutaneous units modified their activity prior to the earliest EMG activity preceding movement (185 msec). In contrast, the activity for most cutaneous units did not change until after the onset of EMG activity.

In conclusion, our results confirm the finding of cutaneous and non-cutaneous regions within MI cortex. More importantly, they reveal striking functional differences between neurons in these two regions. These results provide evidence for the existence of two different functional areas in MI.

REFERENCES

STRICK PL, PRESTON JB (1978) Multiple representation in the primate motor cortex. Brain Res 154:366-370

TANJI J, WISE SP (1981) Submodality distribution in sensorimotor cortex of the unanesthetized monkey. J Neurophysiol 45:467-481

Area 4 Cell Activity During Learning of a New Amplitude of Movement

B. Maton, Y. Burnod, and J. Calvet

Laboratoires de Physiologie du Travail du CNRS et de l'EPHE, CHU Pitié Salpêtrière, 91, bd de l'Hôpital, 75634 Paris Cedex 13, France

INTRODUCTION

Monkeys can learn very precise movements of the arm by a temporal linkage between these movements and a reward. Discharge patterns of Area 4 cortical cells have been extensively studied in such conditioned animals. It has been found that the activity of Area 4 cells is predictive of force or velocity of movement rather than displacement (CHENEY and FETZ, 1980 ; EVARTS, 1968 ; HUMPHREY et al., 1970). However, these patterns of discharge concerned only overtrained animals, and we have shown that the activity of some Area 4 and Area 5 cells may change during operant conditioning (BURNOD et al., 1982). This led us to pose the following questions : are these changes of activity specific of one or another characteristic of the movement ? and, what changes can be expected during learning of a new amplitude of movement ? The answer to this latter question may be of interest in the understanding of both the learning process and the relation between Area 4 cell discharge and amplitude of movement.

METHODS

These experiments were performed on fascicularis macaques. During each experiment the monkey was restrained in a primate chair. The animal was taught to perform flexion movements in a horizontal plane from a constant starting position (50° from the full extension of the elbow) to an arrival angular zone imposed by the conditioning program but not materialized by a visual cue. Two different angular zones of arrival (75° $\pm$ 10° and 105° $\pm$ 10°) were used. As soon as the animal had learned to perform one amplitude of movement, the conditioning program was changed so that the monkey had to perform the other amplitude of movement in .order to be rewarded. Movements were carried out against a constant torque of 1 N.m. A screen prevented the monkey from seeing its rotating forearm and hand. Movements were self-initiated, i.e., there was no start signal. The reward was a small piece of fruit given automatically on a tray in front of the free left hand of the animal. Movement was quantified by recording displacement, velocity and acceleration. The surface elctromyograms of the biceps and triceps brachii were also recorded and integrated. Integrated EMG output was in the form of impulses which are analyzed in the same way as cellular discharges. Unitary activity of motor cortex was recorded by means of platinum microelectrodes. Mean firing rates were computed during successive periods of 3 mn. on 10-20 successive trials with a bin width of 20 msec. These averages were triggered from the onset of the position ramps. Automatic quantification of the relations between cellular activity and movement was obtained by means of a model previously described (BURNOD et al., 1982). Cellular firing frequency and integrated EMG were represented by trapezoids fitted to the perihisto- grams. The values of the plateaus and the time of onset of the ramps relative to onset of movement defined, respectively, the lower level of activity (AB), the higher level (AB + AR) and the latency of activity (DI) (see insert of Fig. 1). Higher level of activity (i.e. AB + AR) will be referred to as peak frequency of discharge (PFD) when applied to cellular activity or peak integrated electromyogram (PIEMG) when applied to muscular activity. Student t test was calculated between AB and AB+AR, and the activity was considered to be tied to the movement when the level of significance of the test was at $p < .001$.

RESULTS

We analyzed the activity of 24 cells whose discharge frequency increased before the onset of active flexion movements and during passive extension movements.

When the frequency of reward increased from the beginning to the end of a conditioning session, as illustrated by Figure 1, the PFD also increased. Nevertheless, there was no point to point correlation between these two parameters. This result was obtained whatever the evolution of the amplitude of the movement. From this point of view it was particularly striking to observe the cell activity while the monkey was learning the small movement after having learned the large one. When the amplitude of the movement decreased, the PFD increased if the frequency of reward increased (Fig. 1).

During the conditioning session the PIEMG did not change in the same way as the PFD. The PIEMG was always strongly correlated with the peak amplitude of the movement.

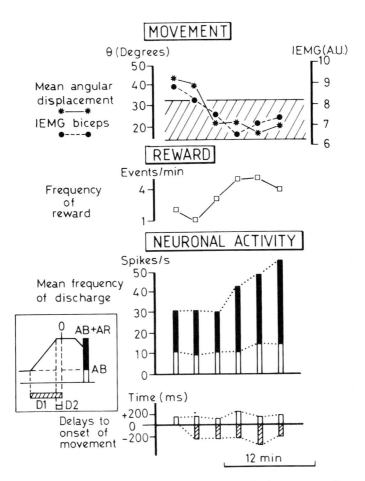

Fig. 1. Evolution of amplitude of movement and frequency of reward and corresponding changes of muscles and cell activities during a conditioning session.
From top to bottom :
Diagram 1 : mean peak amplitude of flexion (degrees) and mean peak amplitude of integrated surface EMG of biceps brachii (IEMG in arbitrary units).
Diagram 2 : mean frequency of reward.
Diagram 3 : mean neuronal peak activity. Open bars indicate the resting level of activity of the cell (AB) and black bars the amount of activity tied to the onset of movement (AR).
Diagram 4 : delay between onset of cell activity and onset of movement (open bars) and between peak of cell activity and onset of movement (hatched bars).
The insert shows the significance of the symbols used in diagrams 3 and 4.
Further explanation in the text

The other question posed by these experiments was, what does the monkey actually learn ? -a final position or an angular displacement ? In some sessions when the animal repeated rewarded movements, we displaced the forearm (20° toward the rewarded zone) prior to the onset of movement and observed the effect upon the following movement. The monkey always failed to reach the rewarded angular zone but achieved a movement of about the same amplitude. Thus, amplitude was the actual parameter which had been learned.

DISCUSSION

In the present experimental conditions (i.e. without any position cue or control of forearm displacement, and without a start signal) amplitude rather than position was the actual parameter which was learned by the monkey. Other studies (POLIT and BIZZI, 1979) have led to the reverse result. This discrepancy can be explained by differences in the experimental conditions, and it stresses that the motor program is mostly adaptative. Thus, the "amplitude" of a movement may be controlled in different ways by Area 4 cell activity.

The main results of this study are the increase of PFD during the learning process and the discrepancy between PFD and PIEMG changes.

The changes of PFD during operant conditioning agree well with the notion of a plasticity of motor cortical cells. This plasticity was evident in the possibilities of reinforcement of particular patterns of discharge as shown, for example, by the experiments of SCHMIDT et al. (1978) or in some other types of conditioning like that used by OLDS et al. (1972). In previous experiments (BURNOD et al., 1982) we have shown that for some Area 4 and Area 5 neurons whose activity was tied either to the movement or to both movement and reward an enhancement of the activity can occur during the shaping of flexion movement. Here it is shown that such a change of activity may occur after the shaping period when a new amplitude of movement is learned even if this amplitude is smaller than the one previously learned. The discrepancy between PFD and PIEMG changes is in agreement with some observations of FROMM and EVARTS (1977). It indicates that the unitary activity of Area 4 is not predictive of the amplitude of the movement due to the constant shift of the PFD during the learning period.

Thus, one may expect that the increase of cell linkage with the movement is a critical factor in conditioning.

SUMMARY

The aim of the present study was to describe how learning of a new amplitude of movement may be due to changes in motor cortex neuronal activity. When the monkey performed repetitively the rewarded movement, a passive displacement of the forearm prior to the onset of the movement led to a movement of quite constant amplitude. Thus, amplitude rather than position was the actual parameter which was learned by the monkey. The peak integrated electromyogram of biceps brachii was strongly correlated with the peak amplitude of the movement. The peak frequency of discharge of most of the cells increased during the learning process as did the frequency of reward, even if the intended movements were smaller than the previously learned one.

REFERENCES

BURNOD Y, MATON B, CALVET J (1982) Neurons in cerebral cortex Area 4 and Area 5 increase their discharge frequency during operant conditioning. Progress in Brain Res 57 (in press)

CHENEY PD, FETZ E (1980) Functional classes of primate corticomotoneuronal cells and their relation to active force. J Neurophysiol 44:773-791

EVARTS EV (1968) Relation of pyramidal tract activity to force exerted during voluntary movement. J Neurophysiol 31:14-27

FROMM C, EVARTS EV (1977) Relation of motor cortex neurons to precisely controlled and ballistic movements. Neurosci Lett 5:259-266

HUMPHREY DR, SCHMIDT EM, THOMPSON W (1970) Predicting measures of motor performance from multiple cortical spike trains. Science 170:758-762

OLDS J, DISTERHOFT JF, SEGAL M, KORNBLITH CL, HIRSH R (1972) Learning centers of rat brain mapped and measuring latencies of conditioned unit responses. J Neurophysiol 35:202-218

POLIT A, BIZZI E (1979) Characteristics of motor programs underlying arm movements in monkeys. J Neurophysiol 42:183-194

SCHMIDT EM, Mc INTOSCH JS, DURELLI L, BAK J (1978) Fine control of operantly conditioned firing patterns of precentral neurons. Exp Neurol 61:340-369

Invertebrate Motor Command During Walking: A Model for the Study of Neuronal Coding

F.Clarac, D.Cattaert, and C.Chasserat

Laboratoire de Neurobiologie Comparée, place Peyneau, 33120 Arcachon, France

Throughout the animal kingdom, the expression of walking behaviour in a single limb involves basically similar kinematics and an alternating pattern of muscular activity in two groups of antagonistic muscles, flexor and extensor, promotor and remotor, which organize each step into two main parts : the return stroke (R.S.) and the power stroke (P.S.). In vertebrates as in invertebrates, there exists the dual role of a central motor program and of proprioceptive and exteroceptive loops interacting with the ongoing movement (GRILLNER, 1975 ; 1981 ; HERMAN et al., 1976).

Invertebrates are particularly suited to locomotion studies due to the relative simplicity of their motor command. In the Decapod Crustacea, for example, only 45 motoneurones innervate an entire walking leg composed of 6 different joints (BEVENGUT, SIMMERS & CLARAC, in prep.).

Although the rock lobster Jasus lalandii possesses 10 legs, it walks on a treadmill using mainly its back legs, particularly the fourth pair. An EMG study of the 2 main antagonistic leg 4 muscles controlling stepping leg movements (promotor and remotor) has been made in conjunction with measurements of the angular excursion of the thoracico-coxal (T-C) joint and the stride length covered by the leg tips (Fig. 1A). Two important extreme positions are defined by the tip of the leg during forward walking : the anterior extreme position (AEP) where the tip touches down onto the belt, corresponding to the onset of the P.S. and the posterior extreme position, (PEP) where the leg tip lifts off the belt corresponding to the onset of the R.S. In each cycle, the relationship between the different parameters recorded allows us to define each stroke more precisely. For example, the onset of the remotor or the promotor discharge always occurs earlier than the onset of the corresponding leg movement ("a" for remotor and "d" for promotor in Fig. 1A). The delay is longer at the end of the P.S. due to inertial forces operating at the time of the change in direction.

Experimental Brain Research, Suppl. 7
© Springer-Verlag Berlin · Heidelberg 1983

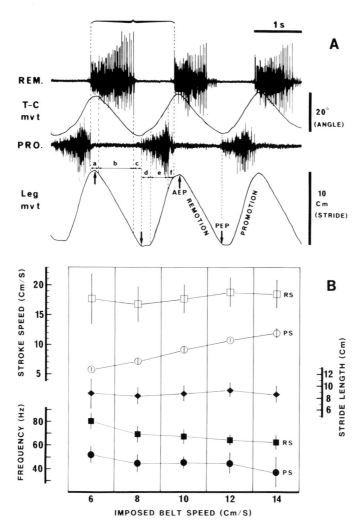

Fig. 1. MOTONEURONAL ACTIVITY DURING WALKING OF THE 4TH LEG OF THE ROCK LOBSTER JASUS LALANDII

(A) 3 consecutive steps monitored by simultaneous recordings of the remotor (rem) and the promotor (pro) EMG's, the thoracico coxal (T-C) joint angle and of the leg movement measured at the tip. The leg movement defines the stride length in cm and indicates the AEP (Anterior Extreme Position) and the PEP (Posterior Extreme Position).

(B) Plots of mean stroke speed (both RS,□ and PS,○), mean stride length (◆——◆) ; mean discharge frequency of a single promotor motoneurone (■) and of a remotor motoneurone (●) all measured at 5 different imposed speeds of a treadmill belt. Each point is the mean value (±SD) over 50 cycles

Due to the very small number of motoneurones innervating the muscles (7 for each) the EMG's in some optimal conditions can display the discharge of a single motoneurone only. In the illustrated record (Fig. 1A), it is clear that the muscular potential of each unit tends to increase in amplitude throughout the ongoing burst corresponding to a marked facilitation in the muscular contraction.

If we systematically change the belt speed from 6cm/s to 14cm/s, the successive steps recorded appear to be characterized by the following (Fig. 1B)

- a stable stride length of about 10 cm/s depending on the size of the animal ; the AEP stays more stable than the PEP.

- a stable promotion time (R.S.). This time is variable from one step to another but shows no clear correlation with the imposed belt speed.

- a remotion time (P.S.) which is strictly inversely proportional to the imposed belt speed.

- the speed ⁄of the promotion movement is always higher than the corresponding remotion even though at slow belt speeds the difference between the two is much greater than at fast belt speeds.

In previous studies (CLARAC, 1982; CLARAC & CRUSE, 1982) these parameters measured during driven walking have been compared to those obtained in free walking ; they are of similar value in those situations where the belt speed corresponds to the free walking range (from 8 to 12 cm/s). However a study of the forces exerted during the P.S. shows that if the belt is at much slower speed than in free conditions, the forces are greater than normal, while at much faster speed they are lower. These changes in forces seem to occur without modification of spatial and temporal parameters and can be explained by the role of the proprioceptors mediating resistance reflexes. These form part of a feedback servo mechanism, the reference input representing the "desired" leg position ; at slow speed a positive error signal increases the force directed posteriorly to ensure that this position is reached. Conversely at fast speeds a negative error signal diminishes the forces.

We have compared the mean burst frequency of a single motor unit of the promotor muscle (R.S.) which moves the leg more or less at constant speed during driven walking, to that of a motoneurone muscle (P.S.) moving the leg at the imposed belt speed (Fig. 1B). The mean burst frequency (60 to 80 Hz) of the promotor unit is of higher value than the remotor unit (35 to 55 Hz). Both units show analogous changes in mean discharge frequency with belt speed ; it is maximum at the slowest belt speed and minimum at the fastest one. At driven speeds analogous to free walking speeds the frequency does not change significantly (between 8 to 12 cm/s). At first approximation, despite the great difference in discharge frequency between the 2 units, it does not seem that these motoneurones are coding the walking speed. But rather, it appears that the frequency is more correlated with the forces exerted (CLARAC & CRUSE, 1982). This absence of correlation between the motor unit burst frequency and the walking speed has already been described in other Crustacea (AYERS & CLARAC, 1978), in insects (BURNS & USHERWOOD, 1979) and in cats (ZAJAC, 1981) ; in decerebrate cat walking above a treadmill, identified motoneurones do not change their discharge frequency with the speed of walking elicited by repetitive stimulation of the mesencephalon.

Two other factors appear to be involved in coding the walking motor program in Crustacea : the number of motoneurones recruited and the patterning of motoneurone bursting in relation to the muscular properties. Further experiments are planned to test these two parameters. In conclusion, this preliminary report serves to demonstrate that the preparation "a rock lobster on a treadmill" provides a suitable model in our attempts to understand how neuronal circuitry can organize the different aspect of motor coding during locomotion.

REFERENCES

AYERS JL, CLARAC F (1978) Neuromuscular strategies underlying different behavioral acts in a multifunctional crustacean leg joint. J comp Physiol 128:81-94

BURNS MD, USHERWOOD PNR (1979) The control of walking in Orthoptera II motor neurone activity in normal free walking animals. J Exp Biol 79:69-98

CLARAC F (1982) Decapod crustacean leg coordination during walking. In: HERREID CF, FOURTNER C (eds) Locomotion and energetics in Arthropods. Plenum Press, New York and London, pp 31-71

CLARAC F, CRUSE H (1982) Comparison of forces developped by the legs of the rock lobster when walking free or on a treadmill. Biol cybern 43:109-114

GRILLNER S (1975) Locomotion in vertebrates, central mechanism and reflex interaction. Physiol Rev 55:247-304

GRILLNER S (1981) Control of locomotion in bipeds, tetrapods and fish. In: BROOKS VB (ed) Handbook of Physiology. Motor Control, Section I, vol II. Williams & Wilkins, Baltimore

HERMAN M, GRILLNER S, STEIN PSG, STUART G (1976) Neural control of locomotion. Plenum Press, New York and London, 822 p

ZAJAC FE (1981) Recruitment and rate modulation of motor units during locomotion. In: DESMEDT JE (ed) Neurophysiology. Karger, Basel (Prog Clin, vol 9 pp 149-160)

Coding of Motor Performance

Muscle Spindle Contribution to the Coding of Motor Activities in Man

J.P. Vedel and J.P. Roll*

C.N.R.S., INP 4, B.P. 71, 13277 Marseille Cedex 9, France
* Laboratoire de Psychophysiologie, Centre St Jérôme, 13397 Marseille Cedex 4, France

INTRODUCTION

The contribution of muscle afferents to the conscious perception of movement and joint position has long been a matter of controversy.

Despite the fact that the discovery by AMASSIAN and BERLIN (1958) that muscle afferent messages project to the cortex has been confirmed by many subsequent authors (OSCARSSON and ROSEN, 1963 ; ALBE-FESSARD and LIEBESKIND, 1966 ; LANDGREN and SILFVENIUS, 1966 ; PHILLIPS et al., 1971), kinaesthesia has nevertheless been classically attributed to joint afferents (BOYD and ROBERTS, 1953 ; ROSE and MOUNTCASTLE, 1959 ; MERTON, 1972 ; SKOGLUND, 1973) or to corollary discharge (SPERRY, 1950 ; von HOLST, 1954).

In 1972 both EKLUND and GOODWIN et al. made observations on the effects of mechanical vibration of tendons which provided an important argument in favour of a contribution to kinaesthesia by muscle, particularly muscle spindle afferents ; their sensitivity to vibratory stimuli had already been demonstrated in animal experiments (BIANCONI and VAN DER MEULEN, 1963 ; BROWN et al., 1967). The first mentioned authors showed that apart from the elicitation of reflex motor activity (tonic vibration reflex, HAGBARTH and EKLUND, 1966 ; DE GAIL et al., 1966), this type of stimulation produces illusory sensations of movement in man. When applied to the tendon of biceps or triceps in a subject unable to see the stimulated arm, vibration elicits a sense of movement in a direction which corresponds to that of a real movement lengthening the vibrated muscle.

The absence of kinaesthetic effects following vibration of bony structures close to tendons (ROLL and VEDEL, 1982) underlines the predominance of muscle afferents in the appearance of this phenomenon. Similarly, MATTHEWS and SIMMONDS (1974) have demonstrated that pulling directly on the tendons of conscious human subjects induces sensations of movement. Finally, neither local anaesthesia nor surgical destruction of articular afferents has any profound effect on position sense (GOODWIN et al., 1972 ; cf. MATTHEWS, 1977) and on vibration induced illusory movements (ROLL, 1981).

Following such observations, it seemed interesting to determine the characteristics of muscle afferent contribution to the encoding of movement by analysing the parameters of both vibration and perceived movement. Demonstration of such a relationship would argue in favour of a quantitative contribution of muscle afferents to kinaesthesia.

By recording single sensory fibres in man it was also possible to determine the sensitivity of different receptors to vibration when various experimental manoeuvres were carried out on the muscle in order to attempt to define the origin and organization of peripheral nerve patterns induced by vibration and responsible for illusory sensations of movement.

Relationship between velocity of illusory movement and frequency of tendon vibration

Vibration was applied selectively to the tendon of biceps, or alternatively to the tendons of biceps and triceps in the mechanically immobilised arm (Fig.1A,A') by an electromagnetic vibrator. The vibration amplitude, which was kept constant throughout each individual experiment, could be varied between 0.2 and 0.5mm. In the absence of visualisation of the stimulated arm, the subjects were asked to reproduce the perceived movement with the other arm ; this was recorded by a potentiometric system (Fig.1B,B'). Bursts of vibration at constant frequency (between 10 and 120 Hz) were applied several times in pseudorandom order.

In all subjects, vibration of the biceps tendon elicited a sensation of forearm extension whose perceived velocity increased as a function of the vibration frequency up to 60-80 Hz (Fig.1C). Above this frequency the apparent velocity decreased progressively until the sensation of movement disappeared. The same phenomenon of increased followed by decreased velocity of illusory movement was observed following vibration of the triceps tendon, except that in this case the illusory movement was one of forearm flexion (ROLL, 1981 ; ROLL and VEDEL, 1982).

Vibration trains of identical frequency applied alternately to biceps and triceps induced a sensation of alternate extension and flexion (Fig.1B'). As

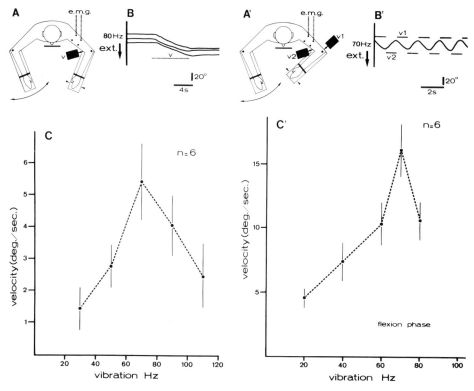

Fig. 1. Quantitative study of illusory movements induced by tendon vibration of Biceps and Triceps in Man.

A-A'. Experimental arrangement for stimulation of a single muscle (A) or of two antagonistic muscles (A'). The elbow joint is mechanically immobilised on the stimulated side.

B-B'. Simulation by the subject's non-vibrated arm of the illusory movements perceived during 80 Hz vibration of biceps (B) and 70 Hz alternating vibration of biceps and triceps (B').

C. Relationship between velocity of perceived extension and vibration frequency of biceps. Mean values obtained from 6 subjects : each point represents 18 trials. Confidence limits calculated at 5%.

C'. Relationship between velocity of perceived flexion and vibration frequency applied alternately to biceps and triceps tendons. Each point represents the mean of 24 trials performed by 6 subjects. Confidence limits of the means have been calculated at 1%

above, the velocity of perceived movement increased linearly with vibration frequency up to a mean value of 70 Hz, then declined progressively (Fig.1C'). On comparing curves C and C' in Figure 1, it may be noted that the maximal perceived velocity in the case of alternate vibration is some three times more rapid than in the case of vibration of a single muscle. However, the maximal attainable apparent velocity, even in the case of alternating stimulation, is relatively slow, the highest speed reached being of the order of 15° per second.

Vibration sensitivity of receptors recorded by microneurography

Using the microneurography technique (HAGBARTH and VALLBO, 1968) on afferent fibres in the anterior compartment of the leg and the dorsal aspect of the foot, the effects of vibration were tested on various classes of receptor. Nerve activity was recorded with tungsten microelectrodes having a resistance between 500kohms and 1Mohms, manually inserted through the skin into the lateral popliteal nerve at the level of the popliteal fossa. In the experiments, the foot of the seated subject was placed on a pedal by means of which voluntary movements could be recorded and also, by using a motor, through which passive movements of varying amplitude and velocity could be imposed. The parameters of ankle movement were recorded potentiometrically. Mechanoreceptors, shown by classical criteria to be muscle spindle primary endings in the tibialis anterior or extensor digitorum longus, were the most sensitive to vibration of the corresponding tendon. These receptors were able to follow high frequencies of vibration (up to 120 Hz) one-for-one, the maximal discharge rate being different for each sensory unit. When they ceased to respond harmonically to vibration, they continued either to do so at subharmonic frequency, or discharged in random fashion. The responses of seven units, considered to be primary endings, to vibratory stimulation are illustrated in Figure 2A. The results confirm those of BURKE et al. (1976a), with the exception that, unlike these authors, we were unable to activate primary endings by vibration of antagonist muscle tendons. This was probably due to the low amplitude of vibration used in our experiments.

Golgi tendon organs also proved sensitive to vibration, but could not follow such high frequencies of stimulation as the primary endings. As noted by BURKE et al. (1976a), it seemed that the degree of tension of the muscle was a determining factor in fixing the extent of sensitivity to tendon vibration.

Muscle afferents identified as muscle spindle secondary endings seemed to show very little if any sensitivity to vibration over the whole range of amplitude (0.2 to 0.5mm.). BURKE et al. (1976a) mentioned the possibility of secondary spindle activation by vibratory stimulation of the tendon, but with an amplitude of 1.5mm.

Many foreleg and foot mechanoreceptors identified as slowly adapting pressure receptors exhibited high sensitivity to vibration, some being able to follow one-for-one up to some 200 Hz. This sensitivity however only became apparent if the head of the vibrator was placed exactly over the receptor site. Similar observations were made on rapidly adapting cutaneous receptors. Under these conditions it may be considered that these two categories of receptor are not concerned with the response to tendon vibration (ROLL and VEDEL, 1982) unless their localisation happens to coincide with the point of application of the stimulus.

Possibility of movement parameters being encoded by the proprioception of the stretched muscle

In animals, the relationship between spindle discharge and muscle length, as well as rate of change of length, is well established (cf. MATTHEWS, 1972). But in order to establish the encoding of movement by these proprioceptors it would be necessary to find a relationship between their discharge rate and the parameters of joint movement. In man, systematic study of primary ending response to plantar flexion of the ankle imposed at constant velocity, and to movements of sinusoidal type (alternating plantar and dorsiflexion) has shown that receptors in the stretched muscle respond throughout the movement by a plateau discharge whose almost constant frequency increases only very slightly between the beginning and end of movement (ROLL and VEDEL, 1982). On this point, it seems that in animals this change in frequency is much more marked when the muscle is stretched directly (cf. MATTHEWS 1972). In man, the mean frequency of spindle discharge calculated throughout a movement in-creased directly with the velocity of angular rotation of the joint ; the extent of increase was very variable as between units (Fig.2B). As has been shown for the dynamic index in animal (BROWN et al., 1965), the mean frequency for the duration of movement seems therefore to express the dynamic sensitivity of the receptor (ROLL and VEDEL, 1982). In man, this type of plateau response of primary endings has been observed both during voluntary movement and during passive movement in the stretched muscle.

During joint movement the discharge of secondary endings increases progressi-vely, the maximal frequency reached at the end of movement rising with the velocity of joint rotation (ROLL and VEDEL, 1982). This feature of secondary

258

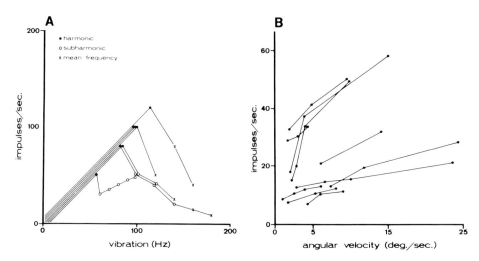

Fig. 2. Human microneurographic muscle spindle responses to tendon vibration (A) and joint movements (B).

A. Responses of 7 muscle spindle primary endings in Tibialis anterior and Extensor digitorum longus at different vibration frequencies. One- for-one responses are shown by solid circles, subharmonic responses by open circles, and random discharges unrelated to vibration frequency by crosses.

B. Relationship between discharge frequency of 10 primary endings in Tibialis anterior and angular velocity of ankle plantar flexion (amplitude 12°). Each point corresponds to the mean frequency of spindle discharge calculated throughout the duration of movement

discharge suggests a more definite relationship both with position and with rate of change of position of the joint than is the case for primary endings during movement.

By virtue of their origin (stretched muscle, i.e. antagonistic muscle) it is evident that muscle afferents yield information on the direction of movement and although it appears to be relatively weak in man (VALLBO, 1974), the static sensitivity of spindle sensory endings nevertheless seems able to encode joint position.

Influence of tendon vibration on primary ending responses to lengthening and shortening of muscle

The application of tendon vibration in man during joint movement has revealed a clear predominance of primary ending response to vibration during muscle lengthening.

During maintenance of a fixed position or during angular movement, tendon vibration at approximately the same frequency as the spindle discharge produces interference between nervous impulses generated by the two types of stimulus. This results in an increase in spindle discharge rate, characterised by large variations in interspike intervals. The tonic discharge, like the phasic, thus appears to be less characteristic of the position and rate of movement of the joint than in the absence of vibration. If the frequency of tendon vibration is above the maximal discharge rate of the primary endings during a given movement, there is complete masking of the spindle response to lengthening and shortening of the muscle by the response to vibration ; this is illustrated in Figure 3. Under these conditions, the response obtained corresponds one-for-one to the vibration frequency, as shown by MATTHEWS and WATSON (1981) in experimental animals during sinusoidal stretching of muscle. This is particularly noteworthy in view of the fact that the illusory movement induced by tendon vibration is increased if a slight rotation in the same direction as the illusory movement is imposed upon the joint. Under these conditions the increase in the perceived sensation is not therefore a consequence of summation of lengthening and vibratory responses, but could be attributed to the greater effectiveness of vibratory stimulation following lengthening of the vibrated muscle (BURKE et al., 1976a). In animals (EMONET-DENAND et al., 1980) it appears that the spindle response to low amplitude stretching increases with the length of the muscle.

It has been shown in man that voluntary isometric muscle contraction is capable of increasing the activity of primary endings (VALLBO, 1970 ; BURKE et al., 1978). This phenomenon, illustrated in Figure 4B, is attributed to fusimotor activation of proprioceptors, and according to BURKE et al. (1976b) has the effect of reinforcing the spindle response to tendon vibration. It may be noted that under these conditions the sensation of movement elicited by vibration is weak or even absent (GOODWIN et al., 1972 ; ROLL, 1981).

In addition to an illusion of movement, vibration applied to tendons can also produce muscle contraction (tonic vibration reflex). When it occurs, this phenomenon usually induces, contrary to what happens on voluntary contraction, a diminution of primary spindle responses to tendon vibration (compare Fig. 4A and 4C). In these circumstances the primary endings generally tend to discharge at a frequency which is a subharmonic of the vibration frequency (Fig. 4C : BURKE et al., 1976b). This kind of effect could explain why illusory movements are less well perceived when tendon vibration also produces simultaneous reflex muscle contraction.

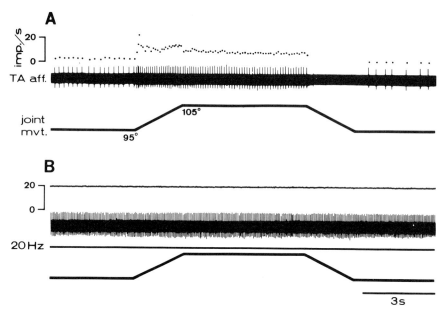

Fig. 3. Influence of 20 Hz vibration of Tibialis anterior tendon on response of a muscle spindle primary ending to 10° plantar flexion and dorsiflexion of ankle.

A. Response of spindle to joint movement in the absence of vibration.

B. Complete masking of spindle response to joint movement by response to tendon vibration at 20 Hz

DISCUSSION

Tendon vibration may be considered as an effective means of activating muscle receptors, particularly muscle spindles. The fact that such stimuli elicit an illusion of movement confers an important role in the conscious perception of movement on these afferents. This function is additional to their reflex activity, which has been studied for many years. The demonstration of a relationship between the parameters of the vibratory stimulus and those of movement sensation suggest further that muscle proprioception could be the source of the quantitative perception of several parameters of movement such as direction, velocity, and amplitude.

Microneurography has made it possible, in man, to demonstrate that corticipetal impulses exhibit, from their point of peripheral origin, information related to the characteristics of a movement performed, at least so far as relatively slow movements are concerned. In this context, a muscle lengthened

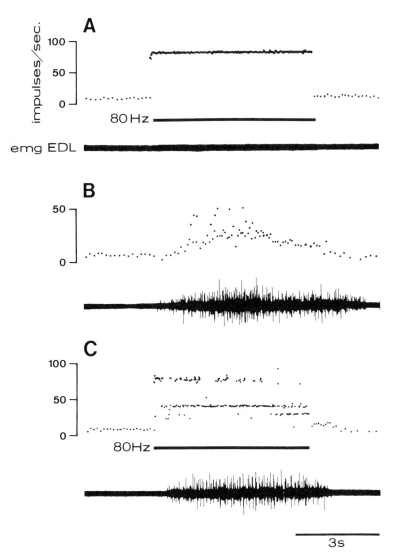

Fig. 4. Responses of a muscle spindle primary ending in Extensor digitorum longus to various parameters of tendon vibration and muscle contraction.

A. One-for-one response to tendon vibration at 80 Hz.

B. Increase of spindle discharge frequency by voluntary isometric contraction of muscle.

C. Diminution of spindle response to vibratory stimulation of tendon in the presence of tonic vibration reflex as a result of movement at a joint takes on particular importance because it is the source of the proprioceptive information which most constantly and representatively characterises the various parameters of movement, whether the latter be voluntarily performed by the subject or passively imposed (ROLL and VEDEL, 1982).

Only the publication of FERREL (1980) attributes the possible encoding of movement to articular receptors, while BURGESS and CLARK (1969) and GRIGG (1975) consider that they only discharge at the extreme positions of joints.

Rather than continue the polemic about the primacy of either articular or muscle receptors in kinaesthesia, it is more profitable, like GARDNER and COSTANZO (1981), to consider that the conscious sense of movement and joint position is due to the concerted activity of the two types of afferent.

Recent work by GARDNER and COSTANZO (1981 ; COSTANZO and GARDNER, 1981) has demonstrated, in the monkey, that unit activity in the somatosensory cortex evoked by joint movement shows considerable analogy in some instances with peripheral proprioceptive messages such as those vehiculated by both muscle spindles and articular receptors. This would appear to indicate that at first sensory information is received at the cortical level with its almost original content before being modified by structures concerned with multisensory integration.

The results concerning the kinesthetic illusions obtained by tendon vibration can be validated by microneurography, which reveals the sensory mechanisms activated by vibration. Microneurography also demonstrates some of the limitations of receptor activation by tendon vibration by revealing the modification of sensory information which occurs when tendon stimulation is applied during activity which is itself capable of modulating muscle afferents. The effects observed in these conditions facilitate the definition of the content of afferent information in various experimental situations and so make it possible better to formulate conclusions or functional hypotheses about illusory movements and the mechanisms responsible for them.

Finally, the exact analysis by microneurography in man of the information contained in peripheral afferent messages of proprioceptive origin and their relationship to kinaesthetic sensation seems to be a useful way to approach an understanding of the nervous mechanisms which underlie the encoding of motor activity.

SUMMARY

In subjects unable to see their forearm, vibration of the biceps or triceps tendon induces an illusory sensation of elbow movement. The perceived direction of movement corresponds to that of a real movement stretching the vibrated muscle. Alternating vibration of biceps and triceps by trains of identical frequency produces sensations of alternating extension and flexion of the forearm.

Successive application of vibration trains from 10 to 120 Hz produce increasing velocity of illusory movement up to 70-80 Hz, but decreasing velocity from 80 to 120 Hz. The maximal perceived velocity is highest when alternating vibration is applied to biceps and triceps.

Microneurographic recording of proprioceptive afferent activity in the tibialis anterior and extensor digitorum longus has shown that, at low amplitude (0.2 to 0.5 mm.), muscle spindle primary endings and Golgi tendon organs are the most sensitive to vibratory stimuli. The secondary endings are only slightly or not at all sensitive to such vibration ; some cutaneous receptors and pressure receptors are able to respond intensely to this type of stimulus, on condition that it is applied directly over the receptor site.

Analysis of primary ending responses to dorsiflexion and plantar flexion of the ankle shows that the discharge of these proprioceptors is able to encode the parameters of the joint movements. Depending on its frequency, tendon vibration can completely mask the response of primary endings to the stretching and relaxation of muscles. When tendon vibration produces reflex muscle contraction (tonic vibration reflex) the response rate of primary endings is reduced.

The results obtained from microneurography are discussed in relation to the characteristics and manner of appearance of illusory movements induced by tendon vibration.

ACKNOWLEDGEMENT

This work was supported by Fondation pour la recherche médicale française grant.

REFERENCES

ALBE-FESSARD D, LIEBESKIND J (1966) Origine des messages somatosensitifs activant les cellules du cortex moteur chez le singe. Exp Brain Res 1:127-146

AMASSIAN VE, BERLIN L (1958) Early cortical projection of group I afferents in the forelimb muscle nerves of cat. J Physiol (Lond) 143:61P

BIANCONI R, VAN DER MEULEN JP (1963) The response to vibration of the end-organs of mammalian muscle spindles. J Neurophysiol 26:177-190

BOYD IA, ROBERTS TDM (1953) Proprioceptive discharges from stretch receptors in the knee-joint of the cat. J Physiol (Lond) 122:38-58

BROWN MC, CROWE A, MATTHEWS PBC (1965) Observations on the fusimotor fibres of the tibialis posterior muscle of the cat. J Physiol (Lond) 177:140-159

BROWN MC, ENGBERG I, MATTHEWS PBC (1967) The relative sensitivity to vibration of muscle receptors of the cat. J Physiol (Lond) 192:773-800

BURGESS PR, CLARK FJ (1969) Characteristics of knee joint receptors in the cat. J Physiol (Lond) 203:301-315

BURKE D, HAGBARTH KE, SKUSE NF (1978) Recruitment order of human spindle endings in isometric voluntary contractions. J Physiol (Lond) 285:101-112

BURKE D, HAGBARTH KE, LOFSTEDT L, WALLIN BG (1976a) The response of human muscle spindle endings to vibration of non-contracting muscle. J Physiol (Lond) 261:673-693

BURKE D, HAGBARTH KE, LOFSTEDT L, WALLIN BG (1976b) The response of human muscle spindle endings to vibration during isometric contraction. J Physiol (Lond) 261:695-711

COSTANZO RM, GARDNER EP (1981) Multiple-joint neurons in somatosensory cortex of awake monkeys. Brain Res 214:321-333

DE GAIL P, LANCE JW, NEILSON PD (1966) Differential effects on tonic and phasic reflex mechanisms produced by vibration of muscles in man. J Neurol Neurosurg Psychiat 29:1-11

EKLUND G (1972) Position sense and state of contraction ; the effects of vibration. J Neurol Neurosurg Psychiat 35:606-611

EMONET-DENAND F, LAPORTE Y, TRISTANT A (1980) Modifications du décours temporel des réponses de terminaisons fusoriales primaires à de petites variations périodiques de longueur produites par un allongement musculaire lent. C R Acad Sc Paris 291:349-351

FERRELL WR (1980) The adequacy of stretch receptors in the cat knee joint for signalling joint angles throughout a full range of movement. J Physiol (Lond) 299:85-99

GARDNER EP, COSTANZO RM (1981) Properties of kinesthetic neurons in somatosensory cortex of awake monkeys. Brain Res 214:301-319

GODDWIN GM, McCLOSKEY DI, MATTHEWS PBC (1972) The contribution of muscle afferents to kinaesthesia shown by vibration induced illusion of movement and by the effects of paralysing joint afferents. Brain 95:705-748

GRIGG P (1975) Mechanical factors influencing the response of joint afferents neurons from the cat knee. J Neurophysiol 38:1473-1484

HAGBARTH KE, EKLUND G (1966) Motor effects of vibratory muscle stimuli in man. In: GRANIT R (ed) Muscular afferents and motor control. Almqvist and Wiksell, Stockholm, 177-186

HAGBARTH KE, VALLBO AB (1968) Discharge characteristics of human muscle afferents during stretch and contraction. Exp Neurol 22:674-694

HOLST E von (1954) Relations between the central nervous system and the peripheral organs. Br J Anim Behav 2:89-94

LANDGREN S, SILFVENIUS N (1969) Projection to cerebral cortex of group I muscle afferents from cat's hind-limb. J Physiol (Lond) 200:353-372

MATTHEWS PBC (1972) Mammalian muscle receptor and their central action. Edward Arnold LTD, London, pp 630

MATTHEWS PBC (1977) Muscle afferents and kianesthesia. Brit Med Bull 33:137-142

MATTHEWS PBC, SIMMONDS A (1974) Sensations of finger movement elicited by pulling upon flexor tendons in man. J Physiol (Lond) 239:27-28P

MATTHEWS PBC, WATSON JDG (1981) Action of vibration on the response of cat muscle spindle Ia afferents to low frequency sinusoidal stretching. J Physiol (Lond) 317:365-381

MERTON PA (1972) How we control the contraction of our muscles. Sci Am 226:30-37

OSCARSSON O, ROSEN I (1963) Projection to cerebral cortex of large muscle spindle afferents in forelimb nerves of the cat. J Physiol (Lond) 169:924-945

PHILLIPS CG, POWELL TPS, WIESENDANGER M (1971) Projection from low threshold muscle afferents of hand and forearm to area 3a of Baboon's cortex. J Physiol (Lond) 217:419-446

ROLL JP (1981) Contribution de la proprioception musculaire à la perception et au contrôle du mouvement chez l'homme. Thèse de Doctorat ès-Sciences, Université d'Aix-Marseille I, pp 400

ROLL JP, VEDEL JP (1982) Kinaesthetic role of muscle afferents in man, studied by tendon vibration and microneurography. Exp Brain Res 47:177-190

ROSE JE, MOUNTCASTLE VB (1959) Touch and kinesthesis. In: FIELD J (ed) Handbook of Physiology, vol. 1. Pentland, Edinburg and London, 387-429

SKOGLUND S (1973) Joint receptors and kinaesthesis. In: IGGO A (ed) Handbook of sensory physiology, vol. 2. Springer, New-York, 111-136

SPERRY RW (1950) Neural basis of the spontaneous optokinetic response produced by visual neural inversion. J comp Physiol Psychol 43:482-489

VALLBO AB (1970) Discharge patterns in human muscle spindle afferents during isometric voluntary contraction. Acta physiol Scand 80:552-566

VALLBO AB (1974) Afferent discharge from human muscle spindles in non-contracting muscles. Steady state impulse frequency as a function of joint angle. Acta physiol Scand 90:303-318

After-Effects of Fusimotor Activity: Long-Lasting Enhancement of the Dynamic Sensitivity of IA Muscle Spindle Afferents Following Stimulation of Dynamic or Static Gamma-Axons

T.K.Baumann, F.Emonet-Denand, and M.Hulliger

Brain Research Institute, University of Zürich, CH-8029 Zürich, and Laboratoire de Neurophysiologie, Collège de France, F-75231 Paris

INTRODUCTION

When fusimotor neurones are activated at high stimulation rates both the onset and termination of their effects on spindle afferents are nearly instantaneous (see e.g. HULLIGER, 1979). Yet, after-effects of fusimotor activity have also been observed. Long lasting stimulation of fusimotor neurones, particularly at high rates, is often followed by a depression of afferent discharge. In contrast, under some conditions the spindle may also be left in a heightened state of responsiveness after stimulation. At constant muscle length the mean discharge rate may be increased above the level of resting discharge prior to stimulation (KUFFLER, HUNT & QUILLIAM, 1951). Also, the initial response at the beginning of a fast stretch ('initial burst') may be augmented after stimulation of either static or dynamic gamma-motoneurones (BROWN, GOODWIN & MATTHEWS, 1969). These effects were of interest for considerations of receptor mechanisms, but their functional significance seemed obscure. However, in recent studies on spindle sensitivity to small disturbances during movements of large amplitude (BAUMANN, EMONET-DENAND & HULLIGER, 1982) we encountered sizable and long-lasting after-effects of fusimotor stimulation, which are likely to be important functionally (see below). These after-effects manifested themselves as an increase in the dynamic response of primary spindle afferents to sinusoidal stretches, which were superimposed on larger triangular movements. Such sensitivity enhancing after-effects were observed following stimulation of dynamic and, remarkably, also static gamma-fibres.

METHODS

The experiments were performed on the soleus muscle of cats anaesthetized with Nembutal. Standard methods were used throughout the experiment (see Baumann et al, 1982). Briefly, gamma-motoneurones were classified conventionally as static or dynamic by their decreasing or increasing effect on the dynamic response of Ia afferents to ramp stretches, using high stimulation rates (70 to 100/s). The responses of these afferents to combined sinusoidal (1 to 4 Hz, up to 0.5 mm half peak to peak amplitude) and slow triangular (2.5 to 4 mm at 0.8 to 6.4 mm/s) stretches were then investigated. Single gamma-fibres were stimulated at low rates (mostly between 15 and 50/s) either at short resting length or during various phases of the triangular movement. The occurrence of after-effects was assessed by comparing post-stimulation responses with pre-stimulation passive controls (see Fig. 2, bottom diagram, also Baumann et al., 1982).

RESULTS

Stimulation at resting length

The responses of primary spindle afferents to ongoing sinusoidal stretches were augmented - compared with passive controls - subsequent to low rate gamma-stimulation at resting length. This was true after stimulation of both dynamic and static (Fig. 1) fusimotor neurones. For sinusoidal oscillations at the same mean length, immediately after stimulation in Figure 1, such enhancement of the dynamic response was moderate and not always manifest. However, it was very pronounced during the lengthening phase of a subsequent slow triangular stretch, but not during the shortening phase (Fig. 1). Also, provided the triangular stretch was in excess of 2 mm (half peak to peak), the enhancement of sinusoidal response was no longer present during the later triangular movements. The duration and the precise timing of stimulation prior to the first triangular movements were not important. The after-effects could be elicited by gamma-stimulation during less than one second. Moreover, as long as no large movements were interspersed, the after-effects following gamma-stimulation during a shortening movement and at resting length persisted throughout the periods tested (up to two minutes). However, the after-effects seen as sensitization of the spindle afferents, were consistently abolished by a single stretch of large amplitude.

Stimulation during movement

When gamma-motoneurones were stimulated, at similarly low rates, during ongoing triangular movements of large amplitude the responses to superimposed sinusoids were also enhanced (compared with the passive controls) during the first, but not during the subsequent triangle cycles following the termination of stimulation. Again the after-effects were pronounced during the

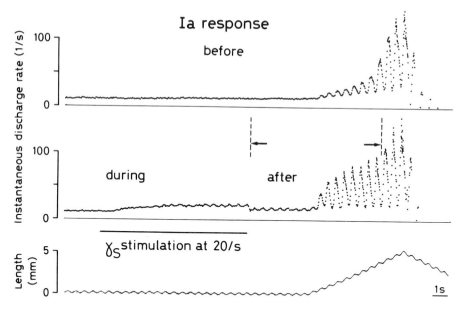

Fig. 1. Sensitivity-enhancing after-effects following low rate stimulation (20/s) of a static gamma-fibre at resting length (0 mm, corresponding to ankle joint angle of 90 deg.). Traces of instantaneous frequency of IA discharge. Top, passive control response of IA afferent. Middle, stimulation and after-effects (arrows) in IA response to sinusoidal stretches at short resting length and during large triangle stretch. Bottom, time course of muscle stretch (length record, retouched)

lengthening and absent during the shortening phase of the slow triangular movement. As with stimulation at resting length such effects were elicited by stimulation of both static and dynamic gamma-fibres.

Further analysis concerning the optimal timing of stimulation relative to the triangular movement cycle showed that the sensitivity enhancing after-effects were readily provoked by stimulation during the shortening phase of the preceding triangle. An example is illustrated in Figure 2, where the timing of stimulation is schematically illustrated in the bottom diagram. After-effects following stimulation of a static gamma-axon at 30/s during muscle shortening (Fig. 2D) are marked in F (arrows). The comparison with the passive controls (B) indicates that the sensitivity for the sinusoidal component of the movement was clearly enhanced at short and intermediate muscle length (0 mm relative muscle length corresponding to an ankle joint

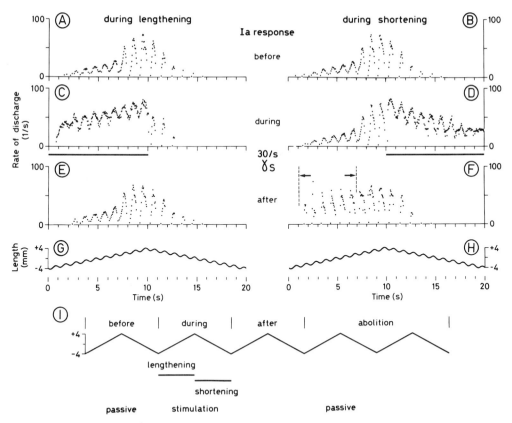

Fig. 2. Sensitivity-enhancing after-effects in separate IA response to sinusoidal stretches, subsequent to static gamma-stimulation during triangular
movement. F, manifestation of after-effects (arrows) during the triangular
extension phase, following stimulation during shortening (D). E, absence of
after-effects following stimulation during extension phase of preceding
triangle movement (C). A and B, passive control responses. A through F,
single sweep average frequency histograms. G and H, schematic illustration of
the time course of muscle stretch. I, overall test sequence with passive
control ('before'), stimulation cycle ('during'), after-effect cycle
('after'), and final passive response cycles ('abolition'). (From BAUMANN et
al. (1982), modified)

angle of 90 deg.). On the few occasions when the matter was tested it was found that even short trains of stimuli, particularly when applied towards the end of the shortening movement, sufficed to provoke effects that were as pronounced as those in Figure 2F.

In contrast, stimulation during the lengthening phase of the preceding triangular stretch failed to provoke such sensitivity enhancing after-effects. This is illustrated for the same primary afferent and static gamma-fibre in Figure 2A (passive control), C (stimulation during lengthening) and E (absence of after-effects, cf.A).

DISCUSSION

Sensitivity enhancing after-effects were seen in more than 2/3 of the sample of gamma-Ia interactions so far investigated (more than 40). They were consistently provoked by gamma-stimulation at low and probably physiological rates. They are therefore likely to be important functionally, either in postural tasks or during rhythmic alternating movements. In either case, they would be pronounced at short muscle length, where sensitivity of passive primary afferents tends to be low (MATTHEWS & STEIN, 1969 ; GOODWIN, HULLIGER & MATTHEWS, 1975 ; BAUMANN & HULLIGER, 1981). In the absence of large movements, as with control of steady posture, short bursts of fusimotor discharge would suffice to set up appreciable spindle sensitivity and so perhaps aid postural reflex responses for rather long periods. Similarly, in rhythmic alternating movements fusimotor activity need not occur during muscle lengthening, especially when the muscle concerned is moved passively by its antagonists. However, even short bursts of fusimotor activity during a preceding active shortening movement would suffice to induce sensitivity enhancing after-effects. These would then be advantageous during the lengthening phase, particularly in the range of short muscle length, where spindle sensitivity might otherwise be poor.

ACKNOWLEDGEMENT

This study was supported by the Fondation pour la Recherche Médicale Française, the Swiss National Foundation (Grant n° 3.225.77), the Dr. E. Slack-Gyr Foundation and the University of Zürich.

REFERENCES

BAUMANN TK, EMONET-DENAND F, HULLIGER M (1982) After-effects of fusimotor stimulation on spindle Ia afferents' dynamic sensitivity, revealed during slow movements. Brain Res 232:460-465

BAUMANN TK, HULLIGER M (1981) The high sensitivity of primary spindle afferents to small stretches is not preserved during larger movements of physiological amplitude, unless they are very slow. Experientia 37:606

BROWN MC, GOODWIN GM, MATTHEWS PBC (1969) After-effects of fusimotor stimulation on the response of muscle spindle primary endings. J. Physiol (Lond) 205:677-694

GOODWIN GM, HULLIGER M, MATTHEWS PBC (1975) The effects of fusimotor stimulation during small amplitude stretching on the frequency response of the primary ending of the mammalian muscle spindle. J Physiol (Lond) 253:175-206

HULLIGER M (1979) The responses of primary spindle afferents to fusimotor stimulation at constant and abruptly changing rates. J Physiol (Lond) 294:461-482

KUFFLER SW, HUNT CC, QUILLIAM JP (1951) Function of medullated small-nerve fibres in mammalian ventral roots : efferent muscle spindle innervation. J Neurophysiol 14:29-54

MATTHEWS PBC, STEIN RB (1969) The sensitivity of muscle spindle afferents to small sinusoidal changes of length. J Physiol (Lond) 200:723-743

A Technique for Reversible Fusimotor Blockade During Chronic Recording from Spindle Afferents in Walking Cats

J.A. Hoffer and G.E. Loeb

Department of Clinical Neurosciences University of Calgary, Faculty of Medicine Calgary, Alberta T2N 1N4, C A N A D A

INTRODUCTION

The functional role of the gamma-motoneuron system in the regulation of muscle spindle afferent discharge during the execution of normal movements remains an elusive but very important topic in the field of motor control. The only records from presumed fusimotoneurons have been obtained either in anaesthesized animals (SEARS, 1964 ; APPENTENG et al., 1980), or in decerebrate preparations (SEVERIN, 1970). In recent years, flexible wire electrodes implanted in cat lumbar dorsal roots or ganglia (PROCHAZKA et al., 1976 ; LOEB et al., 1977) have provided records of discharge patterns of spindle afferent endings during unrestrained locomotory movements. Stable recordings from intact alpha-motoneuron axons coursing along ventral roots have also been achieved (HOFFER et al., 1981b). To date, however, implanted wire electrodes have not rendered proven records from gamma-motoneuron axons, which are of finer caliber and consequently generate much smaller extracellular currents.

As an alternative to direct recording, fusimotor firing patterns may be inferred from the normal discharge patterns of spindle afferents, when compared to the "passive" spindle response to similar limb movements in the absence of fusimotor bias. We present here a method for selective blockade of fine-caliber fibers, which has allowed us to monitor the discharge of single spindle Ia fibers in normal cats walking in a treadmill, through periods of progressive functional spindle deefferentation and subsequent reefferentation. The method relies on the well-known differential sensitivity of peripheral nerve fibers of different diameters to sodium-channel blocking anaesthetics. Infusion of a weak solution of procaine has previously been reported to cause conduction blockade in gamma motoneurons with sparing of the much larger Group Ia afferent fibers, in acute cat experiments (MATTHEWS, RUSHWORTH, 1957) as well as in conjunction with microneurography in humans (HAGBARTH et al., 1970).

We used a cuff electrode, which was installed around the femoral nerve of cats for recording purposes (HOFFER et al., 1981a), to gain access to the perineural space via an implanted catheter. Infusion of a 0.3% solution of sodium xylocaine in small doses over several minutes caused progressive conduction blockade of small myelinated fibers, leading to concomitant changes in the discharge patterns recorded from individual spindle afferents. The progressive functional deefferentation of spindles was gradually reversed after flushing with mammalian saline solution.

METHODS

Design and surgical implantation of devices.

Experiments were performed in 17 cats of both sexes, weighing 3.0-5.5 Kg. Prior to surgery, cats were trained to walk on a motorized treadmill at a range of speeds and continuously for periods of up to 30 min. Implantation of devices was performed aseptically under deep pentobarbital anaesthesia. Analgesic drugs were administered if postsurgical pain or discomfort was apparent. The cats were allowed to recover for 3-7 days before recording sessions during locomotion were started, by which time they generally walked with normal load bearing and no visible limping.

Figure 1 shows schematically the "backpack" connector and the pertinent electrodes and devices that were implanted chronically, some of which have been described in detail previously (LOEB et al., 1977 ; 1979 ; 1981 ; HOFFER et al., 1980 ; 1981a ; 1981b). Up to a dozen flexible wire electrodes were implanted in the fifth lumbar dorsal root or dorsal root ganglion (L5 DRG), to record the activity of single Group Ia spindle afferents. The femoral nerve recording cuff was made of silicone elastomer tubing 15-30 mm long, inside diameter 2.5 mm (Extracorporeal 250), slit longitudinally. Three or five Pt-10%Ir (Medwire 10Ir 9/49T) Teflon-coated, stranded-wire recording electrodes, sewn circumferentially along the inside wall, were connected in one or two tripolar arrangements for differential recording (HOFFER et al., 1981a ; 1981b).

The xylocaine infusion catheter, about 200 mm long, emerged percutaneously just lateral to the spine. It was made of Silastic tubing 1.0 mm inside diameter (ID), 2.1 mm outside diameter (OD ; Dow Corning 602-205). The distal portion of the catheter consisted of finer tubing 0.5 mm ID, 1.0 mm OD (Dow Corning 602-135), which penetrated a hole punched through the nerve cuff wall about half-way along the length of the cuff. The finer tubing also served as

274

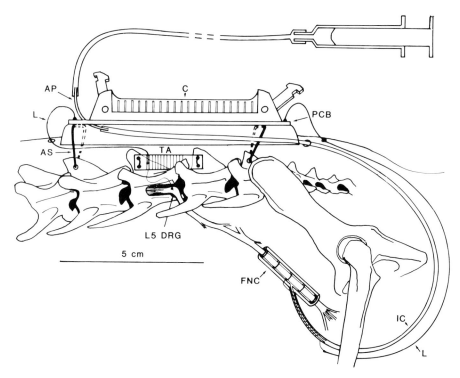

Fig. 1. Schematic diagram of devices implanted in the lumbar region and left hindlimb of cats. Up to a dozen "hatpin" microelectrodes (HOFFER et al., 1981a & b) were implanted in the L5 ganglion (L5 DRG) through a laminotomy. The flexible wire leads (one is shown) were soldered to stranded steel wires inside a Silastic tube array (TA) anchored with sutures to the L5 and L6 spines. The femoral nerve cuff (FNC) contained five electrodes and a flexible catheter which emerged percutaneously and ended in a stainless steel access port (AP) mounted on the "backpack" connector. The backpack was external to the skin, and was anchored to the animal by two sutures (AS; Mersilene size 5) which coursed through holes drilled in the L4 and L7 spines. A total of 40 stranded stainless steel lead wires (L) originating from implanted devices emerged percutaneously in bundles and were soldered to individual pads on a printed circuit board (PCB) on which was mounted a standard 40-pin computer ribbon connector (C; 3M Scotchflex No. 3432). A syringe was connected via a long flexible tube to the catheter access port in order to deliver a solution of xylocaine to the femoral nerve while the cat was walking

a core around which the five fragile Pt-Ir lead wires were wound helically to form a flexible cable. A piece of tubing 1 mm ID, 1.5 mm OD (Sil-Med 40-60) was expanded by immersion in toluene for about 2 min and slipped over the fine tubing and wound wires to provide a protective cover. Silastic Medical Adhesive (Dow Corning 891) was injected between the tubes to insure mechanical strength and impermeability. The Pt-Ir lead wires emerged from the coiled cable portion and were soldered to Teflon-coated stranded stainless steel

wires (Bergen Wire Rope 03.48), which coursed subcutaneously and were soldered to pads on the saddle connector printed circuit board.

The emerging catheter was fitted over a stainless steel hypodermic tube, 1.1
mm outside diameter, bonded with epoxy to the saddle connector (see Fig. 1).
The catheter access port was normally capped with tight-fitting Silastic
tubing with one end sealed. To prevent plugging, the catheter was flushed
every two days with 1.0 ml of a sterile solution of sodium heparin (50
units/ml) in mammalian Ringer's.

Unitary recording and characterization protocol.

The typical preparation was maintained 5-6 weeks. On a typical recording day,
the cat was first walked on the treadmill at several speeds. Data from active
microelectrodes and ancillary data from peripheral nerve and muscle electrodes, as well as muscle length and force (HOFFER, LOEB, 1980) were recorded on
FM tape. The movements were videotaped using two cameras. Spindle afferents
were tentatively identified by their response to passive limb manipulations,
behavior during voluntary movements, and conduction velocity obtained from
spike-triggered averaging (HOFFER et al., 1981a) ; definitive characterization (see LOEB, DUYSENS, 1979) had to await the conclusion of the recording
session, when deep pentobarbital anaesthesia was induced via a second implanted catheter leading to an external jugular vein. If any unit was presumed to
be a Group Ia spindle afferent, its behavior during a xylocaine blockade run
was recorded next. The cat was made to walk at a constant speed, interspersed
with brief periods at other speeds or gaits. After a few minutes of control
walking, a 0.3% solution of xylocaine in sterile mammalian Ringer's, warmed
to 37°C and contained in a 3 ml syringe, was infused via a 30 cm long tube
connected to the catheter access port. A total of 2.0-2.5 ml of solution was
infused in 0.5 ml increments delivered about once per minute, while the cat
continued to walk. The discharge pattern of the presumed spindle afferent was
monitored on a loudspeaker and by an oscillographic display of the instantaneous firing rate.

RESULTS

In general, the bursting pattern of a spindle afferent underwent several
discrete changes as the fusimotor blockade progressed, which suggests that
the several fusimotor fibers innervating the spindle were blocked sequentially. Each incremental infusion caused either no change in spindle activity, or
one or two relatively sudden changes in spindle afferent firing, each taking

place only during a particular phase of limb motion. By 5-12 min a final activity pattern was usually reached. Ten to 15 min later, the catheter was infused with a 37°C solution of mammalian Ringer's to wash out the xylocaine and reverse the block. Since the delivery tube and catheter (with combined volume of approximately 0.5 ml) still contained xylocaine, the initial response to infusion of saline was sometimes in the direction of increased blockade. The blockade sometimes extended from gamma- to alpha-range motor fibers, evidenced by a more pronounced yield at the knee joint during the stance phase and by changes in the EMG of knee extensor muscles. In rare occasions the progression of blockade also involved the axon of the recorded IA afferent, which stopped firing abruptly and did not recover until the xylocaine was washed out.

Additional 0.5 ml increments of saline wash solution brought about a progressive restoration to control conditions over the next 10-30 min. The discharge pattern of the Ia afferent typically recovered in discrete steps, suggesting that fusimotor neurons returned to function sequentially, in a roughly symmetric fashion to the sequence of blockade onset (see Discussion).

An example of changes in the discharge pattern of a sartorius pars medialis Group Ia spindle afferent (conduction velocity = 94 $\pm$ 5 m/s) caused by xylocaine infusion is shown in Figure 2. The left half (Part A) shows typical activity during three normal steps, with the cat walking at 0.44 m/s. This ending typically exhibited two periods of activity during each step cycle : a sharp burst late in the swing phase (arrows), which started as the muscle reached minimum length, lasted about 50 ms with a peak rate of about 150 pps, and ended abruptly ; and a smoothly accelerating burst that lasted over most of the stance phase, when the muscle was lengthening, and reached peak values of 100-120 pps. In addition, the afferent fired a few spikes during the flexion phase (in spite of rapid muscle shortening). The amplitude of the sharp burst was not well correlated with velocity of lengthening. The smoothly accelerating burst appeared related primarily to muscle length.

Xylocaine infusion had a dramatic effect on the sharp burst, whereas the second burst was relatively unaffected (Fig. 2B). Ninety seconds after xylocaine infusion, with the cat walking at the same speed on the treadmill, the sharp burst was no longer present at the predicted time in each step cycle (arrows). However, all the recorded kinesiological parameters (muscle length, velocity, force at the patellar ligament, and EMG of the sartorius pars medialis as well as vastus medialis) were virtually unchanged. At this time, the activity of the ending during the extension phase was also not much

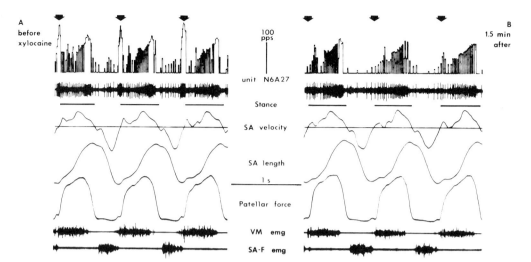

Fig. 2.

A : Activity recorded from a Ia afferent supplying a spindle in the proximal part of sartorius pars medialis, during three consecutive steps. Traces show : instantaneous frequencygram and raw microelectrode record from afferent unit ; bars indicating stance phase of gait ; electronically derived velocity of sartorius ; length of sartorius, obtained from an implanted length gauge (HOFFER, LOEB, 1980) ; force generated at the patellar ligament, obtained from an implanted transducer (HOFFER, LOEB, 1980) ; and electromyograms from indwelling bipolar electrodes sampling vastus medialis (VM) and the medial portion of sartorius (SA-F). Arrows above indicate the times of occurrence of a sharp burst in each step cycle.

B : Activity recorded from the same Ia fiber ninety seconds after xylocaine infusion via the femoral nerve catheter. Note the disappearance of the sharp bursts at the end of the swing phase, unaccompanied by any major changes in the kinesiological parameters monitored. Figure reproduced from HOFFER, LOEB, 1981. Further description in text

affected. A few minutes later the block progressed further, causing a reduction in the amplitude of the smoothly accelerating burst, to 60-80 pps. Activity of this fiber returned to normal some 20 min after the xylocaine was flushed out with saline. We interpret these observations to indicate that this spindle ending was normally under the influence of strong static gamma bias during the swing phase. Dynamic fusimotor activity appeared to have only a moderate role in influencing the stretch sensitivity during the stance phase.

DISCUSSION

The method of progressive nerve fiber blockade with xylocaine infusion has demonstrated directly that fusimotor neurons can have marked effects on the discharge patterns of individual Group Ia spindle afferents during normal locomotion. The discrete changes observed after xylocaine infusion are consistent with the sequential blockade of several fusimotor fibers influencing a spindle ending. The order in which different fusimotor axons cease to conduct presumably depends on the inherent sensitivity of each fiber to the anaesthetic, which is related to the inverse of the fiber diameter. In the case of a large peripheral nerve like the cat femoral (about 2 mm in diameter), the diffusion rate of the drug through the tissue must also be taken into account. Superficial fibers can be expected to block earlier than fibers of similar diameter that lie deeper in the nerve. Some blockade of the smallest alpha-motoneurons may occur, particularly if fusimotor blockade must include the intermediate-sized beta-motoneurons. Interestingly, this loss appears to be fully compensated, since limb trajectory is preserved despite a significant alteration in cutaneous as well as proprioceptive feedback.

Detailed observation of the changes in firing patterns of seven Group Ia endings from sartorius have suggested to us that, in general, the functional removal of one fusimotor fiber affects either the activity burst during flexion or the activity burst during extension, but not both simultaneously. Thus, fusimotor neurons innervating sartorius appear to be organized into at least two distinct functional pools (HOFFER, LOEB, 1982 ; see also LOEB, 1981 and LOEB, HOFFER, 1981). This type of analysis of the discharge patterns of spindle endings in the presence and in the absence of fusimotor blockade is expected to reveal further details about the functional organization of fusimotor neurons and about their patterns of activation during normal movements.

ACKNOWLEDGEMENTS

We thank Dr. CA PRATT, who participated in pilot experiments, and M. O'MALLEY, who trained cats and fabricated devices for implantation.

REFERENCES

APPENTENG K, MORIMOTO T, TAYLOR A (1980) Fusimotor activity in masseter nerve of the cat during reflex jaw movements. J Physiol 305:415-431

HAGBARTH KE, HONGELL A, WALLIN G (1970) The effect of gamma fibre block on afferent muscle nerve activity during voluntary contractions. Acta Physiol Scand 79:27-28

HOFFER JA, LOEB GE (1980) Implantable electrical and mechanical interfaces with nerve and muscle. Annals Biomed Engr 8:351-360

HOFFER JA, LOEB GE (1981) Effect of fusimotor blockade on discharge patterns of cat hindlimb spindle primaries during walking. Neurosci Abstr 7:408

HOFFER JA, LOEB GE (1982) Fusimotor actions on sartorius spindle primary discharge patterns during cat locomotion. Neuroscience 7:S95

HOFFER JA, LOEB GE, PRATT CA (1981a) Single unit conduction velocities from averaged nerve cuff electrode records in freely moving cats. J Neurosci Methods 4:211-225

HOFFER JA, O'DONOVAN MJ, PRATT CA, LOEB GE (1981b) Discharge patterns of hindlimb motoneurons during normal cat locomotion. Science 213: 466-468

LOEB GE (1981) Somatosensory unit input to the spinal cord during normal walking. Canad J Physiol Pharmacol 59:627-635

LOEB GE, BAK MJ, DUYSENS J (1977) Long-term unit recording from somatosensory neurons in the spinal ganglia of the freely walking cat. Science 197:1192-1194

LOEB GE, DUYSENS J (1979) Activity patterns in individual hindlimb primary and secondary muscle spindle afferents during normal movements in unrestrained cats. J Neurophysiol 42:420-440

LOEB GE, HOFFER JA (1981) Muscle spindle function during normal and perturbed locomotion in cats. In: TAYLOR A, PROCHAZKA A (eds) Muscle Receptors and Movement. Macmillan, London, pp 219-228

MATTHEWS PBC, RUSHWORTH G (1957) The relative sensitivity of muscle nerve fibers to procaine. J Physiol 135:263-269

PROCHAZKA A, WESTERMAN RA, ZICCONE SP (1976) Discharge of single hindlimb afferents in the freely moving cat. J Neurophysiol 39:1090-1104

SEARS TA (1964) Efferent discharges in alpha and fusimotor fibres of intercostal nerves of the cat. J Physiol 174:295-315

SEVERIN FV (1970) The role of the gamma motor system in the activation of the extensor alpha motor neurones during controlled locomotion. Biophysics 15:1138-1145

Neural Control Drives a Muscle Spring: A Persisting yet Limited Motor Theory

L.D. Partridge

University of Tennessee, Memphis, TN 38163, USA

If motor control is accomplished by mechanical effects of muscle, any spring-like properties of muscle will influence that control. To be spring-like requires only that muscle force change with muscle length - a property of contractile proteins themselves. With primitive equipment and advanced insights, WEBER in 1846 clearly demonstrated an exchange between force and length in muscle and described it as spring-like*. Further he showed that excitation adjusted this spring and moved loads to positions which were dependent on both load size and on stimulus. The exchange between force and position is further adjustable by neural drive to the muscle in a smooth but non-linear way (BUCHTHAL, 1942)*. In motor control this exchange between force and position partially compensates for effects of changes in load, much like a position feedback (PARTRIDGE, 1965). In any case, the spring-like interaction with loads - excitation dependent, non-linear and in some ranges even negative - is well studied and described in terms of length-tension effects (Fig. 2). Since different slopes of the length tension curves do not extrapolate to the same intercept on zero force level, a bias of force value as well as the slope are necessary specifications to describe local muscle properties. Moreover, unlike a spring, muscle's length dependent forces represent mostly metabolic energy instead of stored potential energy from previous stretch.

By the end of the XIX century, spring of muscle had been studied extensively, perhaps most thoroughly by BLIX (1893-1895)*. WEBER's tables* showed (apparently unknown to him) that the relationship between force and length depended also on recent mechanical history of muscle. BLIX was quite explicit that response in twitches was markedly influenced by load dependent details of the paths taken over the force-length plane. The spring description of muscle

---

*See PARTRIDGE and BENTON 1981 for a collection of figures from the indicated citations

Experimental Brain Research, Suppl. 7
© Springer-Verlag Berlin · Heidelberg 1983

fell into disrepute because of these complications. Those problems also influence modern muscle research in the expectation that mechanical treatment of muscle will be carefully standardized to avoid "artifactual" variability of response. Muscle is clearly not a simple spring with an invariant neural adjustment of either length or stiffness.

Any spring description of muscle mechanics is inadequate without including velocity dependent characteristics. First, to account for observed transient responses in muscle, HILL and associates found that, in addition to spring-like properties, it was necessary to postulate a viscous element (LEVIN and WYMAN, 1927). The described property, now known as the force-velocity curve, was subsequently studied almost entirely during shortening. Second, a spring-like muscle would require damping to produce stable control. Even with joint friction, a purely spring-like muscle attached to an inertial limb would oscillate intolerably after any transient. Force-velocity properties of muscle which, like stiffness and tension change with excitation (JOYCE and RACK, 1969)*, provide the needed damping action (PARTRIDGE, 1965)*. The inclusion of velocity effects is justified by success in predicting moving length in muscle twitches as a combined effect of excitation change, force and velocity (ABBOTT and WILKIE, 1953). Thus, tension-bias and velocity dependent as well as elastic properties which characterize excited muscle are inseparable in either their dependence on neural drive or in the way they influence load movement.

In the four-dimensional activation-force-velocity-position space where mechanical properties of muscle fall on activation dependent response surfaces, the elastic and viscous properties and steady force caused by a load could be shown as a characteristic plane. For controllable loads, that plane would intersect muscle response surfaces at the locus of all null torques for the system (Fig. 1). Neural drive to muscle affects the response surface and thus location of this null line. Null loci of any moment penetrate the zero velocity plane at all current lengths for static equilibrium, while in regions of finite velocity this line of intersecting surfaces marks conditions in which the system might pass through $\emptyset$ acceleration. When operating off the null line the force differences accelerate any inertial parts of the load. Although the relationship between instantaneous response surface and load plane determines all movements in an unambiguous way, selection of a response surface is dependent in a complex way on present and past mechanical input and just past and earlier history of muscle excitation. This is because of lag and hysteresis in muscle response to nerve action (PARTRIDGE, 1966) and hysteresis to mechanical input*. Thus in spite of load compensation by

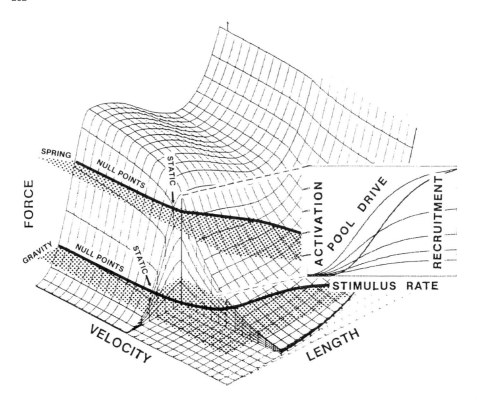

Fig. 1. Illustration of often assumed interaction between a "well behaved muscle" and two different loads. Shaded planes represent force-length-velocity relationships for two different loads ; horizontal plane - isotonic (gravity) load, tilted plane - spring load. Force surface for a muscle, marked by the grid lines, shows dependence on length and velocity. The edges of lower surfaces that can be seen through the "window" in the maximum surface show forces at lower levels of activation resulting either from less recruitment or lower stimulus rate or both as represented by small inserted graph. Heavy lines where muscle surface intersects load plane show all points of balance between visco-elastic plus force load and muscle force. Static equilibria would occur where (↓) null force coincides with zero velocity with location quite dependent on load. Where muscle response is below load plane acceleration of inertial part of load is in direction of load force ; where above toward muscle force. In this schema, since neither muscle lag and hysteresis to stimulus nor hysteresis and velocity dependence on movement are represented, graphs follow common assumption that a fixed relationship exists between activity in a muscle nerve and load dependent mechanical result. An appreciably more accurate model would result from addition of effects of these factors

muscle, (PARTRIDGE, 1966 ; 1967) to program the neural drive that will obtain
a particular response requires that the signal be adjusted for these complications, a problem not simplified by elastic muscles and only partially
reducible by reflex feedback (PARTRIDGE, 1972).

In a single muscle the trade offs between muscle length and delivered force
and between force and velocity can be called spring-like (WEBER, 1846) and
viscous-like (LEVIN and WYMAN, 1927) respectively. In combination they have
been called mechanical impedance or like compensated negative feedback
(PARTRIDGE, 1967). The muscle properties are in fact more effective as a
feedback than is the stretch reflex. Applying d'ALEMBERT's principle, the
neurally controlled force balance among muscle, load and external forces can
be described in a nonlinear partial differential equation (PARTRIDGE, 1972).
These alternate representations all describe a system giving stable equilibria with various loads at points dependent on many factors.

To avoid difficult interpretation in muscle studies, complex internal structures or combinations of muscles have generally been avoided : much muscle
research was on frog sartorius. However, in most limbs (motor control is
usually described for limbs) individual complex muscles work together in
combinations often inappropriately described as if they were simple antagonist pairs acting over a hinge joint. This drastic simplication has also been
used in constructing Figure 2 and 3.

Study of antagonists by SHERRINGTON's group (CREED et al., 1932) led to the
concepts that different balances in tonus of antagonists are the basis of
different postures and that movement is a continuous change of posture. While
a low level activity of motor nerves was called tonus, tonus was commonly
measured as mucle force. However, a force description of position is not
valid. Although differential equations of motor control were not used in this
context, it seems reasonable that Newtonian mechanics was assumed. Then if a
steady change in force-balance (torque) occurred, the result would accelerate
inertial loads moving around the joint. For normal movements, steady torque
inbalances cannot continue but must be dissipated, in fact they must be
reversed long enough to stop each movement. Only in spring-like muscles,
where tonic force trades with tonic displacement, would tonus control position, appearing first as a torque, but soon exchanged for the resulting
displacement. Thus, although not specifically discussed, spring-like properties of antagonistic combinations were intrinsic to the Sherringtonian view
of tonus control of posture and movement.

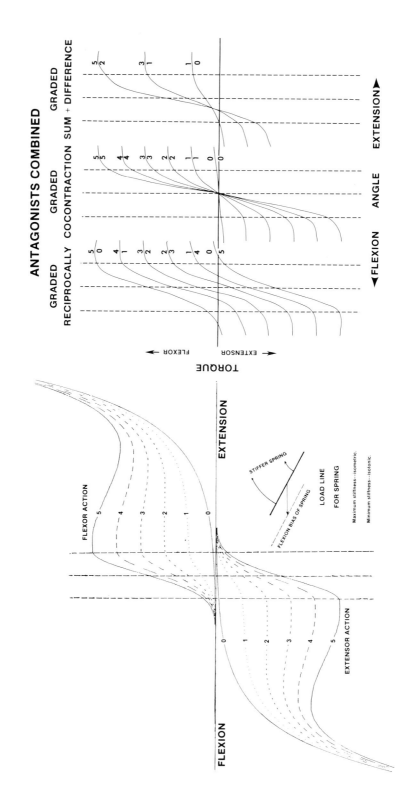

When the actions of antagonistics are combined (SHERRINGTON, 1894 ; POLIT and
BIZZI, 1978 ; COOKE, 1980 ; FELDMAN, 1980), the two muscle torques subtract
while the muscle impedances add (BENTON and PARTRIDGE, 1981 ; PARTRIDGE and
BENTON, 1981). The combination is as much a feedback system (with higher gain
and damping) or as much a mechanical impedance (stiffer and more viscous) as
is the single muscle. The position at which cocontracting antagonists deliver
equal torques has no special significance except as the balance point for
those rare loads that introduce no torque themselves.

The interaction between a load plane and a combined response surface from
antagonists has the same significance as in the single muscle case. A set of
cross sections of 15 different response surfaces, as they would appear when
cut on the zero velocity plane, are illustrated in Figure 2. Each surface was
derived graphically by summing forces expected from a different combination
of activities in an antagonist pair of muscles. Three groups of surfaces were
chosen to show the expected effect of reciprocal adjustment, co-contraction
adjustment and co- and recriprocal-adjustment together. If examined as force
balance equations of loaded antagonists, they would differ from the single
muscle form (PARTRIDGE, 1972) only in that each individual term would be
replaced by the sum of weighted sub-terms, one for each muscle.

◄ Fig. 2. Graphic construction of expected joint torques (isometric) from
length tension effects in simple antagonists. Left graph shows separately the
assumed individual muscle responses. Lines on upper half of graph represents
length tension curves from one muscle in terms of angle and torque of an
associated joint. Numbers label response lines for different levels of muscle
activation. Lower family of lines show corresponding effects from a matched
antagonist muscle with sign of torque and angular direction of stretch
reversed. Vertical interupted lines identify 3 reference angles of the joint.
Joint torque at any particular time is the sum of activation and length
dependent torques of the two muscle. Torque angle exchange for 15 different
combinations of activation in antagonist and agonist are graphed in three
groups at right. Interupted vertical lines again mark reference angles. Pair
of numbers associated with each combined response line identifies relative
static activation of flexor (above) and extensor (below) muscles. Families of
reciprocally adjusted response curves are generated by the rule that changed
activation of flexor, F, is associated with equal but opposite change of
extensor activation, E, thus F + E = K, a constant. It is demonstrated that
reciprocal grading alters angle- torque bias of response curve over mid-range
of angles. A reciprocal change in joint activity shifts the response surface
from one of these lines to another. Grading of coactivation, instead,
involves equal and parallel changes in flexor and extensor activation, thus,
F - E = K producing slope (stiffness) changes in the mid-range of the response curve. No combination of positively sloped individual response curves
produces a negative slope in the combined response. Static angle-torque
combination at equilibrium for any response curve depends on load line as
with a single muscle

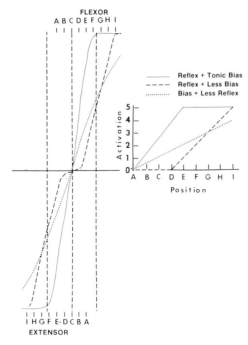

Fig. 3. Graphic model of effects of reflex "gain" and bias when acting on antagonistic muscles. Response lines were derived as in figure 2 by addition of torques produced by antagonist muscles at different angles but in this case each line was derived with a length dependent level of reflex activation of each muscle. Three different rules (shown in insert graph) define reflex conversion of angle (letters) to activation (numbers) of each muscle and were used with figure 2 to generate the corresponding response curves. Separate and inverse scales of angles defined points on reflex conversion graphs for flexor and extensor muscles. These response graphs each contain tonic and reflex contributions to static stiffness (slope)

By either description, antagonist muscles add an inverse range of muscle torques, increase maximal impedance, and make possible separation of control of torque and impedance (BENTON and PARTRIDGE, 1981 ; PARTRIDGE and BENTON, 1981), but would neither eliminate load dependence, history dependence nor the need for damping in converting a particular neural output into a motor response. Except for the increases in ranges of response available and separability of torque and stiffness, the antagonist complicates, rather than simplifies, the problem for direct neural control by adding the variables of the second muscle and reflex and introducing effects of overlap of antagonist actions into the transformation of neural signals into response.

DISCUSSION ADDED TO COMPARE FELDMAN'S STUDY OF ANTAGONIST INTERACTION

While editing this paper Dr. MASSION brought to my attention the related analysis by FELDMAN (1980). A comparison and contrast of the two presentations is instructive.

Both synthesize joint effects from antagonist actions but originated with different data bases. FELDMAN's human data, from an elbow with intact reflex function, was measured starting with either flexor, or extensor active or both, followed by a quick load change, a previously described measurement (ASRATYAN and FELDMAN, 1968). The result, a family of static torque-angle graphs named "invariant characteristic(s) of muscles", IC, has an initial conditions parameter. The current report, instead, is based on experiments on individual cat muscles with severed nerve subjected to constant stimulation rates and operated at either constant or changing muscle lengths. The basis for this treatment, collected length-velocity-force data is a set of graphic surfaces with an activation parameter.

Both studies employ the same, conventional, and graphic treatment of the balance between muscle and load properties. The present paper adds velocity effects to the position effects and is the graphic equivalant of a previous mathematical treatment (PARTRIDGE, 1972).

Bypassing usual difficulties in defining cocontraction of antagonists when reciprocal activity is present, FELDMAN was able to show that the two types of action are used together and controlled separably in the elbow. Further, the coordinates of co- and reciprocal-control were shown to be rotated with respect to the coordinates representing agonist and antagonist activation.

FELDMAN found the elbow IC with cocontraction of antagonists is steeper (stiffer) than with a single muscle contracted, then showed graphically that this might be explained as superposition of separate ICs from antagonist muscles. Independently PARTRIDGE and BENTON (1981) have predicted the same effect from a simple mechanical treatment of antagonist interaction, stating for the two muscles "...torques subtract while stiffnesses add...". The dynamic parts of the impedance were also indicated to add. The easily observed increase of elbow stiffness, with voluntary cocontraction of elbow muscles, was cited as evidence. The present paper provides the corresponding graphic derivation for stiffness (Fig. 2).

The graphs in the two studies of antagonist interaction look quite similar but the present one deals with static activation of muscles whereas FELDMAN suggests the IC curves are primarily generated by reflexly altered activation of muscle. Clearly the stiffness measured from an intact muscle system can contain both reflex and tonic muscle contributions (PARTRIDGE, 1972). (FELDMAN described variable overlap of reflex actions of antagonists in terms of the length, β, at which reflex activation started. In analizing length effects on reflex action PARTRIDGE (1972) described a similar variable in terms of a different measure, the "tonic" force at a reference length). However, neither of these studies derived direct evidence concerning the relative importance of reflex and tonic effects in either IC determination or any other motor action.

Figure 3 has been added to relate the present discussion to FELDMAN's. Applying the assumption that specific angles of the joint reflexly drive the two muscles to particular activation levels to the antagonist graphs of Figure 2 provides basis for a graphic prediction of a stretch reflex effect. (Hysteresis to mechanical and stimulus inputs are ignored in both this model and FELDMAN's study.) In this model the length tension effect is explicitly included within the reflex. The graphic combination shows, in agreement with

FELDMAN, overlaping reflexes would make the system stiffer than when the reflex actions did not overlap. Further this figure brings out the fact that reciprocal reflex action could produce a particular static stiffness with less total muscle activation than required for that stiffness from tonic cocontraction, presumably a metabolic economy. It is also demonstrated that, depending on reflex gain, the reflex might either extend or shorten the range of positions over which the system shows a stiffness like property. (The modeled gains were made high to emphasize reflex action.) The nonlinearity due to non-overlaping in one reflex model (dashed curve) could also have been produced by a non-overlap assumption in the simple tonic model but which ever its source the result is suggestive of a nonlinearity shown in a graph from an earlier IC measurement (ASATRYAN and FELDMAN, 1965). In the static case discussed here, tonic muscle action of antagonists and reflex actions can have similar results.

FELDMAN results and analysis combined with demonstrations of Figure 2 and 3, allows the conclusion that independence in direct and reflex control of co- and reciprocal- contraction of anatagonists are likely mechanisms for the easily demonstrable overlaping but independent control of the output dimensions, torque and stiffness. Thus, instead of just providing control of torque with either sign, antagonist motor pools drive two output dimensions. However, in that action the rotation of the control coordinates with respect to the muscle coordinates produces a functionally indivisible motor component with a two dimensional output. I suggest that the joint based dimensions ; torque and stiffness (including dynamic stiffness) are a step closer to biologically meaningful motor control than are the dimensions often studied, namely the individual muscle responses.

Neither FELDMAN's nor the present study defines the relative importance of the similar static effects of reflex and tonic muscle properties in the immediate interactions between muscles and load. While reflex actions without an influence of the length-tension and force-velocity effects are improbable in any controlled movement, either tonic activity or tonic with reflex activity could determine the force and mechanical impedance of a joint involved in a motor action. The point is made that grading of either reflex or tonic activity in an antagonist pair of muscles introduces the separable control of stiffness and torque which is not available from one muscle. Moreover, these functions half determine the motor response at a joint.

Ultimately, any motor response is a neurally modifiable Newtonian interaction among elastic and other mechanical properties of muscles, external forces, and total load. Each of these factors is subject to large variations during normal physiologic activity. Successful motor control results when neural output modifies muscles properties so that acting with the load, they bend the system's trajectory in an acceptable direction. Except for well practiced action sequences with unusually dependable load rules, the choice of best neural signals to accomplish a desired result can not be played back from a long established and stored program. In all other cases, variable state of muscle and load requires corresponding adjustment of the neural signals which set those spring-like and other mechanical properties of muscles that together are the direct controller of motor response. Visco-elastic muscles seem to provide an easier substrate for neural control than would force motors. While antagonists (compared to single muscles) increase flexibility of control they can not reduce motor control to control of motoneurons followed by a fixed output transformation into mechanical result. No high gain feedback pathway is known which would eliminate the considerable errors to be expected from variable muscle responses.

It would appear that the high quality motor control which is commonly demonstrable is not explained by a single simple principle. Ultimately all motor control accomplished by the nervous system is indirect, acting through control of the mechanical properties (response surfaces) of muscle systems which then interact with the loads to produce motor effects. Clearly the drive signals from higher centers which call particular mechanical sequences are in many cases the result of long practice, acting with adjusted precompensation for predictable problem complexities. Errors in controlled responses caused by unpredictable load changes or extraneous forces would often be reduced by known feedback like effects of both reflexes and muscle response surfaces. Total error of control would be minimized if involved response surfaces were all appropriately biased and adjusted to slopes appropriate for the transient local conditions. In view of the basic involvment of these surfaces in determining all response, the demonstrated adjustability of the response surfaces, the importance of the form of these surfaces to compensation of unpredictable disturbances, and the drifting and complexity of local conditions in motor control : it is proposed that in addition to long term and to automatic types of adjustment, motor control also is likely to involve a short term and continuous trimming of that reflex and tonic muscle activity setting the bias and slopes of the response surfaces, thereby introducing a simple compensation for complex muscle and load properties, reducing long term response error and probably also improving automatic adjustments by tuning feedback like effects toward a fit to the local requirements.

ACKNOWLEDGEMENT

The authors is indebted to R. KNELLER for voluntary assistance in physical preparation of illustrations.

REFERENCES

ABBOTT BC, WILKIE DR (1953) The relation between velocity of shortening and the tension-length curve of skeletal muscle. J Physiol (London) 120:214-223

ASRATYAN DG, FELD'MAN AG (1965) Functional tuning of nervous system with control of movement or maintenance of a steady posture. I. Mechanographic analysis of the work of the joint on execution of a postural task. Biofizika 10:837-846

BENTON LA, PARTRIDGE LD (1981) Two muscles are better than one. Fed Proc 39:969

BLIX M (1892-1895) Die Länge und Spannung des Muskels. Skand Arch Physiol 3:295-318 ; 4:399-409 ; 5:150-172, 173-206

BUCHTHAL F (1942) The mechanical properties of the single striated muscle fibre at rest and during contraction and their structural interpretation. Dann Biol Medd Kbh 17:1-140

COOKE JD (1980) The organization of simple skilled movements. In: STELMACH G, REQUIN J (eds) Tutorials in Motor Behavior. Elsevier, Amsterdam

CREED RS, DENNY-BROWN D, ECCLES JC, LIDDELL EGT, SHERRINGTON CS (1932) Reflex activity of the spinal cord. Oxford University Press, London

FELDMAN AG (1980) Superimposition of motor programs. I. Rhythmic forearm movements in man. Neuroscience 5:81-90

JOYCE GC, RACK PMH (1969) Isotonic lengthening and shortening movements of cat soleus muscle. J Physiol (London) 204:475-492

LEVIN A, WYMAN J (1927) The viscous elastic properties of muscle. Proc R Soc London 101B:218-243

PARTRIDGE LD (1965) Modifications of neural output signals by muscles ; a frequency response study. J Appl Physiol 20:150-156

PARTRIDGE LD (1966) Signal-handling characteristics of load-moving sheletal muscle. Am J Physiol 210:1178-1191

PARTRIDGE LD (1967) Intrinsic feedback factors producing inertial compensation in muscle. Biophys J 7:853-863

PARTRIDGE LD (1972) Interrelationships studied in a semibiological "reflex" Am J Physiol 223:144-158

PARTRIDGE LD, BENTON LA (1981) Muscle the Motor. In: BROOKS VD (ed) Motor control. Handbook of Physiology. The Nervous System. Bethesda MD. Am Physiol Soc Sec 1, Vol II, pt 1, chap 3, p 43-106

POLIT A, BIZZI E (1978) Processes controlling arm movements in monkeys. Science 201:1235-1237

SHERRINGTON CS (1894) Experimental note on two movements of the eye. J Physiol 17:27-29

WEBER E (1846) Muskelbewegung. In: WAGNER R (ed) Handwörterbuch der Physiologie. Braunschweig, Bieweg, vol III, pt 2, p 1-122

Functional Organization of Claw Protrusion in the Cat

R.A. Westerman, D. Sriratana, and D.I. Finkelstein

Physiology Department, Monash University, Clayton, Victoria 3168, Australia

INTRODUCTION

In any animal the final problems in the complex sequence of neural coding of motor performance relate to skeletal muscles and their lower motor neurones. The importance of this peripheral substrate is evident in the climbing agility shown by cats : this depends largely upon their precise adjustment of retractable crampons - that is, claw protrusion. Therefore they possess special arrangements of the toe-joints, phalanges and the muscles controlling toe actions (SRIRATANA et al., 1981 ; SRIRATANA and WESTERMAN, 1982). In addition, there is a specially powerful independent inhibitory reflex control of flexor digitorum longus (FDL) and flexor hallucis longus (FHL) in the cat shown by AOKI and McINTYRE (1975). Although, as illustrated in Figure 1, the long digit flexor muscle in the cat consists of a smaller medial head (FDL) with tibial origin and a larger lateral, i.e., fibular head (FHL), they have shared insertions by a conjoined tendon and a common function has been assumed. The difference between these two muscle heads and the heterogeneity within each will be considered in relation to the function of claw protrusion in the cat.

METHODS

In cats under pentobarbitone anaesthesia (40 mg/kg), 152 single motor units in the FDL and 150 in FHL were isolated by finely splitting the L6, L7 or S1 ventral roots after totally denervating the hindlimb (BAGUST et al., 1973) and identified in terms of the "sag" and "fatigue" criteria described by BURKE et al. (1973), who classified single motor units of medial gastrocnemius muscle into fast fatiguable (FF), fatigue resistant (FR) and slow (S) types according to their isometric mechanical responses to unfused tetanic stimuli. Because optimum lengths for twitch or tetanic contraction are not always the same for either the whole muscle or motor units, and because the

Experimental Brain Research, Suppl. 7
© Springer-Verlag Berlin · Heidelberg 1983

response to BURKE's test is affected by muscle length, an isometric length : tension curve and optimum length was determined for each motor unit.

The test procedure applied to identify units was identical to that of BURKE et al. (1973) except that tetanic tension and "fatigue index" were measured at optimum length for tetanic contraction for each unit, and the "say test" and estimates of twitch contraction time were made at optimum length for a twitch. Subsequent histochemical identification of fibre types and of some individual units was based on serial sections stained for glycogen (periodic acid schiff), phosphorylase, succinic dehydrogenase, and myosin adenosine triphosphatase at pH 4.3, 4.6 and 9.4. Histochemical profiles of identified motor units from both FDL and FHL muscle were examined at various levels along the muscle using the glycogen depletion technique of EDSTROM and KUGELBERG (1968). This permitted correlation of physiological and histochemical properties and the reconstruction and determination of fibre area, specific tension and distribution within the muscle belly (SRIRATANA and WESTERMAN, 1982). The final behavioural observations of claw protrusion during walking, jumping and climbing were photographed on 16 mm cine film one week after performing various tenotomies, FDL or FHL or both, on the plantar aspect of the foot (the results are illustrated in Fig. 2).

RESULTS

Some characteristics of the two muscles FDL and FHL are given in Table 1. The FHL muscle is longer and heavier than FDL, but has shorter fibres (c.f. Fig. 1C,D). The twitch contraction speed and maximum tetanic tension of the muscle, both greater for FHL than FDL, are determined by the proportions and characteristics of the different types of units, also given in Table 1. The predominant type of unit in FDL was FR 47%, and in FHL was FF 56%. The fast units, both FF and FR, in FHL had shorter contraction times than corresponding units in FDL, while type S units had slightly longer contraction times. In both muscles, motor units were found to be widely distributed. That is, muscle fibres belonging to single motor units of all three histochemical and physiological types (FF, FR and S) were found to be scattered through territorial volumes occupying a large fraction of the total muscle volume in both FDL and FHL muscle bellies. The cross-sectional area of individual fibre types was measured (SRIRATANA and WESTERMAN, 1982). Using mean fibres area, the number of fibres in FDL (23,000) and FHL (85,000) was calculated from the cross sectional area of the whole muscle. The mean cross-sectional areas of FF, FR and S motor units in FHL are larger than those of corresponding unit types in FDL. Similarly, the number of muscle fibres in identified motor unit

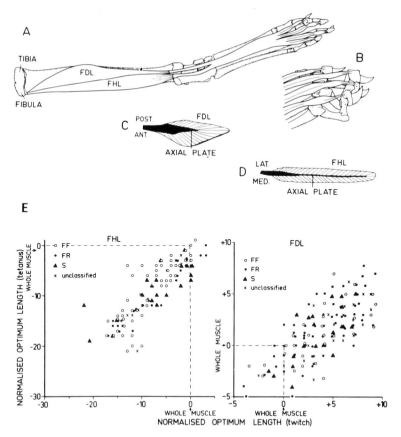

Fig. 1. (A) shows the tendons of FDL and FHL uniting as the deep plantar aponeurosis, inserting (B) into the terminal phalanges of digits 2-5. Both muscles are bipennate, FDL (C) having a greater mean muscle fibre length and sarcomere length than FHL (D) (See Table 1). (E) compares isometric contractions of FDL and FHL whole muscles with classified motor units obtained from each. Each point represents the values for one individual motor unit of types FF, FR, S or unclassified shown by the symbol key ; graphs illustrate the scatter of motor unit optimum lengths in FHL and FDL, respectively. The abscissae shows the optimum length for motor unit twitch measured relative to the optimum length for the whole muscle twitch. The ordinate shows the optimum length for motor unit tetanic tension measured relative to the optimum length for whole muscle tetanic tension. All lengths in mm

Table 1

CHARACTERISTICS OF MUSCLES AND FIBRES IN FDL AND FHL

Muscle	Length (mm) (mean $\pm$ SD)	Weight (g)	Fibre length (mm)
FDL	73.5 $\pm$ 2.0	1.50 $\pm$ 0.03	17.4 $\pm$ 3.3
FHL	103.9 $\pm$ 1.1	4.93 $\pm$ 0.15	16.7 $\pm$ 2.8

CHARACTERISTICS OF 3 TYPES OF CLASSIFIED MOTOR UNITS

N° of units	Percentage of Physiological Types		
	FF	FR	S
FDL (152)	36%	47%	17%
FHL (150)	56%	25%	19%

CONTRACTION TIME (ms) OF MOTOR UNITS

(Mean $\pm$ SD)	FF	FR	S
FDL	22 $\pm$ 5	25 $\pm$ 4	41 $\pm$ 11
FHL	20 $\pm$ 2	24 $\pm$ 3	42 $\pm$ 12

TETANIC TENSION (mN) OF MOTOR UNITS

(Mean $\pm$ SD)			
FDL	462 $\pm$ 192	139 $\pm$ 98	53 $\pm$ 28
FHL	550 $\pm$ 272	330 $\pm$ 212	182 $\pm$ 160

types was counted directly and estimated indirectly from the number of motor units in the muscle. The FHL motor units have a larger number of muscle fibres (200-500) than FDL motor units (60-400). Thus, the innervation ratio appeared to be higher in motor units of FHL than FDL, and in both muscles was higher in type FF units than in type FR and S. From the tetanic tensions as shown in Table 1, the specific tension of muscle fibres within individual motor unit types was also calculated. For the FHL muscle, FF units (3.9 kg cm^{-2}) had a higher specific tension than either FR (3.8 kg cm^{-2}) or S (2.0 kg cm^{-2}) type units. In FDL muscle the specific tensions for the corresponding motor unit types exhibited the same relative size ranking, i.e. FF FR S, but were all smaller than for motor units in FHL (3.6 kg cm^{-2} ; 3.3 kg cm^{-2} ; 1.5 kg cm^{-2}, respectively). In both FDL and FHL muscles a number of motor units with intermediate properties were found, which could not be fitted into the 3 types of BURKE et al. (1973). Such non-classified units amounted to 11.7% of the FHL sample and 16% of the FDL sample. In figure 1E, for both FHL and FDL the isometric contraction of each whole muscle was compared with that of their constituent motor units. Most FDL units exhibited an optimum length for twitches much longer than for tetani, and frequently were longer than for whole FDL muscle. In contrast to these findings, the optimum lengths for most motor units in FHL tended to be strikingly shorter than for the whole muscle. No systematic differences between FF, FR and S motor unit types were detected.

DISCUSSION AND CONCLUSIONS

The fact that optimum length of motor units from FDL and FHL were not the same as for the parent muscles may depend partly on the different muscle fibre arrangement, sarcomere lengths and the location of motor units intramuscularly. Although the physiological action of both muscles is the same (viz., digit plantar flexion and claw protrusion) by way of the shared tendon of insertion, the range of optimum lengths for the motor unit populations of these muscles differs and it is large compared with the physiological range of muscle lengths or mean muscle length. This variation would result in flattening of the whole length : tension curve. The behavioural observations after various tenotomies, analysed from cine (see Fig. 2) as well as whole muscle and joint angle measurements indicate that FHL has its optimum tension range at joint angles < 90°. This, together with its preponderance of FF fibres (56%), suggests that a major function for FHL is eliciting strong phasic digit plantar flexion and claw protrusion such as occurs in crouching or climb positions. By contrast to FHL, the behavioural and length optima data show that the smaller FDL is most effective at ankle angles > 90° up to the extremes of plantar flexion. Also the higher content of FR units (47%) in FDL would be consistent with more tonic contraction roles such as stance, grooming and perhaps some aspects of climbing or walking. EMG data recorded by telemetry during walking in unrestrained cats indicates FDL is active (O'DONOVAN et al., 1980), but activity of FHL in crouching and climbing remains to be confirmed. Finally, the activation of forelimb afferents (Groups II and III) and also cortical stimulation causes a unique and powerful inhibition restricted to motoneurones of the ipsilateral FDL and FHL muscles (AOKI and McINTYRE, 1975). As AOKI and McINTYRE suggest, this long spinal inhibition of both muscles probably has a role in reducing claw protrusion during the flexor phase of stepping and perhaps while standing. It might also represent a mechanism to ensure release of claw-grip at the onset of each flexor phase during the act of climbing.

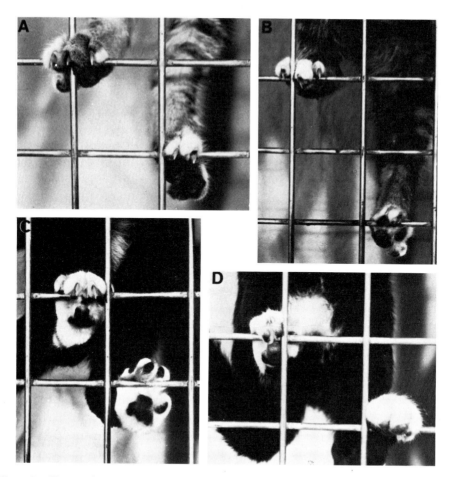

Fig. 2. Shows the extent of claw protrusion during climbing one week after various tenotomies. A : upper left-shows claw protrusion in a normal cat ; B : upper right-bilateral FDL tenotomy-right ankle semiflexed appears almost normal, but left leg is more extended and shows reduced claw protrusion ; C : lower left-both FDL and FHL tenotomised in left leg only-which exhibits absence of claw protrusion ; D : lower right-bilateral FHL tenotomy almost abolishes claw protrusion during climbing

REFERENCES

AOKI M, McINTYRE AK (1975) Cortical and long spinal actions on lumbo-sacral motoneurones in the cat. J Physiol (Lond) 251:569-587

BAGUST J, KNOTT S, LEWIS DM, LUCK JC, WESTERMAN RA (1973) Isometric contractions of motor units in a fast twitch muscle of the cat. J Physiol (Lond) 231:87-104

BURKE RE, LEVINE DN, TSAIRIS P, ZAJAC FE (1973) Physiological types and histochemical profiles in motor units of the cat medial gastrocnemius. J Physiol (Lond) 234:723-748

EDSTROM L, KUGELBERG E (1968) Histochemical composition, distribution of fibres and fatiguability of single motor units. J Neurol Neurosurg Psychiat 31:424-433

O'DONOVAN MJ, PINTER MJ, DUM RP, BURKE RE (1980) Activity patterns of cross-reinnervated flexor digitorum longus and soleus muscle in the cat during unrestrained movement. Abstracts Society for Neurosciences N° 291.1

SRIRATANA D, FINKELSTEIN D, WESTERMAN RA (1981) Functional distinctions and motor unit properties of flexor digitorum longus and flexor hallucis longus in the cat hindlimb. Proc Aust Physiol Pharmacol Soc 12(2):194p

SRIRATANA D, WESTERMAN RA (1983) The morphology and function of the muscle fibres and identified motor units in the long digital flexors in the cat. J Anat Submitted

Discharge Patterns of Cerebellar Cortical Neurons During the Co-Activation and Reciprocal Inhibition of Forearm Muscles

A.M.Smith, R.C.Frysinger, and D.Bourbonnais

Centre de Recherche en sciences neurologiques, Département de Physiologie, Faculté de Médecine, Université de Montréal, C.P. 6128, Succ. A, Montréal, Québec, Canada H3C 3J7

Controlling the balance of activity in opposing muscle groups is an important function of the motor control system of the brain. Reciprocal inhibition and antagonist coactivation are normal but mutually incompatible modes of muscular action. Although the neuronal circuits directly producing reciprocal inhibition and antagonist coactivation probably reside within the spinal cord as suggested by HULTBORN (1972 ; 1976), the selection of one mode or the other appears to be a supraspinal process involving the cerebellum. The movement disorders associated with cerebellar lesions, such as ataxia, dysmetria and adiakokinesis were considered as various forms of asynergia, first by BABINSKI (1899 ; 1902 ; 1909) then later by TILNEY (TILNEY and PIKE, 1925) THOMAS (1925) and WIESENBERG (1927) and can be grouped together as dysfunctions in agonist-antagonist coordination. Although this interpretation was disputed by HOLMES (WIESENBERG, 1927 ; HOLMES, 1939) there is nevertheless considerable evidence to support the asynergic hypothesis (see review by SMITH, 1981).

A recent study of the activity of single neurons in the cerebellar cortex of monkeys trained to exert an isometric precision grip showed that during the coactivation of antagonist muscles, the majority of Purkinje cells decreased their activity (SMITH and BOURBONNAIS, 1981). In contrast, the majority of non-Purkinje neurons of the cerebellar cortex increased firing during prehension. These neurons could include basket, stellate and Golgi cells which have the common property of either inhibiting or disfacilitating activity in Purkinje cells. It was hypothesized that Purkinje cell discharge leads to inhibition of antagonist muscles and that during voluntary co-contraction the Purkinje cells themselves are inhibited by cerebellar cortical interneurons.

In order to test this hypothesis it was decided to examine Purkinje cell discharge in the awake monkey during voluntary reciprocal inhibition and synchronous coactivation of antagonist muscles.

Experimental Brain Research, Suppl. 7
© Springer-Verlag Berlin · Heidelberg 1983

METHODS

Two Macaca fascicularis monkeys were first trained to exert a lateral isometric pinch on a force transducer for one second in the manner described in an earlier publication (SMITH and BOURBONNAIS, 1981). A study of individual forearm muscle activity indicated that all antagonist muscle pairs co-contract during this precision grip (SMITH, 1981). When the monkeys were sufficiently skilled in this task, they were taught to flex and extend the wrist with the fingers extended and to maintain a fixed wrist position for 1.0 or 1.5 seconds. In some cases wrist position was maintained against a force generated by a torque motor but in most instances flexion and extension were exerted against a mechanical stop. The torque generated by the wrist muscles on the manipulandum was measured in most recording sessions.

A detailed study of the forearm muscle activity was conducted because of its critical importance to the interpretation of the results. Intramuscular recordings were made from pairs of 50 μ Teflon-insulated stainless steel wires inserted through the skin into the target muscle. Electrical stimulation at threshold was used to verify the position of each electrode pair. Figure 1 illustrates the trivial but essential point that the three wrist flexors were active during maintained flexion. However, flexor carpi radialis and palmaris longus were clearly more active than flexor capri ulnaris. All three flexor muscles were inactive during maintained extension and extensor carpi ulnaris was the only tonically active wrist extensor. That is, in this animal there was a radial vector to the wrist displacement during flexion and an ulnar vector during extension.

Figure 2 illustrates the contraction pattern of eight reciprocally active muscles of the hand and forearm. These muscles, none of which are prime movers of the wrist, nevertheless showed reciprocal activity to the extent that they contracted with displacement in one direction and were silenced or remained silent during displacement in the opposite direction. In contrast, Figure 3 illustrates the bidirectional activity of 8 additional muscles during the movement phase of the task. However, these muscles were active in both directions only during movement and none of these muscles were tonically contracted in both isometric maintained flexion and extension.

Upon the completion of training on the second task the animals were prepared for chronic unit recording in the manner described by EVARTS (1965). Unit recording began one or two days after surgery and a preliminary search was made for that part of the intermediate zone along the primary fissure where

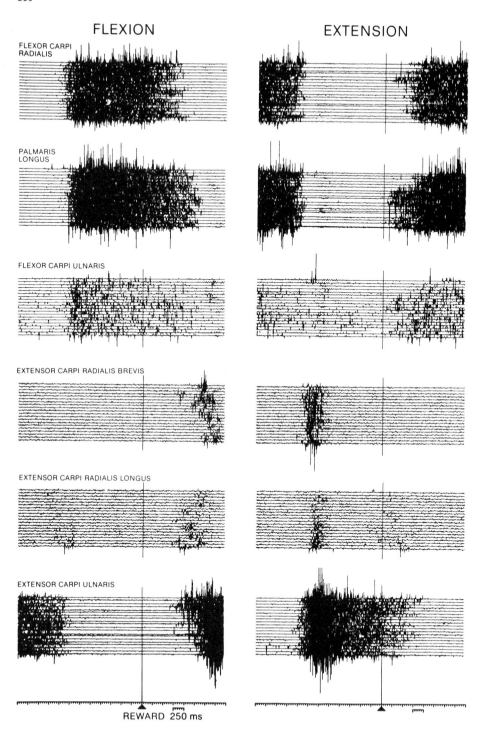

Fig. 1. The EMG traces of the six prime mover muscles of the wrist. Twenty trials have been aligned on the reward delivered after the flexion (at left) and extension (at right) positions were maintained for 1.5 seconds

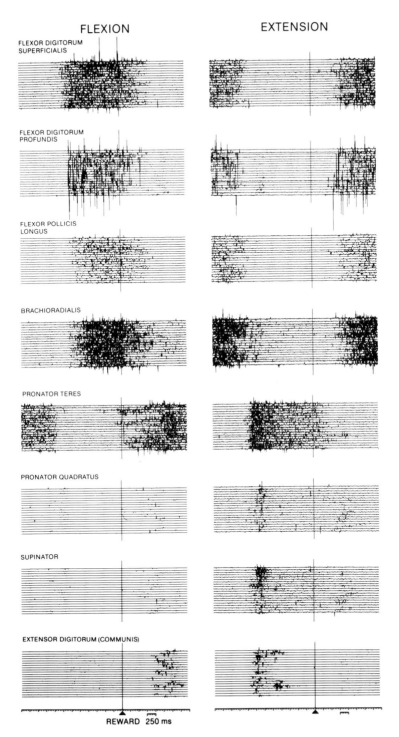

Fig. 2. The activity of 8 reciprocal synergist muscles aligned as in Fig. 1

Table 1

Purkinje cells

Activity during Reciprocal Inhibition	Activity during Co-contraction		
	Increase	Decrease	
Reciprocal	8	9	17
Bi-directional	1	2	3
No change	2	5	7
	11	16	27

Unidentified Cells

Activity during Reciprocal Inhibition	Activity during Co-contraction		
	Increase	Decrease	
Reciprocal	13	6	19
Bi-directional	5	0	5
No change	4	0	4
	22	6	28

neurons responded to cutaneous and proprioceptive stimulation of the hand and forearm. Single neurons recorded in this region of the cerebellar cortex were classified as Purkinje cells if a clear complex climbing fiber discharge could be identified. Units not showing the climbing fiber discharge were grouped together as unidentified neurons. The activity of each neuron was recorded, first during prehension, then during successive wrist displacements. This activity along with the other experimental parameters were recorded on magnetic tape for later analysis performed with the aid of a laboratory computer.

RESULTS

The detailed analysis of activity in individual forearm muscles during isometric maintained flexion and extension of the wrist showed clearly that all the muscles of the forearm studied here were alternately active and relaxed. The generation of static isometric torque in either flexion or extension by muscles which are prevented from shortening appears to be an effective means of inducing reciprocal activity in forearm muscles.

A total of 55 neurons including 27 Purkinje and 28 unidentified neurons were found to either increase or decrease discharge frequency during maintained prehension. The activity of these same units was subsequently evaluated in the wrist flexion and extension task. Table 1 summarizes the activity changes for both Purkinje and non Purkinje cells in each of these two tasks. A slight majority (16/27) of Purkinje cells decreased discharge frequency during the coactivation of antagonist muscles accompanying prehension. In contrast, a greater number of unidentified neurons (22/28) increased activity during the precision grip.

Of the 55 units demontrating activity changes in prehension, only 44 showed modulated discharge during wrist flexion and extension. Eleven units had no consistant changes in firing frequency during wrist displacement and it was thought that these units were related either to muscles activated during prehension only or were specifically recruited by the conditions of muscular co-contraction. However, all of the remaining 44 units including 20 Purkinje and 24 unidentified neurons displayed reciprocal discharge patterns during maintained isometric flexion and extension. That is, the discharge frequency increased with isometric contraction in one direction and decreased for static contraction in the opposite direction. Even the 9 Purkinje cells which increased discharge frequency during the coactivation accompanying prehension had reciprocal discharge patterns during maintained wrist flexion and exten-sion.

Eight neurons either increased or occasionally decreased activity during movements in both directions. The activity of one such bi-directional unit is shown in Figures 4 and 5. This unit belonged to the unidentified category and it increased discharge during the antagonist co-contraction accompanying prehension (Fig. 4). A significant correlation was found between discharge frequency and rate of force change (r= .52 n= 34) during the precision grip. The activity of this same unit in wrist flexion and extension is shown in Figure 5. The peak activity for this unit occurred during movements of the

304

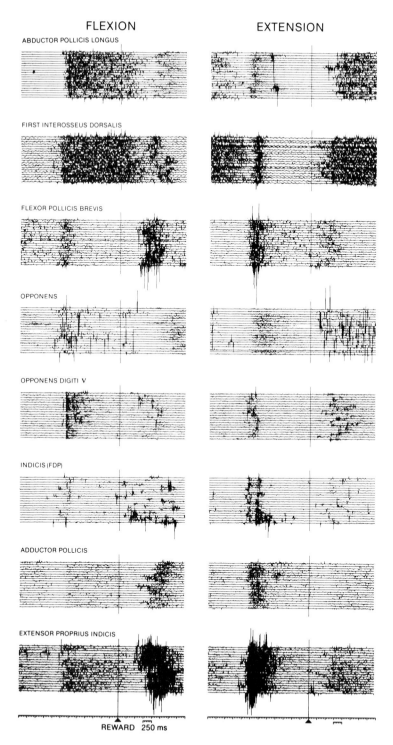

FLEXION   EXTENSION

ABDUCTOR POLLICIS LONGUS

FIRST INTEROSSEUS DORSALIS

FLEXOR POLLICIS BREVIS

OPPONENS

OPPONENS DIGITI V

INDICIS (FDP)

ADDUCTOR POLLICIS

EXTENSOR PROPRIUS INDICIS

REWARD 250 ms

Fig. 3. The activity of 8 bidirectional synergist muscles aligned as in Fig. 1

UNIT 502

N = 17

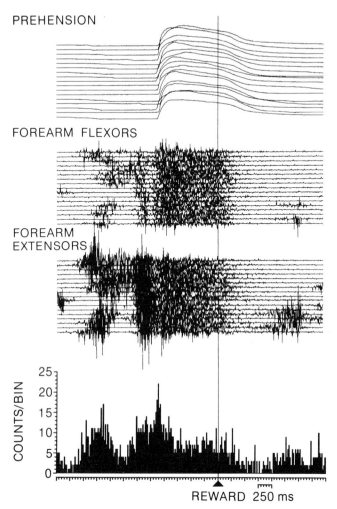

Fig. 4. The histogram at bottom illustrates the activity of an unidentified unit in cerebellar cortex during prehension. Above are shown the forearm surface EMG traces and prehension forces

UNIT 502

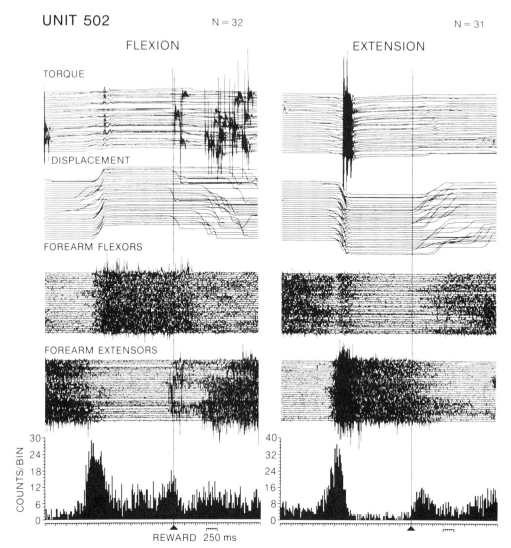

Fig. 5. For the same unit shown in Fig. 4 the histograms show summed activity during flexion (left) and extension (right). Wrist torque and displacement traces show upward deflection for flexion and downward for extension. The large peaks in the torque traces are due to bounces of the manipulandum against the mechanical stops. EMG traces are surface recordings as in Fig. 4

wrist either in flexion or extension. However, the static discharge for the 1.5 seconds preceeding the reward was increased only for isometric flexion and significantly decreased during isometric extension. When the static torques in flexion were expressed as positive values and static extension torques as negative values, a significant correlation between firing frequency and wrist force was demonstrated for this unit (r= .52 n= 63). Correlation coefficients between discharge frequency and flexion and extension torques calculated separately were not significant.

DISCUSSION

Taken together, the observations on Purkinje and unidentified neuron discharge during muscular coactivation and reciprocal inhibition support the hypothesis that the cerebellum plays an important role in selecting the appropriate pattern of muscular contraction. This hypothesis assumes that the activity of a population of Purkinje cells within an individual parallel fiber network is directed to inhibiting a particular muscle in a manner analogous to the Ia inhibitory interneuron. The Purkinje cells which in general decrease discharge frequency during antagonist coactivation have activity which is directionally related to reciprocal muscular contraction. That is, their discharge frequency went up for movements in one direction and down for movements in the opposite direction. The decrease in activity was approximatively the same for opposite direction movements as in antagonist coactivation. The fact that the unidentified neurons which increased activity during antagonist coactivation also showed reciprocal responses to isometric wrist flexion and extension was somewhat surprising. It had been hypothesized (SMITH and BOURBONNAIS, 1981 ; SMITH, 1981) that afferents from both members of an antagonist muscle pair would converge on these presumed inhibitory interneurons of the cerebellar cortex. Instead the data from the present study indicate that the unidentified neurons increase firing in one direction and decrease activity in the other. This implies that there may be separate populations of inhibitory neurons driven by separate parallel fiber afferent networks for movements involving each agonist muscle. During coactivation the inhibitory output of both populations would converge upon a particular population of Purkinje cells to attenuate their discharge and permit the antagonists to maximally stiffen the joint.

It is well known that when external resistance prevents muscle shortening by the prime mover muscles, the antagonists relax (DEMENY, 1890). In the present study, holding the wrist against the stops reliably produced reciprocal EMG activity in both the prime mover muscles and in all synergist muscles as well. However, some synergist muscles contracted with wrist movement in both the flexion and extension directions but contracted tonically in only one of the maintained isometric wrist positions. In addition some neurons of the cerebellar cortex showed bi-directional changes in activity which is in agreement with the results of MANO and YAMAMOTO (1980). However, these same bi-directional units had distinctly different static discharge frequencies during maintained flexion and extension. It is therefore our opinion that the bi-directional activity changes of both the Purkinje cells and the unidentified neurons are related to those muscles which are active during movements in both directions. During isometric wrist flexion or extension, when the muscles were demonstrated to behave reciprocally, all of the Purkinje cells discharged reciprocally, thereby corroborating the link between unit discharge and the activity in specific muscles for the intermediate zone of the cerebellar cortex.

REFERENCES

BABINSKI J (1899) De l'asynergie cérébelleuse. Rev Neurol 7:806-816

BABINSKI J (1902) Sur le rôle du cervelet dans les actes volitionnels nécessitant une succession rapide de mouvements (Diadococinésie). Rev Neurol 10:1013-1014

BABINSKI J (1909) Quelques documents réfletifs à l'histoire des fonctions de l'appareil cérébelleux et de leurs perturbations. Revue Médicale de Médecine Interne 1:113-129

DEMENY G (1890) Du rôle mécanique des muscles antagonistes. Arch Physiol 2:747-761

EVARTS EV (1965) Relation of discharge frequency to conduction velocity in pyramidal tract neurons. J Neurophysiol 28:216-228

HOLMES G (1939) The cerebellum of man. Brain 62:1-30

HULTBORN H (1972) Convergence on interneurons in the reciprocal Ia inhibitory pathway to motoneurons. Acta Physiol Scand Suppl 375:1-42

HULTBORN H (1976) Transmission in the pathway of reciprocal IA inhibition to motoneurons and its control during the tonic stretch reflex. In: HOMMA S (ed) In understanding the stretch reflex. Progress in Brain Research vol 44. Elsevier/North Holland Biomedical Press

MANO NI, YAMAMOTO KI (1980) Single spike activity of cerebellar cortex related to visually guided wrist tracking movements in the monkey. J Neurophysiol 43:713-728

SMITH AM (1981) The coactivation of antagonist muscles. Can J Physiol and Pharmacol 59:733-747

SMITH AM, BOURBONNAIS D (1981) Neuronal activity in cerebellar cortex related to control of prehensile force. J Neurophysiol 45:286-303

THOMAS A (1925) Pathologie du cervelet. In: ROGER GH, WIDAL F, TESSIER LJ (eds), Nouveau Traité de Médecine. Masson, Paris

TILNEY F, PIKE FH (1925) Muscular coordination experimentally studied in its relation to the cerebellum. Arch Neurol Psychiatry 13:289-334

WEISENBERG TH (1927) Cerebellar localization and its symptomatology. Brain 357-390

Activity of Feline Motor Cortical Units to Cutaneous Stimuli During Locomotion and Lifting, Falling and Landing

C.I.Palmer, W.B.Marks, and M.J.Bak

Laboratory of Neural Control, National Institute of Neurological and Communicative Disorders and Stroke, Bethesda, Maryland 20205, USA

Many cells in the feline motor cortex receive cutaneous afferent information (BROOKS et al., 1961 a, b ; BUSER and IMBERT, 1961). The cutaneous receptive fields of these cells are often small and stable. From the extent of the cutaneous input to the motor cortex and the specificity of its information, one could assume that this modality has an important role to play in this region. In this study an attempt has been made to examine to what extent cutaneous peripheral information is available to cells in the motor cortex during movements. This problem was investigated in unanaesthetized freely moving cats during locomotion and a sequence in which the animal was repeatedly lifted and dropped from 20 cm.

The animals were chronically implanted with floating microelectrodes (SALCMAN and BAK, 1976) in the motor cortex, and stimulating electrodes in the pyramidal tract. As the microelectrodes could not be moved, the units they recorded were distinguished from each other by the shape of their action potentials, the size and location of their receptive fields, the latency and duration of their response to cutaneous electrical stimulation, and for PT units, the latency and threshold at which they could be antidromically invaded from pyramidal tract stimulation. Cutaneous stimuli were delivered via an electrode implanted in the forepaw. A cuff electrode (HOFFER et al., 1981) was implanted around the median nerve to record the peripheral cutaneous volley. The reproducibility of forelimb activity during these movements was determined from recordings of forelimb muscles which were chronically implanted with EMG electrodes and from the elbow joint angle recorded with an implanted length gauge.

Cortical units were selected for this study if they had stable cutaneous receptive fields which included the forepaw. The cells had to be consistently activated by weak electrical stimulation from the implanted electrodes when the animals were sitting quietly, and give responses similar to those

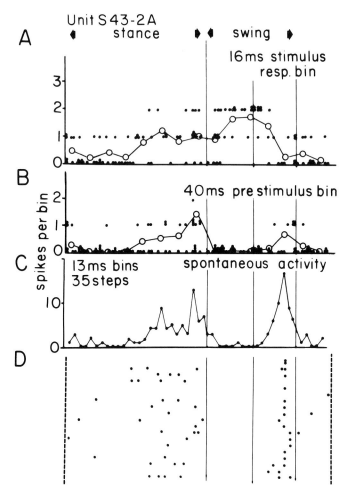

Fig. 1. Profile of a PT unit's response to cutaneous stimulation and profile of its spontaneous activity during a step cycle :

A : Profile of the units stimulus response during a step. The number of action potentials occurring at the time of each of 119 cutaneous stimuli is plotted against where the stimuli were delivered in the step cycle. The stimulus response bin for this unit was 8 to 24 ms after the time of cutaneous stimulation. This value is obtained from the time of the beginning and end of the cortical units post-stimulus histogram peak. The open circles joined by a line are the average of all the points in bins centered on the open circle.

B : Profile of the unit's pre-stimulation activity during a step. The number of action potentials occurring in a 40 ms time bin immediately prior to each of the 119 cutaneous stimuli is plotted against where the stimuli were delivered in the step cycle. Each stimulus response plotted in A is accompanied by a pre-stimulus activity point plotted in B. The open circles are the average number of action potentials occurring during the prestimulation period in a bin centered on the open circles

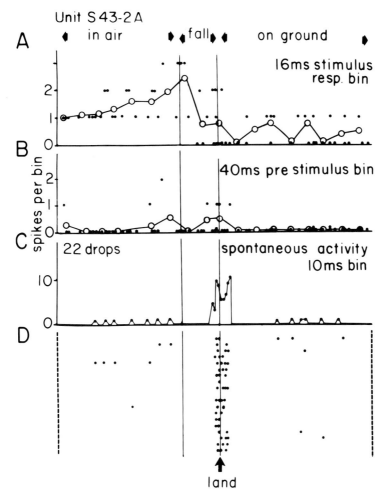

Fig. 2. Profile of a PT unit's response to cutaneous stimulation and profile of its spontaneous activity during the lifting and dropping cycle. Graphs A and B have been constructed in the same way as for figure 1 from 65 stimuli given at 1 per second to the same cell as in figure 1 during the lifting and dropping cycle. C and D have been made by triggering from the foot contact signal obtained on landing, both C and D have the same time scale

C : Profile of the unit's spontaneous activity during a step cycle. Action potentials from 35 steps of similar length have been plotted against where they occurred in the step cycle and the result summed with an average bin width of 13 ms. Before histogramming or rastering the time in each phase of the movement was dilated or contracted so that each normalized phase had the duration of the mean phase. This was almost always less than a 20% adjustment.

D : Spontaneous activity of the unit during 19 steps of similar length. Each line is a step and the action potentials have been plotted against where they occurred in the step cycle, the average bin width is 13 ms

produced by tapping the skin. They also had to fire in a predictable way during locomotion and the lifting and dropping sequence. When a unit was selected its spontaneous activity was first recorded during these movements, then while the animal repeated them during the application of peripheral cutaneous electrical stimulation given once every one or two seconds.

Results were obtained from 22 cortical neurons recorded from 3 cats. Graph A in Figure 1 shows the typical profile of a PT unit's response to cutaneous stimulation during a step cycle. A post-stimulus histogram was first constructed for this unit combining all the stimulation data. The stimulus-response time bin is the time after stimulation between the beginning and end of the post-stimulus histogram peak. The stimulus response is obtained by counting the number of action potentials occurring in the stimulus response time bin for each stimulus. This has been plotted against where each stimulus occurred in the step cycle. To obtain this plot 119 stimuli were given at a rate of one every 2 seconds during locomotion. The inflection points of the elbow joint angle record were used to divide the step into three phases : stance, flexion part of swing and extension part of swing. The phase-related change in the cell's stimulus response shown in graph A Figure 1 is typical of results found for other cortical units. As shown the stimulus response is greatest at the end of stance and beginning of swing and least during the end of swing and beginning of stance. Graph A Figure 2 shows the profile of the same PT units stimulus response during a lifting and dropping cycle. To obtain this plot 65 stimuli were given at a rate of one per second while the animal was repeatedly lifted and dropped. The stimulus response was plotted against its place of occurrence in the cycle. The phases of this cycle were divided using video film of the movements and a pulse produced when the animal's forelimb landed on a platform. The phase-related change in the unit's stimulus response during this cycle is also similar to that found for other units. Thus the response is greatest when the animal is held in the air and immediately after release and least just before and at landing, and while the animal is supporting its weight on the ground.

The cell's stimulus response profile during locomotion and the lifting and dropping cycle cannot be interpreted in terms of a phase-related occlusion of the unit's stimulus response from phase-related increases in the unit's spontaneous firing. In Figure 1 and Figure 2 graph B shows the profile of the unit's pre-stimulation activity during a cycle of the movement. The number of action potentials occurring in a 40 ms time bin immediately prior to each stimulus has been plotted against where they occurred in the movement cycle. Each point in graph A corresponds to a point in graph B. It is clear from comparing graphs A and B that a reduction in the stimulus response is not accompanied by an increase in the unit's spontaneous activity preceding the stimulus.

The cell's stimulus response profile during these movements cannot be due to a modulation in the level of excitability of the cortical cell as ascertained from its spontaneous activity cycle during these movements. If this had been the case then graph A and C in both movements would have a similar profile. When this cell has a high probability of firing, such as at the time of landing or at the end of swing, the peripheral stimulus would then be expected to produce its greatest response if the cortical cell's excitability is the determining factor. However the stimulus response of this cell was less during these periods than at other times during the cycle. The rasters in D of Figures 1 and 2 show that the unit was modulated reproducibly during each step and each lifting and dropping cycle. The probability of firing at the end of swing is the same in each step thus a stimulus given during this period could be assumed to occur when the cortical cell is at a level of excitability which is reproduced during every repetition of this phase of the movement. A comparison of graphs B and C suggests that the prestimulus activity was modulated in the same way as the unstimulated spontaneous activity in C. It was found that the stimulus response was limited to a few milliseconds after stimulation. Thus stimulation did not produce any long-term changes in the excitability of the unit which would have altered its activity cycle during the movement and prevented the drawing of any conclusions from a comparison of graphs A and C.

The stimuli were of low current and short duration, and in the example given in Figures 1 and 2, in which 1 mA pulses of .1 ms duration were used, this stimulus elicited no muscle reflex responses. During locomotion these are known to be linked to phases of the step cycle (FORSSBERG, 1979 ; DUYSENS and LOEB, 1980) however in this case there was no phase-dependent proprioceptive input reaching the cortex.

The cutaneous afferent volley produced with electrical stimulation in the periphery was recorded from the median nerve and found to be constant. Thus the stimulus response profiles of the cortical cells were not due to phase dependent fluctuations in the peripheral input.

Twelve of the 22 cortical units had changes in their stimulus response profiles which could not be accounted for by occlusion of the stimulus response with the unit's spontaneous firing, or by excitability changes of the cells during the movement. This was determined statistically using the x^2 test on pairs of graphs constructed for each cell in a similar way to those shown in Figure 1 and Figure 2. The stimulus response profiles of the cells were similar to those shown in these figures though the units were each spontaneously active at different times during the movements. Six of the 12 were PT units.

Cutaneous information is able to influence motor cortical cells during movement but the response of the cells to cutaneous electrical stimulation changes with different phases of the movement. Since these changes are not dependent on the level of excitability of these cells the afferent input must have already been modulated before reaching them. During locomotion the cortical cells were least responsive to this stimulus at the end of swing and beginning of stance and most responsive at the end of stance and beginning of swing. During the lifting and dropping cycle the response was least just before and at landing and also while the animal was held in the air and immediately after release. Thus there appears to be a movement-phase-related gating of cutaneous afferent input to some cortical cells.

ACKNOWLEDGEMENTS

We wish to thank Mr G. DOLD, Ms C. JACKSON and Ms M. CHAPMAN for excellent technical assistance and encouragement during the course of these experiments, and Dr. G.E. LOEB who generously allowed us the use of his laboratory facilities for the major part of this work.

REFERENCES

BUSER P, IMBERT M (1961) Sensory projections to the motor cortex in cats : a microelectrode study. In: ROSENBLITH WA (ed) Sensory communication. Wiley, New-York, pp 601-626

BROOKS VB, RUDOMIN P, SLAYMAN CL (1961a) Sensory activation of neurons in the cat's cerebral cortex. J Neurophysiol 24:286-301

BROOKS VB, RUDOMIN P, SLAYMAN CL (1961b) Peripheral receptive fields of neurons in the cat's cerebral cortex. J Neurophysiol 24:302-325

DUYSENS J, LOEB GE (1980) Modulation of ipsi- and contralateral reflex responses in unrestrained walking cats. J Neurophysiol 44:1024-1031

FORSSBERG H (1979) Stumbling corrective reaction : a phase-dependent compensatory reaction during locomotion. J Neurophysiol 42:936-953

HOFFER JA, LOEB GE, PRATT CA (1981) Single unit conduction velocities from averaged nerve cuff electrode records in freely moving cats. J Neurosci Meth 4:211-225

SALCMAN M, BAK MJ (1976) A new chronic recording intracortical microelectrode. Med Biol Eng 14:42-50

Neural Coding of Force and of Rate of Force Change in the Precentral Finger Region of the Monkey

M.-C. Hepp-Reymond and R. Diener

Brain Research Institute, University of Zürich, CH-8029 Zürich, Switzerland

INTRODUCTION

The research on neuronal correlates of dynamic parameters - force (F) and rate of force change (dF/dt) - in precentral neurons concerns the oldest problem of coding specificities in area 4 neurons. Since EVARTS' (1968 ; 1969) first demonstration that discharge patterns of certain PT neurons in the precentral arm region can specify active force exerted about a joint and the rate of force change, several investigations of similar and different movements have confirmed EVARTS' findings. The best correlations have been shown between firing rate and isometric static force in precentral finger and jaw neurons (HEPP-REYMOND et al., 1978 ; HOFFMAN and LUSCHEI, 1980) and in cortico-motoneuronal (CM) cells projecting to wrist muscles during auxotonic and isometric torque responses (CHENEY and FETZ, 1980). Indeed all three studies indicate that precentral neurons (PT, CM and non identified) can increase their discharge monotonically, and even linearly over a specific force or torque range, either with biting strength, wrist torque or force in the precision grip. Less convincing evidence has been supplied for the specification of the first derivative of force by the firing rate of phasically discharging neurons. Since EVARTS' observation that PT neurons modulate their firing rate with dF/dt, support was supplied by HUMPHREY et al. (1970) for wrist movement against isotonic loads and by SMITH et al. (1975) for isometric finger muscle contractions. SCHMIDT et al. (1975), however, found only one neuron whose activity could be related to dF/dt, and this parameter was poorly specified in the discharge patterns of CM neurons whose firing rate was well related to static force (CHENEY and FETZ, 1980).
In this paper we will present more evidence for the coding of force in the precentral finger region and raise some questions about the specification of the rate of force change by the neuronal firing in this region.

Experimental Brain Research, Suppl. 7
© Springer-Verlag Berlin · Heidelberg 1983

METHODS

Four monkeys (Macaca fascicularis) were trained to control isometric force on a transducer held between thumb and index finger. The details of the training paradigm have been described previously (HEPP-REYMOND et al., 1978), as well as the force transducer, its fixation and calibration (HEPP-REYMOND and WIESENDANGER, 1972 ; SMITH et al., 1975). Briefly the monkeys initiated the trials by closing their fingers on the transducer, first producing a force ramp, reaching a low force threshold and maintaining it within narrow limits (0.1-0.3 or 0.4 N) for 1.5 s. At the end of the holding period a light instructed the monkey to increase force and reach a second higher force window (0.4 to 0.9 N, or 0.5 to 1.0 N). This second holding time was fixed at 0.8, 1 or 1.1 s depending on the monkey. An idealized force curve is shown on the right side of Figure 3A. The limits set for the upper force window could be shifted to higher values. A tone signalled the entry into the force window and served as feedback during the holding period : a low frequency tone for the lower force level, higher pitched ones for the higher levels. In two monkeys, visual feedback on an oscilloscope, mounted 40 cm in front of the monkey, was also provided. Two horizontal bars on an oscilloscope screen were used to indicate the upper and lower bounds of the force windows, and the force exerted on the transducer was displayed as an excursion of a bright dot. The monkeys were not trained to make fast reactions to the light signal since they had more than 1 second to increase from the low to the high level, but precision in the force control was required. Implantation and recording were made following standard procedures (EVARTS, 1968) using varnished tungsten microelectrodes. Microstimulation (1-15 μA) was applied through the recording microelectrode to verify the recording site. Data were stored on magnetic types for off-line data analysis.

RESULTS

From over 400 neurons recorded in 4 monkeys in the finger region of area 4, only 171 neurons closely related to the task were retained for analysis. From those, 139 displayed during the force ramp and hold period, one of the 4 basic types of firing patterns which were described in previous reports (SMITH et al., 1975 ; HEPP-REYMOND et al., 1978). Most common (32%) were tonic neurons which discharge only during the hold periods, and increase their firing rate with force. Phasic-tonic neurons, which show increase of their firing rate during both force ramp and force hold period, were less numerous in our sample (18%). A third large group of precentral neurons (28%) was found which showed a consistent decrease of the firing rate with force.

Their activity looked like mirror images of either of the two first classes mentioned. The remaining (21%) were phasic neurons whose activity consists of either a phasic burst or an increase of the firing rate on a tonic background before and during the force increase ramp. In two of the 4 monkeys, this sample of discharge patterns included additional neurons which solely increased their activity before, during and after the reward in temporal relation to the release of force on the transducer. These so-called "release" neurons represented 15% of the total neuron population retained in these two monkeys, whereas another 10% was classified as "atypical" because they did not correspond to any of the classes described above. Only the first four classes (phasic, tonic, phasic-tonic and decreasing) have been quantitatively analysed.

In order to test the neuronal correlates of force and/or dF/dt, a trial pro trial quantitative analysis was performed. To check the specification of force, time segments during hold periods were selected from individual trials. Care was taken to choose segments with stable force and little variation to avoid contamination with possible dF/dt related modulation (HEPP-REYMOND et al., 1978). Both force and firing rate were averaged over time for each segment and displayed in scatter diagrams as shown in Figure 1C and 1D for two phasic-tonic neurons, whose firing rate and related force curves are shown in the top part of the figure. Linear regression coefficients, calculated on these diagrams for 33 neurons (19 tonic and 14 phasic-tonic) yielded values from 0.5 to 0.94, all statistically significant ($p < 0.01$). For the phasic-tonic and tonic neurons whose firing rate decreased with force, a trial pro trial analysis was made for 15 neurons, whose activity decreased monotonically with force increase. The regression coefficients varied between -0.4 and -0.75, and all but one reached statistical significance ($p < 0.05$). A large number of decreasing neurons could not be analysed on a trial pro trial basis, as they were totally inactivated at the higher force level. From the regression lines an index of force sensitivity - increment of firing rate per unit of force - was calculated for both groups of neurons. Mean rate-force slope for 33 neurons which showed an increase firing rate with force was 66.5 Hz/N with a large range (12 Hz/N to 163 Hz/N). For the 15 decreasing neurons the average negative rate-force slope was -21 Hz/N (from -7 to -33 Hz/N). The difference in mean slope between the increasing and decreasing neurons can be attributed to the limited firing range of the decreasing neurons, e.g. from 0.2 N decreasing neurons changed their mean discharge rate of 22.5 Hz to ca. zero at 1 N, whereas increasing neurons changed from 24 Hz at 0.2 N to much higher values at 1 N.

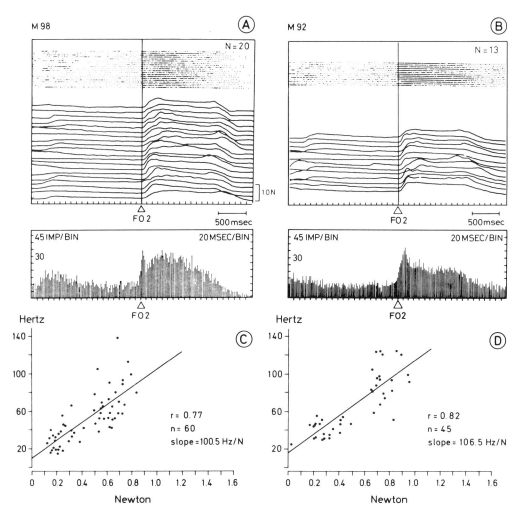

Fig. 1. Example of two phasic-tonic neurons increasing their discharge
frequency with increase of force.
A and B : At the top, raster of unit activity and underneath the associated
force traces aligned on the onset of force change from the low to the high
force level (FO2). Below, peri-response time histograms constructed from the
raster aligned on FO2. Bin width : 20 ms. Display time : 4 s.
C and D : scatter diagrams displaying the relation between mean force and
mean discharge frequency for the 2 neurons displayed in A and B. r : linear
regression coefficient. n : number of measurements. slope : rate-force slope,
see text

Phasic and phasic-tonic neurons displayed a clear burst or activity increase before and during the force ramps, as can be seen on the peri-response time histograms of Figure 1. Because the relation of neuronal discharge to dF/dt is still controversial (SCHMIDT et al., 1975 ; SMITH et al., 1975 ; CHENEY and FETZ, 1980) we decided to check this coding property in a more detailed trial pro trial analysis, which also takes into account delays between the increase in firing rate and onset of force change. We tested a selection of variables on a group of 10 phasic neurons and on a sample of 6 representative phasic-tonic neurons.

All 10 phasic neurons chosen had sharp, delimited bursts of activity. We tried to relate mean firing rate, number of action potentials and duration to mean or peak dF/dt, or to force during the ramp. Only 4 phasic neurons had significant regression coefficients between mean firing frequency and mean dF/dt ($p < 0.05$). Neither the duration of the burst nor the number of spikes in the burst yielded significant correlations. However, in all ten neurons the burst onset was tightly coupled to the onset of force change.

Six phasic-tonic neurons which showed a significant peak in their pe-ri-response time histograms aligned on the change of force from the low to the high force level (F02, see Fig. 1) were chosen for the detailed parametric analysis. The mean or peak firing rate, or the number of spikes during the ramp were correlated to either peak dF/dt, mean dF/dt, peak force or mean force during the ramp (Fig. 3C, interval a). The same could be done for different time intervals, for example for a 60 or 100 ms duration preceding peak dF/dt (Fig. 3C, b and c). These 6 phasic-tonic neurons all had high regression coefficients between their discharge rate and static force. For 4 of these neurons a positive correlation was also found between mean firing frequency and mean force in the ramp, when all the force values (the low ones for the first force step and the higher ones for the second force step) were pooled. This correlation is shown for two neurons in Figure 2B. For the same 4 neurons the mean firing rate in the ramp was also signi-ficantly correlated with the peak dF/dt, but only when the dF/dt values of the first and second force steps were pooled (Fig. 2A). For a fifth neuron the activity in a 100 ms interval before peak dF/dt was related to peak dF/dt, but not to peak force. Finally the last neuron of the sample, although it had a very clear activation during the force ramp, was neither related to force nor to dF/dt. During the high force ramp alone a significant positive correlation between mean firing rate and dF/dt was found in a single neuron. During the low force ramp two neurons showed only correlations between dF/dt and mean firing rate in a 60 ms interval before force onset. An important

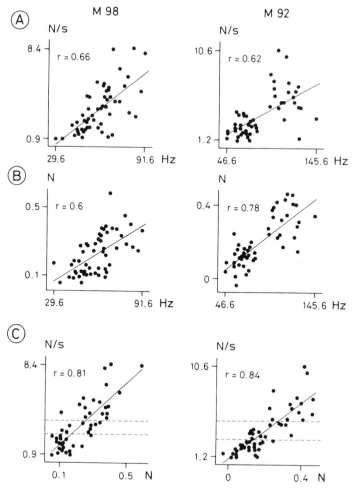

Fig. 2. The scatter diagrams reflect the analysis of the two neurons of figure 1. They display the relation of mean discharge frequency in the force ramp with peak dF/dt (A) and mean force in the ramp (B). C shows the relation between force and dF/dt for the values displayed in A and B. r : linear regression coefficient. Number of measurements in A, B and C is 54 for neuron M98 and 53 for neuron M92

finding for the interpretation of the data is displayed in Figure 2C and was observed in 5 of the 6 neurons : the correlation between force and dF/dt in the analysed values is quite high (0.61, 0.84, 0.75, 0.81 and 0.7 respectively). In other words low dF/dt values correspond to low force values and high dF/dt to high force.

Because of these observations we posed the question which of the two parameters, force or dF/dt, was mainly responsible for the activity increase during the force ramps. In order to dissociate the two parameters we checked within narrow selections of dF/dt values (dashed lines in Fig. 2C) if the selected values had significant relation to force. The same procedure could also be applied to selected narrow force ranges for checking the relation to dF/dt. The result of this analysis for the two neurons displayed in Figures 1 and 2 disclosed for one neuron (M92) high correlation between firing rate of the selected values and force (0.89). For the other neuron (M98) the values within the narrow range selected did not have any correlation to force, whereas the values within a selected force range (not shown in Fig. 2C) yielded a good correlation with dF/dt (0.71), and similar relations were found for the other 3 neurons. These data from a preliminary analysis suggest that in the phasic-tonic neurons the increase of firing frequency in the ramp cannot be simply related to either force or dF/dt alone, but may depend on both to various degrees for different cells.

Finally a consistent finding was that the relation of the discharge frequency during the ramp (or before) and peak dF/dt was highly variable, depending on the strategy used for the generation of force. This could best be observed for the first force step when the monkey initiated the trial. One of the 4 monkeys developed two strategies shown in Figure 3A and C : in one case he was controlling precisely the isometric force necessary to reach the boundaries of the required range. These "controlled" force curves have characteristically a slow monotonic increase of force (Fig. 3A and C, right side). In the other case he was generating a strong uncontrolled pulse of force which overshot the force window. These "ballistic" force curves are characterized by an abrupt onset and a fast increase with high dF/dt values as shown on the left of Figure 3A and C. In this second situation the burst of neuronal activity occurred earlier than in the controlled one. However, the firing rate - neither during the force ramp (a) nor during various intervals before the peak dF/dt (b and c in Fig. 3C) - correlated positively with peak or mean dF/dt. In Figure 3B are scatter diagrams displaying for one neuron the relation between dF/dt and discharge frequency in the ballistic (left) and controlled (right) force ramps. The linear regression coefficient which is significantly positive for the controlled situation ($p < 0.01$) yielded a negative value for the ballistic force ramps. A clear negative trend was found in one phasic-tonic and in two phasic neurons for which both types of force ramps could be reliably dissociated. In four other phasic-tonic neurons for which positive correlations had been found between mean firing rate and peak dF/dt or mean force in the controlled force ramps, the regression coefficients were no longer significant when the ballistic values were mixed with the controlled ones. These data suggest that the neuronal activity in

322

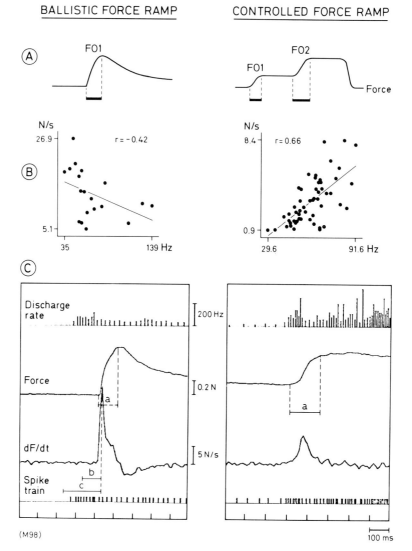

BALLISTIC FORCE RAMP

CONTROLLED FORCE RAMP

Fig. 3. Differences in the firing patterns of one neuron during fast ballistic and slow controlled force ramps (drawn schematically in A). In B scatter diagrams display the relation between dF/dt and discharge frequency for the values measured during the first force ramp (F01 in A), or during both force ramps (F01 and F02 in A) for ballistic and controlled force increase respectively. Number of measurements is 19 for ballistic and 54 for controlled force ramps. In C two examples of single trials are shown with instantaneous frequency, force, rate of force change (dF/dt) and the spike train from top to bottom. a, b and c indicate the intervals for which the firing rate was computed. r : linear regression coefficient

the time variation of force (or dynamic phase in CHENEY and FETZ' nomenclature) is highly modifiable, showing a better relation to force parameters during precise controlled movements. Since the distinction between controlled and ballistic ramps is not always sharp the effect just reported could possibly explain the difficulties in establishing a correlation between firing rate and dF/dt in phasic and phasic-tonic neurons.

DISCUSSION

On the basis of the present data, which extend our previous observations, the following conclusions can be drawn :

Firstly, for a group of precentral neurons the firing rate represents closely the force exerted in the precision grip, which requires the cocontraction of many muscles (SMITH, 1981). The monotonic increase of the discharge frequency is linear only over a limited force range. These data are comparable to those of CHENEY and FETZ (1980) for torque applied at the wrist and to those of HOFFMAN and LUSCHEI (1980) for the jaw musculature. The force sensitivity of the neurons represented by their rate-force slopes, i.e. the increase of firing frequency per unit of force, has a wide scatter with the mean being 66 Hz/N for 33 neurons in the finger area. For 11 wrist flexor and 14 extensor CM neurons CHENEY and FETZ (1980) reported rate-torque slopes of 2.5 Hz/N.cm and 4.8 Hz/N.cm respectively. HOFFMAN and LUSCHEI (1980) have classified their force sensitive neurons into two groups, one with 8 neurons had steep mean rate-force slope (2.5 Hz/N) over a small force range before reaching saturation, whereas the other group of 7 neurons increased their firing rate over the whole force range tested, with a mean slope of 0.6 Hz/N. If one compares these three sets of data, it is evident that the firing rates of the neurons are similar when related to maximal force development in three different muscle groups. Indeed, for estimates of maximal force in the different tasks (72 N for HOFFMAN and LUSCHEI, 15 N.cm for CHENEY and FETZ and ca. 1 N in our situation) the mean firing of the neurons in the three experiments is 79.5 for CHENEY and FETZ (1980), 81 Hz for HOFFMAN and LUSCHEI (1980) and 79.6 Hz for our own data. The resemblance of the behavior of the neurons under these three conditions suggest that they may belong to the same population of CM neurons.

Our second conclusion is related to whether dF/dt may be a parameter coded in motor cortex. The experimental evidence gathered so far seems to indicate that only a small percentage of pure phasic neurons increase their firing rate with an increase of the first derivative of force. According to SMITH et al. (1975) the activity of 18 precentral (PT and non-identified) neurons out of 76 could be related to dF/dt (7 of 12 dynamic, 11 of 31 mixed). We found in our two force steps paradigm, which requires a much smaller and more precise force increment, no improvement of this correlation, although many more variables were tested. The finding that the firing frequency of phasic neurons does not always correlate with dF/dt is not surprising, since this type of neuron could not be identified as a CM neuron (FETZ and CHENEY, 1980) and might give temporal but not always parameter-specific signals to the spinal motor apparatus. Of course these neurons could also project to muscles less directly involved in the precision grip task. As to the significance of the increase of discharge of phasic-tonic neurons during the force ramp, our simple two parameter analysis has disclosed that this increase cannot be always related to dF/dt alone. From our restricted sample of representative neurons, all of which had high regression coefficient to static force, the following can be summarized : some neurons show modulation of activity mainly related to dF/dt, some mainly relate to the force developed during the ramp and some have no relation to either parameter. In view of the large fluctuations in the firing rates of precentral neurons, it is not clear that other methods which have been used with success in various sensory systems and in the oculomotor system (ROBINSON, 1981) are applicable to our experimental situation. Our observation on the phasic-tonic neurons confirms those of CHENEY and FETZ (1980) who found a positive relation between a dynamic index (SMITH et al., 1975) and dF/dt only in 5 of 13 phasic-tonic CM cells. In two neurons they even found negative correlations which fits well with our finding in one neuron.

Finally the third observation is the dissociation in the specification of dF/dt by phasic and phasic-tonic neurons, which occurs when fast ballistic force ramps are generated instead of controlled ones. This finding suggests that the phasic-tonic force and dF/dt sensitive neurons are well related to those parameters only under precisely controlled situations. Other neuronal populations in the cortex or subcortical structures might participate in the control of fast ballistic and powerful force generation. Our data are in agreement with CHENEY and FETZ' observations (1980) on certain phasic-tonic CM cells which became virtually inactive during ballistic alternating movement of the wrist.

In other experimental paradigms it has already been suggested that these two movement strategies can influence differently the discharge of PT neurons, by modifying the afferent input to these neurons (EVARTS and FROMM, 1977 ; FROMM and EVARTS, 1977). However, in their situation the PT (pyramidal tract) neurons investigated were showing similar maximal discharge rates for fast ballistic or slow controlled movements, therefore being related neither to the amplitude nor to the velocity of the movements. In precentral neurons, the correlation of firing rate with velocity, which according to LAMARRE et al. (1978) is significant for ballistic flexion-extension movements of the forearm, was very poor for controlled flexion and extension of the wrist in a visual tracking task (HAMADA and KUBOTA, 1979). All these observations suggest that the coding of movement parameters and of dF/dt in motor cortical neurons is conditional, depending on the strategies or motor programs involved.

ACKNOWLEDGEMENTS

The authors gratefully acknowledge the assistance provided by the technical staff of the Brain Research Institute and in particular by R. GYSIN, M. PADUA and C. WUEST.

This research was supported by the Swiss National Science Foundation grants n° 3.585.79 and 3.505.79, the Slack-Gyr-Foundation in Zürich and the Sandoz-Foundation, Basel.

REFERENCES

CHENEY PD, FETZ EE (1980) Functional classes of primate corticomotoneuronal cells and their relation to active force. J Neurophysiol 44:773-791

EVARTS EV (1968) Relation of pyramidal tract activity to force exerted during voluntary movement. J Neurophysiol 31:14-27

EVARTS EV (1969) Activity of pyramidal tract neurons during postural fixation. J Neurophysiol 32:375-385

EVARTS EV, FROMM C (1977) Sensory responses in motor cortex neurons during precise motor control. Neurosci Lett 5:267-272

FETZ EE, CHENEY PD (1980) Postspike facilitation of forelimb muscle activity by primate corticomotoneuronal cells. J Neurophysiol 44:751-772

FROMM C, EVARTS EV (1977) Relation of motor cortex neurons to precisely controlled and ballistic movements. Neurosci Lett 5:259-266

HAMADA I, KUBOTA K (1979) Monkey pyramidal tract neurons and changes of movement parameters in visual tracking. Brain Res Bull 4:249-257

HEPP-REYMOND M-C, WIESENDANGER M (1972) Unilateral pyramidotomy in monkeys : effects on force and speed of a conditioned precision grip. Brain Res 36:117-131

HEPP-REYMOND M-C, WYSS UR, ANNER R (1978) Neuronal coding of static force in the primate motor cortex. J Physiol (Paris) 74:287-291

HOFFMAN DS, LUSCHEI ES (1980) Responses of monkey precentral cortical cells during a controlled jaw bite task. J Neurophysiol 44:333-348

HUMPHREY DR, SCHMIDT EM, THOMPSON WD (1970) Predicting measures of motor performance from multiple cortical spike trains. Science 170:758-762

LAMARRE Y, BIOULAC B, JACKS B (1978) Activity of precentral neurones in conscious monkeys : effects of deafferentation and cerebellar ablation. J Physiol (Paris) 74:253-264

ROBINSON DA (1981) The use of control systems analysis in the neurophysiology of eye movements. Ann Rev Neurosci 4:463-503

SCHMIDT EM, JOST RG, DAVIS KK (1975) Reexamination of the force relationship of cortical cell discharge patterns with conditioned wrist movements. Brain Res 83:213-223

SMITH AM, HEPP-REYMOND M-C, WYSS UR (1975) Relation of activity in precentral cortical neurons to force and rate of force change during isometric contractions of finger muscles. Exp Brain Res 23:315-332

SMITH AM (1981) The coactivation of antagonist muscles. Can J Physiol Pharmacol 59:733-747

Spatial Coding of Movement: A Hypothesis Concerning the Coding of Movement Direction by Motor Cortical Populations

A.P.Georgopoulos, R.Caminiti, J.F.Kalaska, and J.T.Massey

The Philip Bard Laboratories of Neurophysiology, Department of Neuroscience, The Johns Hopkins University, School of Medicine, Baltimore, MA 21205, USA

How are movements in a particular direction made ? We studied this problem by recording the discharge of single neurons in the motor cortex of monkeys while the animals performed two-dimensional arm movements on a plane working surface. These movements started from the same point and were of the same amplitude, but their directions differed at intervals of 45°.

Experimental procedure

An apparatus was used (GEORGOPOULOS et al., 1981) in which a light-weight handle could be moved freely and with low friction in the two (X-Y) dimensions across a plane working surface. Monkeys were trained to move the handle and capture (within a circle attached to it) lighted targets in a reaction-time task. Of 9 targets, one was at the center and 8 around it on a circle of 8 cm radius. In a typical trial, the animal first captured the center light and held there for a variable period of time (control period), then a peripheral light came on and the animal had to move the handle to capture that target to receive a liquid reward. Since the 8 targets were arranged equidistantly around the circumference of the circle, the directions of the movements made from the center to the target covered the whole circle at 45° intervals. Motor behavioral data concerning performance in this task have been described elsewhere (GEORGOPOULOS et al., 1981). Families of trajectories of movement made by a well trained animal are shown in Figure 1.

Glass-coated platinum-iridium microelectrodes were advanced through the dura into the cortex of rhesus monkeys. The action potentials of individual neurons were recorded extracellularly using standard electrophysiological techniques (GEORGOPOULOS et al., 1982). The experiment was controlled through a PDP 11/20 minicomputer. The XY position of the manipulandum was sampled at 100/sec. Neuronal data were collected as interspike intervals with a sampling density of 10^4/sec and analyzed off-line using standard display and statisti-

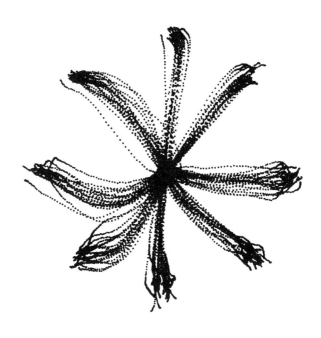

PA35TR.001   ⌐⌐ 10 MM

Fig. 1. Families of trajectories of movements made in 8 directions by a well trained monkey from the center of the plane to peripheral targets

cal techniques. Methods appropriate for the analysis of directional data were employed (MARDIA, 1972) where needed.

Single cell discharge and movement direction

Sixty nine penetrations were made into the proximal arm area (WOOLSEY et al., 1950) of the motor cortex of rhesus monkeys (area 4 and posterior strip of area 6, see WIESENDANGER, 1981). Three hundred and twenty three task-related cells were recorded (5 hemispheres, 4 monkeys). All of these cells discharged in association with movements of the contralateral arm at the shoulder and/or elbow.

The frequency of discharge of 241/323 (74.6%) of cells studied varied in an orderly fashion with the direction of the movement ("directionally tuned cells"). Almost all of these cells showed changes of activity in association with more than one, and commonly with all, movement directions. However, discharge was most intense with movements in a preferred direction and was

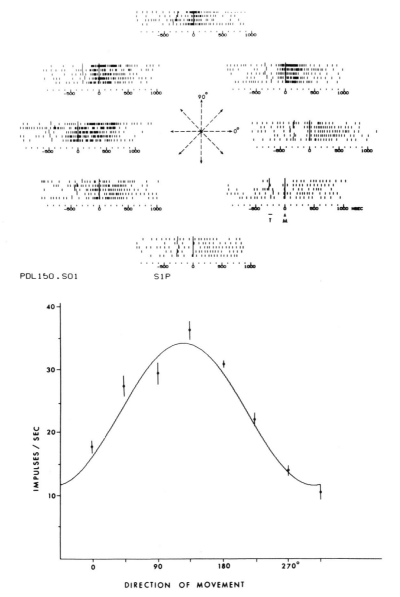

Fig. 2. Orderly variation in the frequency of discharge of a motor cortical cell with the direction of movement. Upper half : Rasters are oriented to movement onset, M, and show impulse activity during five movements in each of the 8 directions indicated by the center diagram. Longer vertical bars in the spike trains indicate the time of target (T) and movement onset for individual trials. Lower half : Directional tuning curve of the same cell. Discharge frequency is for "total experimental time", i.e. from the appearance of the target to the end of the movement (approximately 500 msec after movement onset). Data points are mean ± SEM. The regression equation for the fitted sinusoidal curve is $D = 23.37 + 9.27 \sin \theta - 6.88 \cos \theta$, , where D is the frequency of discharge and θ the direction of movement ; or, equivalently, $D = 23.37 + 11.54 \cos (\theta - \theta_o)$, where θ_o is the preferred direction ($\theta_o = 126.6°$

reduced gradually with movements made in directions farther and farther away
from the preferred one (Fig. 2). This resulted in a directional tuning curve.
These curves were bell-shaped, and in 75% of cells they were sinusoids ; that
is, the frequency of discharge was a sinusoidal function of the direction of
movement. An exemple is illustrated in Figure 2. Preferred directions differed for different cells so that the tuning curves partially overlapped.
Similar results were obtained when the relations were analyzed between
movement direction and cell discharge during the reaction time, movement
time, total experimental time (TET, from the appearance of the target to the
end of the movement), and also during the period preceding the earliest
changes in electromyographic (EMG) activity (ca. 80 msec before movement
onset). A detailed analysis of the directional properties of motor cortical
cells has been described elsewhere (GEORGOPOULOS et al., 1982).

Coding for the direction of movement in motor cortex : a population code ?

A salient finding of this study was that although individual cells in the
motor cortex possessed directional preference, they lacked extreme directional specificity ; that is, virtually no cells discharged during movement in a
particular direction without also discharging during movements in other
directions. Indeed, it was found that movements in a certain direction
engaged neurons with overlapping directional tuning curves. These results
indicate that the direction of movement is not subserved by cells uniquely
related to a particular direction but is instead encoded in a directionally
heterogeneous population of cells.

We discuss below a possible mechanism by which movements in a given direction
could be generated by populations made up of cells possessing both directional preference and directional spread. We call it the "vector hypothesis" ;
it is illustrated in Figure 3. In (A) the tuning curve of a neuron is shown
as a polar plot. Discharge frequency is for TET. Notice that the cell
discharged most in a preferred direction (at $0°$), and that the frequency of
discharge was less for directions away from this preferred one. The circle
indicates the average frequency of discharge during these movements. In (B),
the first of two main assumptions underlying this hypothesis is illustrated.
This assumption comprises the three following postulates. 1) For all movements, a cell exerts a directional influence (vector) which is along the axis
of the cell's preferred direction(e.g. at $0° - 180°$ in Fig. 3); 2)the direction
of this vector is in the cell's preferred direction(at $0°$)for an increase(+) of
discharge above the average level, or in the opposite direction (at $180°$) for a
decrease (-) in discharge (shaded area, Fig. 3A) ; and 3) the magnitude of

A)

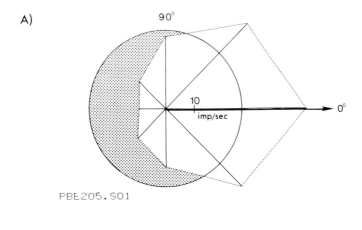

PBE205.S01

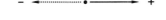

B)

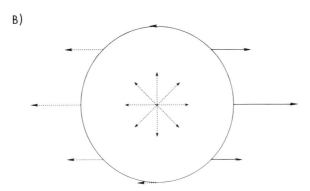

Fig. 3. Vector hypothesis. See text for explanation. The interrupted lines at the center in B indicate the 8 directions of movement tested

that vector is proportional to the change in discharge from the average level. The second assumption (not illustrated) is that for a given movement direction individual cell contributions as defined above are summed linearly as vectors.

Figure 4 shows the result of the application of this hypothesis to data obtained for movements in the 8 directions tested. For each direction of movement (indicated by interrupted lines at the center of the figure) the vector contributions of each of the 241 directionally tuned cells are displayed. Each line represents a vector which denotes the directional

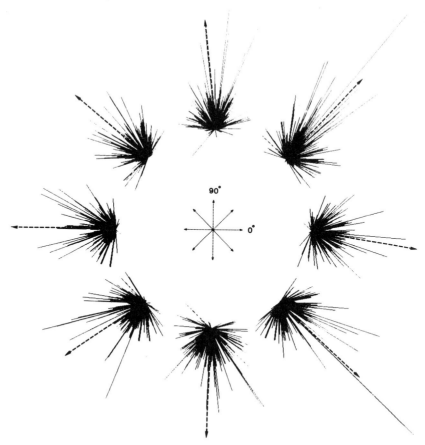

Fig. 4. Vector contributions of 241 directionally tuned motor cortical cells are shown for each of the 8 movement directions tested. Notice the spatial congruence between the direction of the vectorial sum (thick interrupted lines in each plot) and the direction of movement (thin interrupted lines at center). See text for explanation

influence of a cell along the axis of its preferred direction, according to the assumption described above. All cell-vectors are directed from center outward. The length of each vector is proportional to the percent change in cell discharge from the average frequency of discharge observed during the 8 movement directions. These vectors were then summed linearly. The direction of the vectorial sum is indicated by an interrupted line (long bars) for each direction of movement. It can be seen that this direction was very close (within 11°) to the actual direction of movement. This range was within the variability of the directions of the actual movement trajectories observed in well trained animals.

These results suggest that the direction of movement might be encoded in the population discharge of directionally tuned motor cortical cells. In the hypothesis discussed above both the preferred direction (direction of cell vectors) and the variation in the frequency of discharge (length of cell vectors) were taken into account to compute the vectorial sum(s) shown in Figure 4. A simpler vectorial model would take into account only the preferred direction. It can be seen in Figure 4 that, in general, these preferred directions were distributed symmetrically around any particular direction of movement (see also Fig. 8 in GEORGOPOULOS et al., 1982), so that the directional influence of the population as a whole was towards that direction of movement. Although this simpler model can account for the data, the fact that the frequency of discharge was a sinusoidal function of the movement direction in 75% of the cells supports the original version of the vectorial hypothesis, as described in the beginning of this section.

Possible relations to muscle events

An important assumption of the hypothesis outlined above is that motor cortical cells exert a directional influence, which is exerted on the same axis (the preferred direction) but varies in magnitude during movements in different directions. We wish now to examine this assumption in the light of known relations between motor cortical cells and peripheral motor structures.

Movements in the task were produced mainly by muscles acting on the shoulder. The intramuscularly recorded EMG activity of these muscles varied with the direction of movement in an orderly fashion, in that it was high during movements in a particular ("preferred") direction and decreased gradually with movements made in directions farther and farther away from the preferred one (MASSEY et al., 1981).

It could be regarded that this orderly variation in EMG activity is associated with similar variation in force exerted by the muscle, since force is related to surface EMG (BOUISSET, 1973), and surface EMG to intramuscular EMG (BOUISSET and MATON, 1972). Although some of these relations are non-linear (BOUISSET, 1973), it is likely that the essence of the tuning curve, i.e., directionality with spread, will be also observed in the force domain. The question then becomes one of interpreting the variation in the force exerted by an individual muscles during movements in different directions. In this context, it is reasonable to assume that the force developed by individual muscles is exerted in a direction determined by the anatomical relations between muscles and bones under specified positions of the skeleton. It is likely that this preferred direction of muscle action will be similar during movements of various directions. For example, the pectoralis major exerts force in a roughly horizontal dimension, so that the upper arm is deviated medially. Accordingly, the "preferred" direction of pectoralis, as determined in our studies, was at 180° (right arm). Nevertheless this muscle was also active, but at a lower intensity, during movements at 135°, i.e. movements that deviated 45° from the muscle's preferred direction toward forward extension of the upper arm. It is reasonable to assume that during this latter movement at 135° the action of pectoralis was still at 180°, although the magnitude of its activation was lower ; and similarly, for other directions. The same sort of analysis could be applied regarding other muscles. A generalization could then be made, namely that the direction of an increase in force exerted by individual muscles is approximately the same during movements in different directions, assuming that the relative position of other parts of the limb does not alter this relation. Another generalization could be made for a decrease in muscle activity, namely that a decrease in the force exerted by a muscle contributes, in fact, a force in a direction opposite to the muscle's preferred direction of action.

The considerations discussed above provide the background for an interpretation of the vector hypothesis, proposed above for motor cortical cells, as follows. For those cells that may relate to individual muscles, cell vectors could have an interpretation along the lines discussed for individual muscles above. However, a divergence exists in the corticospinal projection (ASANUMA et al., 1979 ; JANKOWSKA et al., 1975 ; SHINODA et al., 1981) so that a motor cortical cell might influence cells in several motoneuronal pools. A functional interpretation of this divergence could be that these motor cortical cells control muscle synergies (EVARTS, 1967). Muscle synergies, in turn, will produce force in a certain direction. This direction will differ depending upon the muscular composition of the synergy and the relative strength of activation of component muscles. An analysis similar to that described above for individual muscles could then be performed for these "synergistic" forces as well. Therefore, the vector hypothesis would apply whether motor cortical cells are regarded as controlling individual muscles or muscle synergies. Finally, it is crucial in this hypothesis that there be a summation point of the individual cell vectors, so that a vectorial sum of the population can be produced. Assuming that these vectors are related to forces produced by muscles or muscle synergies, a summation point could ultimately be the joint ; more specifically for the task used in the present study, the shoulder joint.

Concluding remarks

A "vectorial hypothesis" was proposed by which motor cortical cells possessing directional preference and directional spread could, as populations, generate movements in particular directions. The main assumptions of this hypothesis are that (a) cells exert a directional influence (vector) along the axis of their preferred direction, (b) this directional influence is on the same axis for all directions of movement, but (c) it is exerted toward the cell's preferred direction when there is an increase above the average discharge level, or toward the opposite direction when there is a decrease in discharge ; and (d) for a particular movement direction, the vectorial components of individual cells sum linearly. Given these assumptions, the population vectorial sum was determined for each of the 8 direction of movement tested using experimentally observed data from 241 directionally tuned motor cortical cells. The direction of this population vector was within 11° from the straight-line movement direction. This was within the range of the directions of the movement trajectories produced by well trained animals. Possible relations between motor cortical cells and individual muscles or muscle synergies were discussed with respect to the hypothesis above. It was argued that the hypothesis would hold under either assumption, i.e. whether motor cortical cells are thought as controlling muscles or muscle synergies, assuming that no changes in the position of parts of the limb occur that would alter fundamentally the directions in which muscles exert their actions.

ACKNOWLEDGEMENT

We thank Dr. K.O. JOHNSON for valuable discussions and suggestions concerning the hypothesis proposed. Supported by United States Public Health Service Grant NS17413.

REFERENCES

ASANUMA H, ZARZECKI P, JANKOWSKA E, HONGO T, MARCUS S (1979) Projection of individual pyramidal tract neurons to lumbar motor nuclei of the monkey. Exp Brain Res 34:73-89

BOUISSET S (1973) EMG and muscle force in normal motor activities. In: DESMEDT JE (ed) New developments in electromyography and clinical neurophysiology. Karger, Basel, p 547-583

BOUISSET S, MATON B (1972) The quantitative relation between surface and intramuscular electromyographic activities for voluntary movement. Amer J Phys Med 51:285-295

EVARTS EV (1967) Representation of movements and muscles by pyramidal tract neurons of the precentral motor cortex. In: YAHR MD, PURPURA DP (eds)

Neurophysiological basis of normal and abnormal motor activities. Raven, New York, p 215-251

GEORGOPOULOS AP, KALASKA JF, MASSEY JT (1981) Spatial trajectories and reaction times of aimed movements : effect of practice, uncertainty, and change in target location. J Neurophysiol 46:725-743

GEORGOPOULOS AP, KALASKA JF, CAMINITI R, MASSEY JT (1982) On the relations between the direction fo two-dimensional arm movements and cell discharge in primate motor cortex. J Neurosci 2:1527-1537

JANKOWSKA E, PADEL Y, TANAKA R (1975) Projections of pyramidal tract cells to alpha-motoneurones innervating hind-limb muscles in the monkey. J Physiol (Lond) 249:637-667

MARDIA KV (1972) Statistics of directional data. Academic Press, New York

MASSEY JT, CAMINITI R, KALASKA JF, GEORGOPOULOS AP (1981) Cortical mechanisms of two-dimensional aimed arm movements. VI. Electromyographic analysis. Soc Neurosci Abstr 7:563

SHINODA Y, YOKOTA JI, FUTAMI T (1981) Divergent projection of corticospinal motoneurons of multiple muscles in the monkey. Neurosci Lett 23:7-13

WIESENDANGER M (1981) Organization of secondary motor areas of cerebral cortex. In: Handbook of Physiology. The Nervous System. Bethesda, Md. Amer Physiol Soc, Sect 1, Vol II, Part 2, p 1121-1148

WOOLSEY CN, SETTLAGE PH, MEYER DR, SPENCER W, HAMUY P, TRAVIS AM (1950) Patterns of localization in the precentral and "supplementary" motor areas and their relation to the concept of a premotor area. Res Publ Assoc Res Nerv Ment Dis 30:238-264

Résumé

R. Porter

The John Curtin School of Medical Research, Australian National University
P.O. Box 334, Canberra ACT 2601 Australia

This conference made it clear, through presentations of both the invited papers and the large number of excellent posters, that the whole nervous system is concerned in control of movement performance. This should not be too surprising when we recognize that the production of movement is the only means available to the brain for expression of all behaviour. Without this output, we can have no knowledge of the behavioural significance of the processing of information within the brain. While it goes without saying that muscles and their afferent and efferent systems are involved in movement performance, and while a great deal of work over a very long period has examined the involvement of the motor areas of the cerebral cortex, the spinal cord machinery for locomotion, the cerebellum and the basal ganglia in motor control, this conference shed new light on each of these areas and also extended the range of subject coverage well beyond them. In particular, new information was presented which renews interest in premotor and prefrontal areas of cerebral cortex, along with parietal and infra-temporal cortical zones, as intimately involved in the management of movement performance. The connections of these with other brain structures and the mechanism of cooperative working of neurons within this extensive sheet of brain substance must now be examined in minute detail.

Moreover, if a given study involves not just the question of regulation of the movement itself, but aspects of the decision to move at all, for example to collect a food reward, then additional brain centres, in the amygdala and hypothalamus may have to be included in the motor physiologists' territory. The centres which have been considered in the past to be involved in drive and motivation may now assume a new significance for movement initiation.

But even when the territories for detailed study have been precisely defined, the problem remains of how to examine the coding of motor performance as it is represented at each of those places. M. PAILLARD reminded the meeting of

Experimental Brain Research, Suppl. 7
© Springer-Verlag Berlin · Heidelberg 1983

the formal definitions that had to be considered if one were required to examine neural events from the point of view of coding of relevant information. He particularly stressed that the behavioural outcome provided the only meaning to a candidate code. In spite of all the presentations in this conference, however, little has been added to knowledge of neural coding as it exists for motor control. Some imaginative, fresh approach may be needed, because the results that are obtained from any experiment are only seen in the context of the particular question that is asked.

It became clear that both the mechanical properties of muscle, "the sole executant" of movement (SHERRINGTON) and the functions of somaesthetic receptors and afferent systems deserve further study. Those who do not work in the field may have taken the view that the functions of muscle spindle receptors and of their efferent supply through fusimotor fibres were fully described. Yet, as more observations are made in man and in animals during the performance of natural movements, the subtlety and the complexity of the relationships between muscle receptor behaviour and movement performance becomes very challenging.

General connectivity in the nervous system is now quite well known. Modern neuro-anatomical tracing methods have greatly increased our knowledge of connections between one part of the brain and another. Moreover, neuro-chemical methods have allowed measures to be made of changes in connectivity at a much more quantitative level. But we are still far from understanding the detailed cell-to-cell connectivity within one brain region or between cells in connected brain regions. Much more information is needed about this at both the anatomical and the physiological levels. With which precise cells in which situations are connections made by the cortico-cortical fibres which enter area 4 of the cerebral mantle ? Are the influences which are exerted on particular receiving cells excitatory or inhibitory ? How do these cellular connections and their influences differ from those which conduct signals from the thalamus conveying coded elements of cerebellar function ? What parts do each of these contribute to the total machinery for movement performance ?

Even within a given brain territory concepts of organization are still evolving. Are the territories which contain the subsets of elements involved in a particular aspect of function localized and segregated or do these territories overlap with one another ? Are functionally related units distributed and over which brain territories do they extend ?

One of the most important ideas which has been achieving greater and greater significance in recent years is that of variability and flexibility in the functional associations between neuronal elements and identified parameters of movement performance. This may have great meaning for the study of the mechanisms of learning of movement skills. It may be that this flexibility confers a capacity on the nervous system for change following lesions of the brain and subsequent recovery of function. Yet neuronal events following imposed disturbance of function caused by brain lesions are only just beginning. Some examples were presented in this meeting.

Many of the attempts to find associations between neural events and movement performance have employed averaging techniques. Yet these may conceal important details of information and possible subtle changes in the code. Trial-by-trial analysis and a study of the changes between trials may be needed and some examples of this were presented at the meeting. In particular, Professor SASAKI's attempts to examine changes occurring in a defined nervous pathway during learning of a motor performance challenge others to consider this philosophy and approach their experiments in this way.

In addition to spatial considerations, temporal factors become exceedingly important in examining the neural events that could be associated with production of a movement. Some early attempts are now being made to examine simultaneous recordings in more than one brain site and to sample the activities within continuously active and reciprocally connected pairs of neurons. Great advances could be made by the further application of these methods and using techniques such as cross correlation analysis. A search must be made for changes which accompany modifications in the movement performance itself.

But even when a functionally connected set of signals is available, the experimenter needs to know more about real decoding systems. Between the train of impulses at low frequency which issues from a motoneuron and the movement of a joint in a monkey's forelimb in a given direction are a number of transforming systems with defined mechanical properties. Synaptic processes within the brain are themselves non-linear in their operation. These non-linear elements need to be included in any considerations of possible decoding systems and the meaning for a receiving cell of a neuron's frequency of discharge can be interpreted only when these transformations are fully understood and quantitatively described.

Finally, knowledge of movement by a conscious, sentient human subject and the subject's quantitative description of this knowledge could give information about the code. Psychophysical contributions to the study of movement provide data not only about the two-way relationships between sensations and movement but they also allow an estimate to be made of the brain's own decoding of the total signals which are interpreted by the subject as knowledge of position and movement in space.

Subject Index

Author Index

Animal Mind – Human Mind

Editor: D. R. Griffin
Report of the Dahlem Workshop on
Animal Mind – Human Mind
Berlin 1981, March 22–27
Rapporteurs: M. Dawkins et al.
1982. 4 photographs, 30 figures, 2 tables.
X, 427 pages.
(Dahlem Workshop Reports – Life Sciences
Research Report, Volume 21)
ISBN 3-540-11330-4

The Aging Brain

Physiological and Pathophysiological Aspects
Editor: S. Hoyer
1982. 52 figures, 66 tables. XIV, 281 pages.
(Experimental Brain Research, Supplement 5)
ISBN 3-540-11394-0

E. Braak

On the Structure of the Human Striate Area

1982. 44 figures. VI, 87 pages.
(Advances in Anatomy, Volume 77)
ISBN 3-540-11512-9

The Cerebellum – New Vistas

Editors: S. L. Palay, V. Chan-Palay
1982. 264 figures, 16 tables. XVII, 637 pages.
(Experimental Brain Research, Supplement 6)
ISBN 3-540-11472-6

Fundamentals of Neurophysiology

Editor: R. F. Schmidt
Translated from the German by
M. A. Biederman-Thorson
2nd revised and enlarged edition. 1978.
137 figures. IX, 339 pages.
(Springer Study Edition)
ISBN 3-540-08188-7

Fundamentals of Sensory Physiology

Editor: R. F. Schmidt
Translated from the German by
M. A. Biederman-Thorson
2 nd corrected edition. 1981. 139 figures.
XI, 286 pages.
(Springer Study Edition).
ISBN 3-540-10349-X

Gonadal Steroids and Brain Function

IUPS-Satellite Symposium, Berlin,
July 10–11, 1980
Editors: W. Wuttke, R. Horowski
1981. 136 figures, 10 tables. XIII, 373 pages.
(Experimental Brain Research, Supplement 3)
ISBN 3-540-10606-5

Human Physiology

Editors: R. F. Schmidt, G. Thews
Translated from the German by
M. A. Biederman-Thorson
1983. 569 figures, most in color.
XXI, 725 pages.
ISBN 3-540-11669-9

G. Palm

Neural Assemblies

An Alternative Approach to Artificial
Intelligence
1982. 147 figures. VIII, 244 pages.
(Studies of Brain Function, Volume 7)
ISBN 3-540-11366-5

The Renin Angiotensin System in the Brain

A Model for the Synthesis of Peptides in the Brain
Editors: D. Ganten, M. Printz, M. I. Phillips,
B. A. Schölkens
1982. 108 figures, 46 tables. XVII, 385 pages.
(Experimental Brain Research, Supplement 4)
ISBN 3-540-11344-4

Springer-Verlag
Berlin
Heidelberg
New York

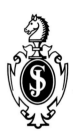

Progress in Sensory Physiology

Editors: H. Autrum, D. Ottoson, E. R. Perl, R. F. Schmidt
Editor-in-Chief: D. Ottoson
This series has gained a lot of friends. It leads the readers to the forefront of ongoing research in sensory physiology. Scientists active in the field open the curtain to their own work, providing a brilliant overview of research in progress.

Volume 1

1981. 72 figures, 6 tables. VII, 179 pages. ISBN 3-540-08413-4

Contents: *G. Westheimer:* Visual Hyperacuity. – *H. W. Kosterlitz, A. T. McKnight:* Opioid Peptides and Sensory Function. – *E. Shapiro, M. Klein, E. R. Kandel:* Presynaptic Facilitation and Presynaptic Inhibition in Aplysia. – *P. Gouras, E. Zrenner:* Color Vision.

Volume 2

1981. 103 figures. V, 187 pages. ISBN 3-540-10923-4

Contents: *R. Necker:* Thermoreception and Temperature Regulation in Homeothermic Vertebrates. – *G. A. Manley:* Auditory Physiology of the Reptiles. – *C. A. Smith:* Structural Correlates of Auditory Receptors.

Volume 3

W. D. Willis, Jr.

Control of Nociceptive Transmission in the Spinal Cord

1982. 51 figures. VI, 159 pages. ISBN 3-540-11510-2

Contents: Introduction: Centrifugal Control of Sensory Pathways. – Behavioral Evidence for Descending Control of Nociceptive Transmission. – Pharmacology of Analgesia Due to Descending Control Systems. – Descending Control of the Flexion Reflex. – Descending Control of Spinal Cord Nociceptive Neurons. – Correlations Between the Descending Control of Spinal Cord Nociceptive Pathways and the Operation of the Analgesia Systems. – References. – Subject Index.

The centrifugal pathways originating in the brain that control pain transmission and the pharmacological, anatomical and physiological evidence concerning the neural mechanisms of the "intrinsic analgesia systems" are reviewed comprehensively in this volume. A thorough survey of the pertinent literature is also included.

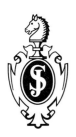

Springer-Verlag
Berlin
Heidelberg
New York